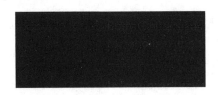

Essential
Medical Terminology

Essential
Medical Terminology

THIRD EDITION

PEGGY STANFIELD, MS, RD/LD, CNS
Dietetic Resources
Twin Falls, Idaho

Y.H. HUI, PHD
Science Technology System
West Sacramento, California

NANNA CROSS, PHD, RD/LD
Cross & Associates
Chicago, Illinois

JONES AND BARTLETT PUBLISHERS
Sudbury, Massachusetts
BOSTON   TORONTO   LONDON   SINGAPORE

World Headquarters
Jones and Bartlett Publishers
40 Tall Pine Drive
Sudbury, MA 01776
978-443-5000
info@jbpub.com
www.jbpub.com

Jones and Bartlett Publishers
Canada
6339 Ormindale Way
Mississauga, Ontario L5V 1J2
Canada

Jones and Bartlett Publishers
International
Barb House, Barb Mews
London W6 7PA
United Kingdom

Jones and Bartlett's books and products are available through most bookstores and online booksellers. To contact Jones and Bartlett Publishers directly, call 800-832-0034, fax 978-443-8000, or visit our website www.jbpub.com.

Substantial discounts on bulk quantities of Jones and Bartlett's publications are available to corporations, professional associations, and other qualified organizations. For details and specific discount information, contact the special sales department at Jones and Bartlett via the above contact information or send an email to specialsales@jbpub.com.

The authors, editor, and publisher have made every effort to provide accurate information. However, they are not responsible for errors, omissions, or for any outcomes related to the use of the contents of this book and take no responsibility for the use of the products and procedures described. Treatments and side effects described in this book may not be applicable to all people; likewise, some people may require a dose or experience a side effect that is not described herein. Drugs and medical devices are discussed that may have limited availability controlled by the Food and Drug Administration (FDA) for use only in a research study or clinical trial. Research, clinical practice, and government regulations often change the accepted standard in this field. When consideration is being given to use of any drug in the clinical setting, the health care provider or reader is responsible for determining FDA status of the drug, reading the package insert, and reviewing prescribing information for the most up-to-date recommendations on dose, precautions, and contraindications, and determining the appropriate usage for the product. This is especially important in the case of drugs that are new or seldom used.

Library of Congress Cataloging-in-Publication Data
Stanfield, Peggy.
  Essential medical terminology / Peggy Stanfield, Y.H. Hui, and Nanna Cross. -- 3rd ed.
      p. ; cm.
  Includes bibliographical references and index.
  ISBN-13: 978-0-7637-4913-2
  ISBN-10: 0-7637-4913-3
  1. Medicine--Terminology. 2. Medicine--Terminology--Problems, exercises, etc. I. Hui, Y. H. (Yiu H.) II. Cross, Nanna. III. Title.
  [DNLM: 1. Terminology--Problems and Exercises. W 15 S785e 2008]
  R123.S678 2008
  610.1'4--dc22
                                        2007013273

6048

Production Credits
Executive Editor: David Cella
Editorial Assistant: Lisa Gordon
Production Director: Amy Rose
Production Editor: Renée Sekerak
Associate Marketing Manager: Jennifer Bengtson
Manufacturing and Inventory Coordinator: Amy Bacus
Cover Design: Kristin E. Ohlin
Composition and Text Design: Shawn Girsberger
Printing and Binding: Malloy Incorporated
Cover Printing: Malloy Incorporated

Printed in the United States of America
13 12 11 10   10 9 8 7 6 5 4 3

Contents

Preface to the First Edition

Essential Medical Terminology is a brief, user-friendly text designed to aid students in mastering the medical vocabulary and terms they will encounter in allied health, nursing, and medical careers. The terms have been selected on the basis of their utility, practical value, and application to the real world of the healthcare work environment.

The intended audience includes students in nursing, nursing assistants/aides, vocational/practical nurses, medical secretaries, medical technologists, medical librarians, medical assistants, physician's assistants, and other persons in the allied health and paramedical fields. This book is designed for use in a one-quarter or one-semester course. It provides students with the basic principles of medical terminology and teaches vocabulary by applying terms in practice examples.

Although many instructors have expressed satisfaction with our 1989 text, *Medical Terminology: Principles and Practices,* others prefer a smaller book because their students need only a general knowledge of medical terminology. Therefore, we were ready when the publishers expressed an interest in a more compact textbook. To accomplish this goal, we have made a careful selection of the most essential terms, exercises, illustrations, and other instructional materials that are of maximum benefit to those students required to take a general survey course of medical terminology.

After much hard work, we have succeeded in producing a book that has fewer than 300 pages. This condensed edition has many unique features that distinguish it from other medical terminology texts:

1. The selection of medical terms is unique, and although some terms are found in other books, many are not.
2. Half of the book is devoted to practice exercises or self-instructional modules.

3. The amount of descriptive text is minimal, allowing students to concentrate on learning the key terms.

4. Although the frame format is common in some texts, we have not adopted that didactic mode. Rather, we present medical terminology as it applies to the major body systems.

5. Students will find that learning by way of the major body systems is a meaningful and unifying method of mastering medical terminology and solidifying previously learned concepts of anatomy and physiology.

The book is organized into five units: Unit I: Word Parts and Medical Terminology (Chapters 1–3); Unit II: Special Root Words (Chapters 4–6); Unit III: General Application and Medical Terminology (Chapters 7–8); Unit IV: Abbreviations (Chapters 9–10); and Unit V: Medical Terminology and Body Systems (Chapters 11–20). With the exception of Chapter 1, all chapters contain two components: Lesson One: Materials to Be Learned, and Lesson Two: Progress Check.

This unique text is accompanied by both traditional and modern supplementary teaching materials.

Instructor's manual. This booklet provides a spectrum of information: clinical case histories, practice tests, and student activities. It serves two important objectives: a wide selection of teaching materials and a reduction in class preparation time. For example, by using clinical case histories to supplement a complex topic in the classroom, the instructor can usually elicit enthusiastic participation and enliven classroom presentations.

Full-color pictures of body systems. We have included a full-color atlas of human anatomy, which details the major body systems, special senses, and skin. It provides an anatomic reference for all the medical terms in the text.

Our intention was to create a textbook that would serve the needs of both instructor and student. We strove to create a text that is both concise and thorough, thematically unified, easy to read, beautifully illustrated, and fully supplemented with supporting material to assure mastery of the material. We hope that both instructor and student will find the book a satisfactory and rewarding experience in teaching and learning medical terminology.

We are especially interested in suggestions for improvement. We want to make this an even better book in the next edition.

Preface to the Second Edition

When we started to write the *First Edition* of this book in preparation for its publication in 1990, we were concerned about the large number of competitors in the market. Our concern was even more intense when we were preparing the *Second Edition*. No fewer than five new competitive books with the same coverage appeared during the 5-year interval. Fortunately for us, though, our method of presentation and the contents in the *First Edition* were preferred by many instructors and their students. This was substantiated by the large number of college adoptions. We are also flattered that many of the features of the *First Edition* have been incorporated into other medical terminology books. Now, with our foot firmly in the door, we present our new edition. We are confident you will find the *Second Edition* of *Essential Medical Terminology* to be an even more useful learning tool.

The new edition includes updated coverage, improved exercises, and a more accurate and uniform presentation. This new emphasis is found throughout the text. The major changes, which are designed to streamline the presentation, are summarized as follows:

1. Objectives are listed for each of the five units.
2. All general word parts are grouped together and presented in Unit I.
3. A review chapter on root words is provided in Unit IV, immediately before the body systems.
4. The content of the body systems chapters in Unit V now more closely matches the content of earlier chapters.
5. Each chapter in Unit V starts with an overview of one of the major body systems.
6. This *Second Edition* includes 100 flash cards, which can be cut out and used by students. A fun way to use these cards is for pairs of students to study together.
7. The bibliography has been updated to include new references.

The book is organized into five units: Unit I: Word Parts and Medical Terminology (Chapters 1–2); Unit II: Root Words, Medical Terminology, and Patient Care (Chapters 3–6); Unit III: Abbreviations (Chapters 7–8); Unit IV: Review (Chapter 9); and Unit V: Medical Terminology and Body Systems (Chapters 10–19). All chapters contain two components: Lesson One: Materials to be Learned, and Lesson Two: Progress Check.

We have retained the full-color atlas of human anatomy, which details the major body systems, special senses, and skin, that appeared in the first edition. It provides an anatomic reference for all the medical terms in the text.

This unique text is accompanied by both traditional and modern supplementary teaching materials.

For the instructor, there is a complete instructor's manual with transparency masters. In addition, a complete video series, *Medical Terminology with Vikki Wetle, RN, MA,* is available to accompany this text. This program includes 14 tapes covering word structure; basic body parts and the body as a whole; abbreviations, diagnosis, and pharmacology; and an in-depth study of the body systems. Please contact your local Jones and Bartlett sales representative or the marketing department.

Our intention was to create a textbook that would serve the needs of both instructor and student. We strove to create a text that is both concise and thorough, thematically unified, easy to read, beautifully illustrated, and fully supplemented with supporting material to assure mastery of the material. We hope that both instructor and student will find the book a satisfactory and rewarding experience in teaching and learning medical terminology.

We are especially interested in suggestions for improvement. We want to make this an even better book in the next edition.

Preface to the Third Edition

We are pleased to be able to provide you with this updated and revised *Third Edition* of *Essential Medical Terminology*. The health professions are the fastest growing career choices today, and we salute those students who choose to offer their services to others.

It is our intention to provide you with the words and descriptions that are the foundation for your practice in the health field.

We have several new additions to this *Third Edition* which we hope will facilitate your learning of the language of medicine.

- Specific learning objectives for each chapter
- Expanded overviews with some reference to anatomy and physiology of each system
- Additional medical terms including many new clinical disorders
- New chapter on cancer medicine
- Extra practice exercises and test questions
- Consolidation of some chapters and rearrangement of others to enable quicker access to certain sections
- New tables, new figures, and new references
- New CD-ROM that includes interactive flashcards, crossword puzzles, and additional exercises.

Your instructors, in addition to their role as educators, are the key professionals who will correct any deficiency in this book.

Peggy Stanfield
Nanna Cross
Y. H. Hui

Acknowledgments

We would like to acknowledge those individuals who have helped move this edition from manuscript to publication. First to Dave Cella and assistant Lisa Gordon, thank you for providing us with assistance, encouragement, and support. Thanks also to the production staff whose dedicated work and professionalism is evident in the quality of their work.

We sincerely thank our reviewers who offered many valuable suggestions. Your comments were very helpful, and we incorporated as many of them into this edition as allocated page space would permit.

We do want to extend our appreciation to many students and their instructors for continued use of *Essentials* through the first two editions. We have tried to provide you with the updates and new information that you have asked for. We hope our mutual relationships continue with this *Third Edition* and beyond.

We also thank Mr. James Keating of Watsonville, Oregon. As the original acquisition editor of the *First Edition*, he gave us an unusual opportunity to educate many students for nearly 20 years. We are indebted to him and his vision.

How to Use This Book

Essential Medical Terminology, Third Edition, fits all types of medical terminology courses. It can be the primary text in either a one- or two-semester course.

One instructional mode other than formal classroom lecturing is as follows. The instructor serves as a supervisor and assigns materials in the text for self-study. The instructor may or may not enforce the following: class meetings between instructor and students, supervised or unsupervised tests, and preparation of tests with questions similar to those in the book.

The text offers a great deal of flexibility to instructors. Our recommendation is to progress through the table of contents as written. In any learning process, studying the information progressively provides sequence of thought and assures that one does not overlook critical information.

The student, especially one studying independently of a formal class lecture, should read each chapter thoroughly and complete all exercises.

GENERAL GUIDELINES

We also offer the following guidelines to both instructors and students:

1. Read the table of contents to determine the syllabus or match up the contents to a prepared syllabus.
2. After studying the basis of pronunciation, students may start with any of the remaining chapters in Units I to IV. The chapters on body systems (10–19) can be taught in any order.
3. For each chapter after Chapter 1, the study procedure is simple. Read the materials to be learned a few times and proceed with the progress check. Students might want to repeat or review chapter materials before taking a test.
4. Once a chapter is started, finish it before proceeding to the next one.
5. Complete each chapter from beginning to end. Do not begin randomly within a chapter.

6. When students begin Unit V, Medical Terminology and Body Systems, they will find that each chapter contains an overview of the body system. Each body system can be studied in more depth from an anatomy and physiology textbook.

7. We encourage students to develop their own methods of memorizing unfamiliar words. Word associations are useful. Flash cards are a useful adjunct to study. Studying in pairs is also helpful for most students.

8. Students should review completed materials as often as possible to refresh their memories.

9. All answers to progress checks are provided in Appendix A. Most instructors prefer that students not look at the answers until they have completed the assigned exercise.

PRONUNCIATION

Instructors vary in their opinions about including pronunciation in a medical terminology text. We believe including the pronunciation for each medical term benefits students. The recognition of a medical term is best accomplished by learning its pronunciation. It is important that students pronounce each new word correctly. Here are a few tips for learning the pronunciation of medical terms:

1. Study the guidelines for pronunciations in Chapter 1. The instructor may or may not assign additional material from outside sources for this chapter.

2. Remember the syllable(s) to be emphasized in each word. This component of the word is underlined in this book.

3. Attend the spelling lesson, if any, conducted by the instructor.

4. Exchange dictating and spelling practice with other students.

ABBREVIATIONS AND MEDICAL DICTIONARY

Instructors should recommend a medical dictionary for students. These dictionaries vary in comprehensiveness and price. The instructor can suggest the dictionaries most suitable for students and their eventual careers.

UNIT I   Word Parts and Medical Terminology

CHAPTER 1 | Word Pronunciations

The pronunciation of each medical term is governed by the following rules. Pronunciation is indicated by a simple phonetic respelling of the term and these diacritical markings:

1. The primary accent is indicated by an underlining, e.g., cerebellum (ser-e-bel-um).
2. The secondary accent is indicated by ('), e.g., ser'e-bel-um.
3. When an unmarked vowel ends a syllable, it is long, e.g., immune (i-mun').
4. When a syllable ends with a consonant, its unmarked vowel is short, e.g., cranial (kra-ne-al).

For ease of interpretation, the phonetic spellings used in this text have no other diacritical markings. However, the following basic rules apply to all pronunciation and are listed here for ease of interpretation of medical terms.

5. An unmarked vowel ending a syllable is *long:* It is indicated by a macron (ˉ), as in the examples below:

   a   urease (u-re-ās); abate (ah-bāt)
   e   electroscope (e-lek-tro-scōp); lead (lēd)
   i   askaracide (as-kar-i-sīd); bile (bīl)
   o   ohms (ōmz); ionophere (i-on-o-phēr); hormone (hor-mōn)
   u   union (ūn-ion); ampule (am-pūl)
   oo oophoron (oo-fōr-on)

6. A short vowel that *is* the syllable or that *ends* the syllable is indicated by a breve (˘):

   a   apophysis (ă-pof-i-sis)
   e   edema (ĕ-dēm-ah); effusion (ĕ-fūs-ion)
   i   immunity (ĭ-mūn-ĭ-te'); oxidation (oks'-sĭ-da-shun)
   o   otic (ŏ-tic); official (ŏ-fish-al)
   u   avoirdupois (av-er-dŭ-poiz)
   oo book (bŏŏk)

3

CHAPTER 2

Word Parts and Word Building Rules

OBJECTIVES

After completion of this chapter and the exercises, the student should be able to:

1. List the basic parts of a medical term
2. Define the terms *word root, combining vowel, combining form, prefix,* and *suffix*
3. State the rules for building medical terms
4. Divide medical words into their component parts
5. Build medical words using combining forms, prefixes, and suffixes
6. Use multiple word roots in a compound word

LESSON ONE MATERIALS TO BE LEARNED

PARTS OF A MEDICAL TERM

Words, including medical terms, are composed of three basic parts: word roots, prefixes, and suffixes. How the parts are combined determine their meaning. Changing any part of a word changes its meaning. Spelling and pronunciation are also very important, as some medical terms sound similar, and some sound exactly alike but are spelled differently, and therefore have different meanings.

For example, the word phagia (fay-jee-ah) means eating or swallowing, and the word phasia (fay-zee-ah) means without speech.

Examples of words that are pronounced exactly alike but spelled differently are the terms ileum (ill-ee-um) and ilium (ill-ee-um). Ileum is part of the small intestine, but ilium is part of the hipbone.

1. Prefix: the word or element attached to the *beginning* of a word root to modify its meaning. Not all medical words have a prefix. A prefix will keep its same meaning in every term in which it is used. **When defining a medical term that has both a prefix and a suffix, define the suffix first, the prefix second, and the word root last.**

Note in the following example how the meaning of the word changes:

Peri = prefix for around, cardi = root word for heart, -itis = suffix for inflammation.

Term: pericarditis
Definition: inflammation around the heart (muscle).

2. Word root: the *meaning* or *core* part of the word. Medical terms have one or more roots.

    By adding prefixes and suffixes to a word root, the meaning of a word is changed. Most medical words have at least one word root, and some have several. Word roots are joined by a combining vowel. A word root will have the same meaning in every word that contains it. When a word root is joined to a suffix, or to other root words to make a compound word, it requires the use of a combining vowel.

3. Combining vowel: usually an o and occasionally an i, used between compound word roots or between a word root and a suffix. Combining vowels make word pronunciation easier. When a vowel is added to a root word, it is called a *combining form*. It is usually marked with a diagonal, e.g., arthr/o.

    Combining vowels are kept between compound words even if the second word root does begin with a vowel, for example, gastr/oentero/logy. Compound words are two or more root words joined with a combining vowel. Compound words may also have a suffix, which is joined to the word by a combining vowel. When the suffix begins with a vowel (usually an i), the combining vowel on the root word is dropped. When the suffix begins with a consonant, the combining vowel is kept. Examples are:

    a. mening/o (root word and combining vowel) and -itis (suffix). The word is spelled *meningitis,* dropping the o. The term means inflammation of the meninges.
    b. hem/o (root word and combining vowel) and -rrhage (suffix). The word is spelled *hemorrhage,* keeping the o. The term means escape of blood from the vessels. If the suffix and the combining vowel have the same vowel, the duplicate vowel is also dropped, for example, cardi/o (root word for heart) and -itis (suffix). The word is spelled *carditis* (only one i is used). It means inflammation of the heart (muscle).

4. **Suffix:** the word part or element attached to the end of a root word to modify its meaning. Not all root words have a suffix, and some words have two suffixes (e.g., psych/o/log/ic/al). When a medical term has two suffixes (as *psychological* does), they are joined and considered one suffix, that is, -ic/al = ical. Some suffixes are attached to a prefix only, e.g., dia (prefix) -rrhea (suffix) or *diarrhea.* When they form a complete word, as in this example (diarrhea), the resulting word may be considered a root word, depending on its use.

The literal meaning of a word may be shortened through usage, by common consent, or when understood without being expressed.

Word parts combine in various ways, as can be seen in the accompanying table.

Please note the following two premises when studying this entire book:

1. Many columns carry the heading "word root." This is taken to mean that items under this column can be the word root itself or a word root with /o, that is, a combining form. This practice is to avoid excess repetition of the term "combining form" throughout the book.

2. About 3–5% of the medical terms in this book are included in the practice exercises that have not been presented in the lessons. This is designed to:

   a. encourage students to use the dictionary, since the practice exercises are all open-book.

   b. provide students an opportunity to practice dividing those words into their respective components according to the rules in the book.

   c. give the instructor a choice whether to include these additional words.

Some textbooks on medical terminology use the same technique; others do not. Feedback from students and instructors will be noted.

Word Parts	Examples	Medical Terms
A prefix + a word root	anti (prefix meaning against) + thyroid (root word for thyroid gland)	Antithyroid literal definition: against the thyroid actual usage: (agent) suppressing thyroid activity
A word root + a suffix	gastr (word root for stomach) + -ic (suffix meaning pertaining to)	Gastric definition: pertaining to the stomach
A combining form (a word root + a combining vowel) + a suffix	cardi (root word for heart) + /o (a combining vowel) + -logy (suffix meaning study of)	Cardiology definition: study of the heart

Word Parts	Examples	Medical Terms
A prefix + a suffix	an- (prefix meaning no, without) + -emia (suffix meaning blood)	Anemia literal definition: without (or no) blood actual usage: decreased number of red blood cells or decreased hemoglobin in the cells
A prefix + a root word + a suffix	epi (prefix meaning above, over) + gastr (root word for stomach) + -algia (suffix meaning pain)	Epigastralgia literal definition: pain above the stomach actual usage: pain in the upper region of the abdomen
A compound word* + a suffix	ot/o (root word for ear) + rhin/o (root word for nose) + laryng/o (root word for throat or larynx) + -logy (suffix meaning study of)	otorhinolaryngology definition: the branch of medicine dealing with diseases of the ear, nose, and throat

*Two or more root words connected with a combining vowel.

LISTINGS OF WORD PARTS

You may or may not know most of the words presented in the table. Do not be concerned if you don't. There will be plenty of opportunity to learn more about them. In the next three sections, you are provided with listings of word parts. Many of the prefixes, combining forms, word roots, and suffixes are indicated. Eventually, you will have to be familiar with all of them. Here are some steps that will help you to learn:

1. Go through the lists of word parts once or twice.
2. Check your knowledge by covering all but the first column and see if you can provide meanings for some of the words.

PREFIXES, WORD ROOTS WITH COMBINING FORMS, AND SUFFIXES

Table 2–1 Prefixes Commonly Used in Medicine

Prefix	Definition	Word Example	Pronunciation	Definition
a-, an-	no, not, without, lack of, apart	anoxia	an-ok'-se-ah	lack of sufficient oxygen in the blood
ad-	toward, near, to	adhesion	ad-he'zhun	union of two surfaces that are normally separate

Prefix	Definition	Word Example	Pronunciation	Definition
bi-	two, double	bicuspid	bi-kus'-pid	having two cusps
de-	down, away from	degenerate	de-jen'-er-ate	to change from a higher to a lower form
di-	two, double	diplopia	di-plo-pe-ah	double vision
dia-	through, between	dialysis	di-al'-i-sis	diffusion of solute molecules through a semipermeable membrane
dif-, dis-	apart, free from, separate	diffusion	di-fu'-zhun	state or process of being widely spread
dys-	bad, difficult, painful	dysfunctional	dis-fungk'-zhun-al	disturbance, impairment, or abnormality of an organ
ec-, ecto-	out, outside, outer	ectoderm	ek-to-derm	outermost of the three primitive germ layers of the embryo
end-, endo	within, inner	endometrium	en-do-me'-tre-um	mucous membrane lining the uterus
ep-, epi-	upon, over, above	epidural	ep-i-du-ral	situated upon or outside the dura mater
eu-	good, normal	euphoria	u-fo're-ah	an exaggerated feeling of mental and physical well-being
ex-, exo-	out, away from	excrete	ek-skreet'	to throw off or eliminate, as waste matter, by normal discharge
extra-	outside, beyond	extrauterine	ek-strah-u'-ter-in	situated or occurring outside the uterus
hyper-	above, beyond, excessive	hypertension	hi-per-ten'shun	persistently high blood pressure
hypo-	below, under, deficient	hypodermic	hi-po-der'mik	beneath the skin
in-	in, into, not	infusion	in-fu'-zhun	steeping a substance in water to obtain its soluble principles
mega-	large, great	megalgia	meg-al-je-ah	a severe pain

Prefix	Definition	Word Example	Pronunciation	Definition
meta-	beyond, over, between, change	metastasis	me-tas'tah-sis	transfer of a disease from one organ to another not directly connected to it
para-	beside, alongside, abnormal	paracolitis	par'ah-ko-li'-tis	inflammation of the outer coat of the colon
poly-	many, much, excessive	polycystic	pol'-e-sis'-tik	containing many cysts
post-	after, behind	postnatal	post-na'-tal	occurring after birth, with reference to the newborn
pre-	before, in front of	premenstrual	pre-men'-stroo-al	preceding menstruation
pro-	before, in front of	prootic	pro-ot'-ik	in front of the ear
super-	above, beyond	supernutrition	soo-per-nu-trish'-un	excessive nutrition
supra-	above, beyond	supracostal	soo-prah-kos'-tal	above or outside the ribs

Table 2–2 Word Roots and Combining Forms for Body Parts

Word Part	Definition	Word Example	Pronunciation	Definition
abdomin/o	abdomen	abdominocystic	ab-dom'-i-no-<u>sis</u>-tic	pertaining to the abdomen and gallbladder
aden/o	gland	adenitis	ad'e-<u>ni</u>-tis	inflammation of a gland
an/o	anus	anaplasty	an'ah-plas-te	plastic repair of the anus
andr/o	men	android	<u>an</u>-droid	resembling a man
angi/o	vessel	angiectomy	an'je'-<u>ek</u>-to-me	excision of part of a blood vessel or lymph vessel
appendage	attached to or outgrowth	appendectomy	<u>ah</u>-pen-dek'-to-me	excision of the vermiform appendix
appendic/o	appendix	appendicolysis	ah-<u>pen</u>-di-kol'-i-sis	surgical separation of adhesions binding the appendix
arteri/o	artery	arteriogram	ar-<u>te</u>-re-o-gram'	an x-ray picture of an artery

Word Part	Definition	Word Example	Pronunciation	Definition
arthr/o	joint	arthrocele	<u>ar</u>-thro-sel	a joint swelling
cardi/o	heart	cardiology	<u>kar</u>-de-ol'ogy	study of the heart
cephal/o	head	cephalic	se'phăl-ic	pertaining to the head
cerebr/o	cerebrum (part of the brain)	cerebral	ser'e-<u>bral</u>	pertaining to the brain
cyst/o	bladder	cystocele	<u>sis</u>-toh-seel	hernia of the bladder into the vagina
cyt/o	cell	cytology	si'toh-lōgy	study of the body cells
encephal/o	brain	encephaloma	en-sef'ah-<u>lo</u>-mah	a swelling or tumor of the brain
enter/o	intestines	enteritis	<u>en</u>-<u>ter</u>-<u>i</u>'-tis	inflammation of the intestine (usually small intestine)
esophag/o	esophagus	esophagism	e-<u>sof</u>-ah-jism	spasm of the esophagus
gastro/o	stomach	gastropathy	gas-<u>trop</u>-ah-the	any disease of the stomach
gloss/o	tongue	glossodynia	glos'o-<u>din</u>-e-ah	pain in the tongue
gyne	woman	gynephobia	jin'e-<u>fo</u>-be-ah	morbid aversion to women
hem/o	blood	hematoma	<u>he-ma</u>-toh'-mah	blood clot in an organ or under the skin
hepat/o	liver	hepatocele	<u>hep</u>-ah-to-sel	hernia of the liver
hyster/o	uterus	hysterolith	<u>his</u>-ter-o-lith'	a uterine calculus (stone)
ile/o	ileum (small intestine)	ileus	<u>il</u>-e-us	intestinal obstruction
irid/o	iris (eye)	iridomalacia	ir'i-do-mah-<u>la</u>-she-ah	softening of the iris
kerat/o	cornea of eye; horny substance	keratorrhexis	ker'ah-to-<u>rek</u>-sis	rupture of the cornea
lamina, lamin/o	thin, flat part of vertebra	laminotomy	lam'i-<u>not</u>-o-me	transection of a vertebral lamina
lapar/o	abdominal wall	laparorrhaphy	lap'ah-<u>ror</u>-ah-fe	suture of the abdominal wall

Word Part	Definition	Word Example	Pronunciation	Definition
lingua	tongue	nigralingua	ni-gra-<u>ling</u>-gwah	black tongue
lob/o	lobe, as of lung or brain	lobotomy	lo-<u>bot</u>-o-me	cutting of nerve fibers connecting a lobe of the brain with the thalamus
mamm/o	breast	mammogram	<u>mam</u>-o-gram	x-ray recording of breast tissue
mast/o	breast	mastitis	mas-<u>ti</u>-tis	inflammation of the breast
my/o	muscle	myocarditis	mi'o-kar-<u>di</u>-tis	inflammation of the heart muscle
myel/o	bone marrow; spinal cord	myelocyte	<u>mi</u>-e-lo-sit'	immature cell of bone marrow
myring/o	eardrum	myringoplasty	mi-<u>ring</u>-o-plas'te	surgical reconstruction of the eardrum
nephr/o	kidney	nephritis	ne-<u>fri</u>-tis	inflammation of the kidney
neur/o	nerve	neuralgia	nu-<u>ral</u>-je-ah	pain in a nerve
oophor/o	ovary	oophorocystosis	o-of'o-ro-sis-<u>to</u>-sis	formation of an ovarian cyst
ophthalm/o	eye	ophthalmorrhagia	of-thal'mo-<u>ra</u>-je-ah	hemorrhage from the eye
orchi/o	testicle	orchiopathy	or'ke-<u>op</u>-ah-the	any disease of the testes
orchid/o	testicle	orchidorrhaphy	or'ki-<u>dor</u>-ah-fe	surgical fixation of an undescended testis into the scrotum by suturing
oste/o	bone	osteoporosis	os'te-o-po-<u>ro</u>-sis	abnormal thinning of the skeleton
ot/o	ear	otitis	o-<u>ti</u>-tis	inflammation of the ear
pancreat/o	pancreas	pancreatogenous	pan'kre-ah-<u>toj</u>-e-nus	arising in the pancreas
pharyng/o	pharynx	pharyngismus	far'in-<u>jis</u>-mus	muscular spasm of the pharynx
phleb/o	vein	phlebotomy	fle-<u>bot</u>-o-me	incision of a vein
pneum/o	lungs (air or gas)	pneumonectomy	nu'mo-<u>nek</u>-to-me	excision of lung tissue
proct/o	rectum	proctodynia	prok'to-<u>din</u>-e-ah	pain in the rectum

Word Part	Definition	Word Example	Pronunciation	Definition
prostat/o	prostate gland	prostatitis	pros'-tah-<u>ti</u>-tis	inflammation of the prostate
pyel/o	pelvis of kidney	pyelectasis	pi'e-<u>lek</u>-tah-sis	dilation of the renal pelvis
rect/o	rectum and/or anus	rectocele	<u>rek</u>-to-sel	hernial protrusion of part of the rectum into the vagina
ren/i	renal (kidney)	reniform	<u>ren</u>-i-form	kidney-shaped
rhin/o	nose	rhinitis	ri-<u>ni</u>-tis	inflammation of the mucous membrane of the nose
sacr/o	sacrum	sacrolumbar	sa'kro-<u>lum</u>-bar	pertaining to the sacrum and loins
salping/o	fallopian tube	salpingocyesis	sal-ping'go-ci-<u>e</u>-sis	development of an embryo in the uterine tube; a tubal pregnancy
splen/o	spleen	splenoptosis	sple-nop-<u>to</u>-sis	downward displacement of the spleen
spondyl/o	vertebra	spondylodymus	spon'di-<u>lod</u>-i-mus	twin fetuses united by the vertebrae
steth/o	chest	stethospasm	<u>steth</u>-o-spasm	spasm of the chest muscles
stomat/o	mouth	stomatomalacia	sto-mah-to-ma-<u>la</u>-she-ah	softening of the structures of the mouth
ten/o	tendon	tendolysis	ten-<u>dol</u>-i-sis	the freeing of tendon adhesions
thorac/a	thorax (chest)	thoracentesis	tho'rah-sen-<u>te</u>-sis	surgical puncture and drainage of the thoracic cavity
thyr/o	thyroid gland	thyroxine	thi-<u>rok</u>-sin	a hormone of the thyroid gland that contains iodine
trache/o	trachea	tracheoscopy	tra'ke-<u>os</u>-ko-pe	inspection of the interior of the trachea
tympan/o	eardrum	tympanum	<u>tim</u>-pah-num	part of the cavity of the middle ear, in the temporal bone

Word Part	Definition	Word Example	Pronunciation	Definition
ureter/o	ureter	ureteropathy	u-re'ter-<u>op</u>-ah-the	any disease of the ureter
vas/o	vessel	vascular	<u>vas</u>-ku-lar	pertaining to blood vessels
ven/i	vein	venipuncture	<u>ven</u>'i-punk-chur	surgical puncture of a vein

Table 2–3 Suffixes Used in Surgery

Suffix	Definition	Word Example	Pronunciation	Definition
-age	related to	tri/age (three)	tre-<u>ahzh</u>	sorting out and classification of casualties to determine priority of treatment
-centesis	surgical puncture	arthro/centesis (joint)	ar'thro-sen-<u>te</u>-sis	puncture of a joint cavity for aspiration of fluid
-cid	kill	germi/cidal (germ)	<u>jer</u>-mi-si-dal	destructive to pathogenic microorganisms
-cis	cut, kill, excise	circum/cision (around)	<u>ser</u>-kum-sizh'un	surgical removal of the foreskin of the penis
-clasis	to break down, refracture	oste/oclasis (bone)	os'te-<u>ok</u>-lah-sis	surgical fracture or refracture of bones
-desis	binding, stabilization	arthr/odesis (joint)	ar'thro-<u>de</u>-sis	surgical fusion of a joint
-ectomy	excision, removal	append/ectomy	ap'en-<u>dek</u>-to-me	excision of the vermiform appendix
-iatry	healing (by a physician)	psych/iatry (mind)	si'<u>ki</u>-ah-tre	healing of the mind
-ion	process	excerebration (brain)	<u>ek</u>-ser-e-bra'shun	process of removal of the brain
-lysis	loosen, free from adhesions, destruction	enter/olysis (intestine)	en'ter-<u>ol</u>-i-sis	surgical separation of intestinal adhesions

Suffix	Definition	Word Example	Pronunciation	Definition
-osis	condition of	necr/osis (death)	ne-<u>kro</u>-sis	death of cells or tissues
-os/tomy	mouth, forming an opening	col/ostomy (colon)	ko-<u>los</u>-to-me	the surgical creation of an opening between the colon and the body surface
-pexy	fixation, suspension	gastro/pexy (stomach)	<u>gas</u>-tro-pek'se	surgical fixation of the stomach
-plasty	formation, plastic repair	rhino/plasty (nose)	<u>ri</u>-no-plas'te	plastic surgery of the nose
-stasis	stop/control	hemo/stasis (blood)	<u>he</u>-mo-sta'sis	stopping the escape of blood by either natural or artificial means
-therapy	treatment	chemo/therapy (drug)	<u>ke</u>-mo-ther'ah-pe	treatment of illness by medication
-tomy	incision, to cut into	phlebo/tomy (vein)	fle-<u>bot</u>-o-me	incision of a vein
-tripsy	to crush	litho/tripsy (stone)	<u>lith</u>-o-trip'se	the crushing of a stone in the bladder

Table 2–4 Suffixes for Diagnoses and Symptoms

Suffix	Definition	Word Example	Pronunciation	Definition
-algia	pain	cephal/algia (head)	sef'<u>a</u>-lal-je-ah	headache
-cele	hernia, swelling	hepat/ocele (liver)	<u>hep</u>-ah-to-sel	hernia of the liver
-dynia	pain	cephal/odynia (head)	sef'ah-lo-<u>din</u>-e-ah	pain in the head
-ectasis	dilation, expansion	bronchi/ectasis (bronchus)	brong'ke-<u>ek</u>-tah-sis	chronic dilation of one or more bronchi

Suffix	Definition	Word Example	Pronunciation	Definition
-emia	blood	poly/cyth/emia (many)	pol-e-si-the′me-ah	increase in total red cell mass of the blood
-gen	producing, beginning	carcin/o/gen (cancer)	car-<u>sin</u>-o-jen	any substance that causes cancer
-gram	record, picture	encephal/o/gram (brain)	en-<u>sef</u>-ah-lo-gram	the x-ray film obtained by encephalography
-graph	instrument for recording	cardi/o/graph (heart)	<u>kar</u>-de-o-graf′	an instrument used for recording electrical activity of the heartbeat
-graphy	process of recording	roentgen/o/graphy	rent′gen-<u>og</u>-rah-fe	x-ray films (roentgenograms) of internal structures of the body
-iasis	abnormal condition, formation of, presence of	chole/lith/iasis (gallstone)	ko′le-li-<u>thi</u>-ah-sis	the presence or formation of gallstones
-itis	inflammation	gastr/itis (stomach)	gas-<u>tri</u>-tis	inflammation of the stomach
-logy	study of	bio/logy (life)	bi-<u>ol</u>-o-je	scientific study of living organisms
-malacia	softening	oste/o/malacia (bone)	os′te-o-mah-<u>la</u>-she-ah	softening of the bones resulting from vitamin D deficiency
-megaly	enlargement	hepat/o/megaly (liver)	hep′aht-o-<u>meg</u>-ah-le	enlargement of the liver
-meter	instrument for measuring	crani/o/meter (cranium)	kra′ne-<u>om</u>-e-ter	an instrument for measuring skulls
-metry	process of measuring	pelvi/metry (pelvis)	pel-<u>vim</u>-e-tre	measurement of the capacity and diameter of the pelvis
-oid	resemble	lip/oid (fat)	<u>lip</u>-oid	fatlike; lipid (resembling a fat)
-oma	tumor	aden/oma (gland)	ad′e-<u>no</u>-mah	a benign skin tumor in which the cells are derived from glandular epithelium

Suffix	Definition	Word Example	Pronunciation	Definition
-osis	abnormal condition	dermat/osis (skin)	der'mah-<u>to</u>-sis	any skin disease, especially one not characterized by inflammation
-pathy	disease	nephr/o/pathy (kidney)	ne-<u>frop</u>-ah-the	disease of the kidneys
-penia	decrease, deficiency	leuk/o/cyto/penia (white) (cell)	loo-ko-sit-o-<u>pe</u>-ne-ah	reduction of the number of leukocytes (white blood cells), the count being 5,000/mm^3 or less
-phagia	eating, swallowing	dys/phagia (difficult)	dis-<u>fa</u>-je-ah	difficulty in swallowing or eating
-phasia	speech	a/phasia (without)	ah-<u>fa</u>-zhe-ah	defect or loss of the power of expression by speech, writing, or signs, or of comprehending spoken or written words
-phobia	fear	acr/o/phobia (extremities or top)	ak'ro-<u>fo</u>-be-ah	morbid fear of heights
-plegia	paralysis	hemi/plegia (half)	hem'e-<u>ple</u>-je-ah	paralysis of one side of the body
-ptosis	prolapse, falling, dropping	hyster/o/ptosis (uterus)	his'ter-op-<u>to</u>-sis	metroptosis; downward displacement or prolapse of the uterus
-rrhage	burst forth, hemorrhage	hem/o/rrhage (blood)	<u>hem</u>-o-rij	the escape of blood from the vessels; excessive bleeding
-rrhea	discharge, flow	men/o/rrhea (menses)	men'o-<u>re</u>-ah	normal menstruation
-rrhexis	rupture	angi/o/rrhexis (blood vessel)	an'je-or-<u>ek</u>-sis	rupture of a vessel, especially a blood vessel

Suffix	Definition	Word Example	Pronunciation	Definition
-sclerosis	hardening	arteri/o/sclerosis (artery)	ar-te're-o-skle-<u>ro</u>-sis	a group of diseases characterized by thickening and loss of elasticity of the arterial walls
-scopy	examination, view	oto/scopy (ear)	o-<u>tos</u>-ko-pe	examination of the ear by means of the otoscope
-spasm	involuntary contraction, twitching of a muscle	blephar/o/spasm (eyelid)	<u>blef</u>-ah-ro-spazm	spasm of the eyelids

In summary, the important elements of a medical term are:

1. The root: the foundation of the term
2. Prefix: the word beginning
3. Suffix: the word ending.
4. Combining vowel: a vowel that links the root word to the suffix or to other root words.
5. Combining form: a combination of the root word(s) and the combining vowel.

The rules for building medical words from these elements are as follows:

1. A prefix is always placed at the beginning of the word.
2. A suffix is always placed at the end of the word.
3. When more than one root word is used, it is a compound word and requires the use of a combining vowel to separate the words, even if the root word begins with a vowel.
4. When defining medical terms, begin with the suffix and read backward.
5. If the word also contains a prefix, define the suffix first, prefix second, and root word(s) last.
6. When using compound words that relate to parts of the body, anatomical position determines which root word comes first.

LESSON TWO   **PROGRESS CHECK PART A**

■ MATCHING

Match the following word elements with their meaning:

F	**1.** aden/o		**a.**	brain
D	**2.** bronch/o		**b.**	uterus
A	**3.** encephal/o		**c.**	abdominal wall
G	**4.** gloss/o		**d.**	bronchus
B	**5.** hyster/o		**e.**	bone
H	**6.** irid/o		**f.**	gland
C	**7.** lapar/o		**g.**	tongue
E	**8.** oste/o		**h.**	iris

■ SPELLING AND DEFINITION

Circle the letter of the correct spelling and then define the combining form:

1. **(a)** oophor/o   **(b)** ophoor/o   **(c)** oorphor/o

Definition: _ovary_

2. **(a)** prosct/o   **(b)** proct/o   **(c)** prost/o

Definition: _rectum or anus_

3. **(a)** neuphr/o   **(b)** neprect/o   **(c)** nephr/o

Definition: _kidney_

4. **(a)** rhinit/o   **(b)** rhin/o   **(c)** rhen/o

Definition: _nose_

5. **(a)** orchi/o   **(b)** oorch/o   **(c)** orche/o

Definition: _testicle_

6. **(a)** salcr/o   **(b)** salp/o   **(c)** sacr/o

Definition: _sacrum_

7. **(a)** salpr/o   **(b)** salping/o   **(c)** salpen/o

Definition: _fallopian tube_

8. **(a)** myring/o   **(b)** mirang/o   **(c)** myleng/o

Definition: _eardrum_

9. **(a)** pharang/o   **(b)** pharyng/o   **(c)** pragyn/o

Definition: _pharynx_

10. (a) spongyl/o   (b) sphondyl/o   (c) spondyl/o

Definition: _Vertebra_

11. (a) urotor/o   (b) uroter/o   (c) ureter/o

Definition: _ureter_

12. (a) chondr/o   (b) cholondr/o   (c) chodol/o

Definition: _cartilage_

13. (a) chost/o   (b) cost/o   (c) costol/o

Definition: _rib_

14. (a) vast/o   (b) vas/o   (c) vein/o

Definition: _vessel_

15. (a) ven/o   (b) vin/o   (c) vein/o

Definition: _vein_

■ DEFINING MEDICAL WORD ELEMENTS

Provide the medical root word for the following terms:

1. man _andr/o_
2. woman _gene_
3. heart _cardi/o_
4. head _cephal/o_
5. chest _steth/o_
6. bone _odont/o_
7. brain _encephal/o_
8. stomach _gastr/o_
9. liver _hepat/o_
10. gallbladder _cholecyst/o_
11. mouth _stomat/o_
12. tongue _lingua_
13. breast _mamm/o_
14. muscle _myos_
15. nerve _neur/o_

■ BUILDING MEDICAL WORDS

Using all word elements necessary, build medical words that mean:

1. Inflammation of a tendon _tendinitis_
2. Removal of the thyroid gland _thyroidectomy_
3. Incision into the trachea _tracheotomy_
4. Any disease of the intestine _enteropathy_
5. Pain in the nerves _neuralgia_
6. Inflammation in the urinary bladder _cystitis_
7. Inflammation in a joint _arthritis_

8. Removal of the spleen _splenectomy_

9. An eye specialist _ophthamologist_

10. An x-ray picture of a blood vessel _angiogram_

11. Stones in the gallbladder _chclelithiasis_

12. An obstructed artery _arteriosclerosis_

13. Removal of a lung _pneumonectomy_

14. An x-ray picture of the spinal cord _myelogram_

15. Instrument for examining the ear _otoscope_

16. Incision into a vein _phlebotomy_

17. Removal of the prostate gland _prostatectomy_

18. Rupture of a vessel in the cerebrum _cerebrovascular accident_

19. Inflammation of the esophagus _esophagitis_

20. Incision into the thorax _thoracotomy_

LESSON TWO   PROGRESS CHECK PART B

■ MATCHING

Match the following word elements with their meaning:

I	1.	-ectomy	a.	tumor
J	2.	-ostomy	b.	abnormal condition
G	3.	-otomy	c.	rupture
H	4.	-rrhaphy	d.	resembling
F	5.	-rrhage	e.	discharge
E	6.	-rrhea	f.	burst forth
C	7.	-rrhexis	g.	cut into
D	8.	-oid	h.	suture
A	9.	-oma	i.	surgical removal
B	10.	-osis	j.	mouth, surgical creation

■ SPELLING AND DEFINITION

Circle the letter of the correct spelling and then define the word element:

1. **(a)** -centesis   **(b)** -centisis   **(c)** -senticis   **(d)** -cinteses

    Definition: _surgical puncture_

2. **(a)** -clysis   **(b)** -clasis   **(c)** -claxis   **(d)** -clasy

    Definition: _to break down / refracture_

3. **(a)** -ectasy   **(b)** -ectosis   **(c)** -ectasis   **(d)** -eclasis

    Definition: _dialate / to expand_

4. **(a)** -malachi   **(b)** -melacia   **(c)** -malazia   **(d)** -malacia

    Definition: _softening_

5. **(a)** -plegia   **(b)** -plagia   **(c)** -phlagia   **(d)** -pelagia

    Definition: _paralysis (stroke)_

6. **(a)** -tosis   **(b)** -ptosis   **(c)** -protosis   **(d)** -tsosis

    Definition: _falling, drooping, prolapse_

7. **(a)** -slerosis   **(b)** -schlerosis   **(c)** -sclerosis   **(d)** -shlerosis

    Definition: _hardening_

8. **(a)** -magaly   **(b)** -mejally   **(c)** -magely   **(d)** -megaly

    Definition: _enlargement_

9. **(a)** -cele   **(b)** -cely   **(c)** -cili   **(d)** -ceal

    Definition: _hernia, swelling_

10. **(a)** -isis   **(b)** -iasis   **(c)** -iatis   **(d)** -iesis

    Definition: _presence of, formation (in abnorm. cond.)_

■ BUILDING MEDICAL WORDS

Using any of the appropriate word elements, build medical words that mean:

1. a headache _cephalgia_

2. taking x-ray films of internal body structures _roentgenography_

3. inflammation of the stomach _gastritis_

4. formation of gallstones _cholelithiasis_

5. increase in red cell mass _polycythemia_

6. softening of the bones _osteomalacia_

7. surgical puncture of a joint _arthrocentesis_
8. removal of blood from a vein _phlebotomy_
9. repair of a broken nose _rhinoplasty_
10. scientific study of living organisms _biology_
11. enlargement of the liver _hepatomegaly_
12. any skin disease _dermatosis_
13. excision of the appendix _appendectomy_
14. healing of the mind _psychiatry_
15. incision into the brain _encephalotomy_
16. treatment of illness by medication _chemotherapy_
17. stopping the flow of blood _hemostasis_
18. a substance that causes cancer _carcinogen_
19. disease of the kidneys _nephropathy_
20. loss of the power of speech _aphasia_

■ DEFINING MEDICAL TERMS

Define the following medical terms:

1. osteoclasis _surgical fracture or refracture of a bone_
2. enterolysis _surgical separation of intestinal adhesions_
3. lithotripsy _crushing of a stone in bladder + washing out the fragments_
4. necrosis _death of cell or tissue_
5. circumcision _removal of foreskin from penis_
6. adenoma _a gland tumor_
7. dysphagia _difficulty in swallowing_
8. leukopenia _reduced number of white blood cells_
9. hemiplegia _paralyzed on one side of the body_
10. acrophobia _morbid fear of heights_

UNIT II

Root Words, Medical Terminology, and Patient Care

CHAPTER 3 Bacteria, Color, and Some Medical Terms

OBJECTIVES

1. List and define the five major types of bacteria.
2. List and define prefixes that deal with color.
3. Change the meaning of a given word root by adding appropriate prefixes.
   Define, spell, and pronounce the new word.
4. Define, spell, and pronounce medical words used in this chapter.

LESSON ONE   MATERIALS TO BE LEARNED

ROOT WORDS FOR BACTERIA

Table 3–1 Root Words for Bacteria

Root Word	Definition	Word Example	Pronunciation	Definition
bacillus*	bacteria that are rod-shaped (plural is bacilli)	streptobacillus	strep'to-bah-<u>sil</u>-lis	rod-shaped bacteria that grow in twisted chains
coccus*	bacteria that are round in shape (plural is cocci, prounced 'coc'seye'	streptococcus	strep'to-<u>kok</u>-us	round bacteria that grow in twisted chains

25

Root Word	Definition	Word Example	Pronunciation	Definition
dipl/o	pairs; bacteria that grow in pairs	diplococcus	dip'lo-<u>kok</u>-us	round bacteria that grow in pairs
staphyl/o	bunches, like grapes; bacteria that grow in clusters	staphylococcus	staf'i-lo-<u>kok</u>-us	round bacteria that grow in clusters
strepto/o	twisted; bacteria that grow in twisted chains	streptococcus	strep-to-<u>kok</u>-us	round bacteria that grow in twisted chains

*Both "bacillus" and "coccus" are Latin and considered regular scientific words. They are neither word roots nor combining forms. Although some consider them suffixes when written as "-bacillus," and "-coccus," others disagree. We are placing them under the heading "root word" because we do not want to start another column or invent another heading.

PREFIXES FOR COLOR

The prefixes used to denote color are very useful. The color of the cells, body fluids and reactions, skin, growths, and rashes are important indications used in diagnosing and treating conditions and diseases. This table contains definitions and examples of some of the more commonly used prefixes for color.

Table 3–2 Prefixes for Color

Prefix	Definition	Word Example	Pronunciation	Definition
alb-	white	albino	al-<u>bi</u>-no	a person with white hair, very pale skin, and nonpigmented iris
chlor/o-	green	chlorophyll	<u>klo</u>-ro-fil	any of a group of green pigments that are involved in oxygen-producing photosynthesis
chrom/o-	color	chromocyte	<u>kro</u>-mo-sit	any colored cell or pigmented corpuscle

Prefix	Definition	Word Example	Pronunciation	Definition
cirrh/o-	orange-yellow	cirrhosis	si-<u>ro</u>-sis	interstitial inflammation of an organ, particularly the liver (cirrhosis of the liver), showing orange-yellow discoloration in organ pigments
cyan/o-	blue	cyanosis	si'ah-<u>no</u>-sis	a bluish discoloration of skin and mucous membranes
erythr/o-	red	erythrocyte	e-<u>rith</u>-ro-sit	a red blood cell or corpuscle containing hemoglobin and transporting oxygen
leuk/o-	white	leukocyte	<u>loo</u>-ko-sit	white cell; a colorless blood corpuscle whose chief function is to protect the body against microorganisms causing disease
lutein/o-	saffron yellow	lutein	<u>loo</u>-te-in	a lipochrome from the corpus luteum, fat cells, and egg yolk
melan/o-	black	melanoma	mel'ah-<u>no</u>-mah	malignant melanoma— "black tumor"
poli/o-	gray	poliomyelitis	po'le-o-mi'e-<u>li</u>-tis	an acute viral disease marked clinically by fever, sore throat, headache, vomiting, and often stiffness of the neck and back. It may attack the gray matter of the central nervous system (CNS) and brain, hence the common name "polio"
rhod/o-	red	rhodopsin	ro-<u>dop</u>-sin	visual purple; a photosensitive purple-red chromoprotein in the retinal rods

Prefix	Definition	Word Example	Pronunciation	Definition
rubi/o-	reddish, redness	rubella	roo-<u>bel</u>-ah	German measles; a mild viral infection marked by a pink macular rash, fever, and lymph node enlargement
xanth/o-	yellowish	xanthochromia	zan'tho-<u>kro</u>-me-ah	yellowish discoloration, as of the skin or spinal fluid

COMMONLY USED PREFIXES

These prefixes are commonly used in medical terminology. Many have been defined previously. They will also appear throughout the text, especially as they relate to body systems. They are included in this chapter for easy reference.

Table 3–3 Commonly Used Prefixes

Prefix	Definition	Word Example	Pronunciation	Definition
a-, an-	without, not	afebrile	a-<u>feb</u>-ril	without fever
		anoxia	an-<u>ok</u>-se-ah	absence of oxygen supply to tissues despite adequate perfusion of the tissue by blood; often used interchangeably with hypoxia to indicate a reduced oxygen supply
acro-	extremities; top or extreme point	acrodermatitis	ak-ro-der'mah-<u>ti</u>-tis	inflammation of the skin of the hands or feet
aero-	air	aerobic	ar-<u>o</u>-bik	produced in the presence of oxygen
		anaerobic	an-ar-<u>o</u>-bik	produced without oxygen
aniso-	unequal	anisocytosis	an-i'so-si-<u>to</u>-sis	presence in the blood of erythrocytes showing excessive variations in size
brady-	slow	bradycardia	brad'e-<u>kar</u>-de-ah	slowness of the heartbeat, as evidenced by slowing of the pulse rate to < 60

Prefix	Definition	Word Example	Pronunciation	Definition
de-	take away, remove	dehydrate	de-<u>hi</u>-drat	remove water from, to dry; to lose water, become dry
dia-	through (as in running through)	diarrhea	di'ah-<u>re</u>-ah	abnormally frequent evacuation of watery stools
dif-, dis-	apart, free from, separate	diffusion	di-fu'-zhun	state or process of being widely spread
dys-	bad, painful, difficult	dystocia	dis-<u>to</u>-se-ah	abnormal labor or childbirth
		dysmenorrhea	dis'men-or-<u>re</u>-ah	painful menstruation
ec, ecto-	out, outside, outer	ectoderm	ek'-to-derm	outermost of the three primitive germ layers of the embryo
emia-	blood: condition of	anemia	an-<u>ne</u>-me-ah	reduction below normal of the number of erythrocytes, quantity of hemoglobin, or the volume of packed red cells in the blood; a symptom of various diseases and disorders
end-, endo-	within, inner	endometrium	<u>en</u>-do-me'-tre-um	mucous membrane lining the uterus
eu-	good, easy	euphoria	u-<u>fo</u>-re-ah	bodily comfort; well-being; absence of pain or distress
		euthanasia	u'thah-<u>na</u>-zhe-ah	easy or painless death; mercy killing; deliberate ending of life of a person suffering from an incurable disease
extra-	outside, beyond	extrauterine	ek-strah-u'-ter-in	situated or occurring outside the uterus
hemi-	one side, half	hemiplegia	hem'e-<u>ple</u>-je-ah	paralysis of one side of the body
hemo-	blood	hemolysis	he-<u>mol</u>-i-sis	separation of the hemoglobin from the red cells and its appearance in the plasma
hetero-	different	heterosexual	het'er-o-<u>seks</u>-u-al	one who is sexually attracted to persons of the opposite sex

Prefix	Definition	Word Example	Pronunciation	Definition
homo-	same	homosexual	ho'mo-<u>seks</u>-u-al	one who is sexually attracted to persons of the same sex
	resembling each other	homogeneous	ho'mo-<u>je</u>-ne-us	of uniform quality, composition, or structure throughout
hydro-	water	hydrotherapy	hi'dro-<u>ther</u>-a-pe	the treatment of disease by the internal or external use of water
		hydrocephalus	hi'dro-<u>sef</u>-ah-lus	a congenital or acquired condition marked by dilation of the cerebral ventricles and an accumulation of cerebrospinal fluid within the skull
hyper-	above normal, excessive, beyond	hypertension	hi-per-<u>ten</u>-shun	persistently high arterial blood pressure; it may have no known cause or be associated with other diseases
hypo-	under, below normal	hypoglycemia	hi'po-gli-<u>se</u>-me-ah	deficiency of glucose concentration in the blood, which may lead to nervousness, hypothermia, headache, confusion, and sometimes convulsions and coma
in-	in, into, not	infusion	<u>in</u>-fu'-zhun	steeping a substance in water to obtain its soluble principles
iso-	equal, same	isotonic	i'so-<u>ton</u>-ik	of equal tension
		isothermal	i'so-<u>ther</u>-mal	having the same temperature
lip-	fat	lipidemia	lip'i-<u>de</u>-me-ah	hyperlipidemia: a general term for elevated concentrations of any or all of the lipids in the plasma
mal-	bad, poor	malaise	mal-<u>az</u>	a vague feeling of bodily discomfort
		malocclusion	mal'o-<u>kloo</u>-zhun	absence of proper relations of opposing teeth when the jaws are in contact
mega-	large, great	megalgia	meg-al'-je-ah	a severe pain

Prefix	Definition	Word Example	Pronunciation	Definition
megalo-	large (enlarged)	acromegaly	ak'ro-<u>meg</u>-ah-le	abnormal enlargement of the extremities of the skeleton—nose, jaws, fingers, and toes
		megavitamin	meg'ah-<u>vi</u>-tah-min	a dose of vitamin(s) vastly exceeding the amount recommended for nutritional balance
meno-	menses (menstruation)	menopause	<u>men</u>-o-pawz	cessation of menstruation
noct-	night	nocturia	nok-<u>tu</u>-re-ah	excessive urination at night
nyct-	night	nycturia	nik-<u>tu</u>-re-ah	excessive urination at night
pan-	all, every	pandemic	pan-<u>dem</u>-ik	a widespread epidemic disease
para-	beside, beyond, accessory to	paracystic	par'ah-<u>sis</u>-tik	situated near the bladder
per-	through	perforate	<u>pur</u>-fo-rat	to make a hole or holes through, as by punching or boring; to pierce, penetrate
peri-	around	peritoneum	per'i-to-<u>ne</u>-um	the serous membrane lining the walls of the abdominal and pelvic cavities
poly-	many, much	polyuria	pol'e-<u>u</u>-re-ah	excessive secretion of urine
post-	following, after	postpartum	post-<u>par</u>-tum	occurring after childbirth, with reference to the mother
		postoperative	post-<u>op</u>-ra-tiv	following surgery
pre-	before	prenatal	pre-<u>na</u>-tal	preceding birth
pro-	preceding, coming before	prognosis	prog-<u>no</u>-sis	a forecast of the probable course and outcome of a disorder
pyo-	pus	pyogenic	pi'o-<u>jen</u>-ik	producing pus
		pyorrhea	pi-o-<u>re</u>-ah	a copious discharge of pus
re-	put back	rehydrate	re-<u>hi</u>-drat	to restore water or fluid content to the body

Prefix	Definition	Word Example	Pronunciation	Definition
super-	above, beyond	supernutrition	soo-per-nu-trish'-un	excessive nutrition
supra-	above, beyond	supracostal	soo-prah-kos'-tal	above or outside the ribs
syn-	going together, united	synthesis	sin-the-sis	creation of a compound by union of elements composing it, done artificially or as a result of natural processes
		syndrome	sin-drome	a set of symptoms occurring together
tachy-	fast	tachycardia	tak'-e-kar-de-ah	abnormally rapid heart rate

LESSON TWO   PROGRESS CHECK

■ MULTIPLE CHOICE

Circle only one answer unless directed otherwise:

1. A bacterium that grows in a twisted chain is called

    a. coccus
    b. diplo
    c. strepto
    d. staphylo

2. Bacteria that are rod-shaped are called

    a. acoccus
    b. diplo
    c. bacillus
    d. staphylo

3. Round bacteria that grow in clusters are called

    a. streptococcus
    b. staphylococcus
    c. streptobacillus
    d. diplococcus

4. Round bacteria that grow in twisted chains are called

    a. streptobacillus
    b. diplococcus
    c. staphylococcus
    d. streptococcus

5. Round bacteria that grow in pairs are called

    a. streptobacillus
    b. diplococcus
    c. staphylococcus
    d. streptococcus

6. Rod-shaped bacteria that grow in twisted chains are called

    a. streptobacillus
    b. diplococcus
    c. staphylococcus
    d. streptococcus

■ MATCHING

Match the terms on the left to their correct color on the right:

H	**1.** erythr/o	**a.**	white
E	**2.** lutein	**b.**	green
J	**3.** chrom/o	**c.**	orange-yellow
I	**4.** poli/o	**d.**	yellowish
F	**5.** melan/o	**e.**	saffron yellow
G	**6.** cyan/o	**f.**	black
A	**7.** albus	**g.**	blue
H	**8.** rhod/o	**h.**	red
C	**9.** cirrh/o	**i.**	gray
D	**10.** xanth/o	**j.**	any color
H	**11.** rubor		
B	**12.** chlor/o		
A	**13.** leuk/o		

■ WRITE IN THE PREFIX

Write in the correct prefix for each term given:

    1. extremities   *acro –*

    2. unequal   *aniso –*

3. different _hetero-_
4. painful _dys-_
5. same _homo-_
6. equal _iso-_
7. poor _mal-_
8. large _megaly-_
9. every _pan-_
10. following _post-_
11. blood _hemo-_

■ DEFINE THE PREFIX

State the meaning of the following prefixes:

1. mal _bad, poor_
2. dys _difficult, painful, bad_
3. megalo _enlarged, large_
4. hyper _excessive, beyond, above normal_
5. tachy _fast_
6. hypo _under, below normal_
7. brady _slow_
8. de _remove, take away_
9. re _put back_
10. hydro _water_
11. para _beside_
12. peri _around_
13. poly _many_
14. pre _before_
15. pro _before, preceding_
16. per _through_
17. syn _together, united_
18. noct _night_
19. nyct _night_
20. dia _through_

CHAPTER 4	Body Openings and Plural Endings

LESSON ONE   MATERIALS TO BE LEARNED

BODY OPENINGS

Table 4–1 Body Openings

Term	Pronunciation	Definition or Usage
aperture	<u>ap</u>-er-chur	an opening or orifice
canal (alimentary)	kah-<u>nal</u>	the musculomembranous digestive tube extending from the mouth to the anus
canal (vaginal)	kah-<u>nal</u>	the canal in the female from the vulva to the cervix uteri that receives the penis in copulation
cavity	<u>kav</u>-i-te	a hollow place or space, or a potential space, within the body or one of its organs
constriction	kon-<u>strik</u>-shun	making something narrow; to contract; to close (an opening)
dilatation, dilation	dil'ah-<u>ta</u>-shun di-<u>la</u>-shun	stretched beyond normal dimensions; the widening of something; expansion, opening
foramen	for-<u>ra</u>-men	a natural opening or passage, especially one into or through a bone
hiatus	hi-<u>a</u>-tus	a gap, cleft, or opening

Term	Pronunciation	Definition or Usage
introitus	in-<u>tro</u>-itus	opening or entrance to a canal or cavity such as the vagina
lumen	<u>loo</u>-men	opening within a hollow tube or organ
meatus	me-<u>a</u>-tus	urinary passage or opening
orifice	<u>or</u>-i-fis	any orifice, such as the anal orifice
os	os	mouth opening; os uteri: mouth of the uterus, or cervix
patent	<u>pa</u>-tent	adjective, meaning open or not plugged, as in "the tube is patent"
perforation	per-fo-<u>ra</u>-shun	a hole in something, e.g., perforation of the stomach wall by a gastric ulcer
stoma	<u>sto</u>-mah	artificial opening established by colostomy, ileostomy, and tracheostomy
ventricle	<u>ven</u>-tri-kul	a small cavity or chamber, as in the brain or heart

PLURAL ENDINGS

Many medical terms have special plural forms. They are based on the ending of the word. Some of them are made plural in the same way you learned in English class. For example:

1. Adding an s to a singular noun. Example: singular, abrasi*on*; plural, abra-sion*s*.
2. Singular nouns that end in s or ch form plurals by adding es. Example: singular, absce*ss*; plural, abscess*es*.
3. Singular nouns that end in y preceded by a consonant form plurals by changing the y to i and adding es. Example: singular, arter*y*; plural, arter-*ies*.

The following rules are commonly used for forming plurals for medical terms. If the word:

1. Ends in a, retain the a and add e. Example: singular, burs*a*, vertebr*a*; plural, burs*ae*, vertebr*ae*.
2. Ends in is, drop the is and add es. Example: singular, cris*is*, diagnos*is*; plural, cris*es*, diagnos*es*.
3. Ends in ix or ex, drop the ix or ex and add ices. Example: singular, ind*ex*, append*ix*; plural, ind*ices*, append*ices*.
4. Ends in on, drop the on and add a. Example: singular, gangl*ion*; plural, gangl*ia*.
5. Ends in um, drop the um and add a. Example: singular, ov*um*; plural, ov*a*.

6. Ends in us, drop the us and add i. Example: singular, nucle*us*, fung*us*; plural, nucle*i*, fung*i*.

There are exceptions to the rules. Some terms have more than one acceptable plural. If in doubt, consult your medical dictionary.

Table 4–2 Plural Endings

Singular	Word Example	Pronunciation	Plural	Word Example	Pronunciation
a	burs*a*	<u>ber</u>-sah	ae	burs*ae*	<u>bur</u>-sae
	vertebr*a*	<u>vur</u>-ta-bra		vertebr*ae*	<u>vur</u>-te-bre
ax	thor*ax*	<u>thor</u>-aks	aces	thor*aces*	<u>thor</u>-a-sez
en	lum*en*	<u>loo</u>-men	ina	lum*ina*	<u>lu</u>-mina
	foram*en*	for-<u>ra</u>-men	ina	foram*ina*	for-<u>ra</u>-mina
is	cris*is*	<u>kri</u>-sis	es	cris*es*	<u>kri</u>-ses
	diagnos*is*	di'ag-<u>no</u>-sis	es	diagnos*es*	di'ag-<u>no</u>-sez
is	femor*is*	fe'<u>mo</u>-ris	a	femor*a*	fe'<u>mo</u>-ra
ix	append*ix*	ah-<u>pen</u>-diks	ices	append*ices*	ah-<u>pen</u>-dises
inx	men*inx*	<u>me</u>-ninks	inges	men*inges*	me-<u>nin</u>-ges
nx	phal*anx*	<u>fa</u>-lanks	ges	phal*anges*	fa-<u>lan</u>-ges
on	spermatoz*oon*	sper'ma-to-<u>zo</u>-on	a	spermatoz*oa*	sper'ma-to-<u>zo</u>-a
um	diverticul*um*	di'ver-<u>tik</u>-u-lum	a	diverticul*a*	di'ver-<u>tik</u>-u-la
	ov*um*	<u>o</u>-vum	a	ov*a*	<u>o</u>-va
us	nucle*us*	<u>nu</u>-kli-us	i	nucle*i*	<u>nu</u>-clei
	thromb*us*	<u>throm</u>-bus	i	thromb*i*	<u>throm</u>-bi
ur	fem*ur*	<u>fe</u>-mur	ora	femor*a*	<u>fem</u>-ora
y	arter*y*	<u>ar</u>-ter-e	ies	arter*ies*	<u>ar</u>-ter-es
	ovar*y*	<u>o</u>-var-e	ies	ovar*ies*	<u>o</u>-var-es

LESSON TWO   PROGRESS CHECK

■ SPELLING AND DEFINITION

Circle the letter of the correctly spelled word and define it:

1. (a) apurchur   (b) aperchur   **(c) aperture**   (d) apurchure

    Definition: _____

2. **(a) constriction**   (b) constrictuve   (c) conscriture   (d) consctrition

    Definition: _____

3. (a) foramine   **(b) foramen**   (c) formanen   (d) formaine

    Definition: _____

4. (a) hitias   (b) hiateus   (c) hitrois   **(d) hiatus**

    Definition: _____

5. **(a) orifice**   (b) orafus   (c) orafice   (d) orifux

    Definition: _____

6. (a) introtoitus   **(b) introitus**   (c) introtois   (d) introices

    Definition: _____

7. (a) ventracle   (b) vintricle   **(c) ventricle**   (d) veintricle

    Definition: _____

8. (a) loomen   **(b) lumen**   (c) louman   (d) lumine

    Definition: _____

■ WORD CONSTRUCTION

The following questions pertain to *plural endings.* For each singular ending listed, write the correct change to make it *plural:*

1. a _ae_ _____
2. ax _aces_ _____
3. en _ina_ _____
4. is _es/a_ _____
5. ix _ices_ _____
6. inx _inges_ _____ or ex _____

7. nx _ges_

8. on _a_

9. um _a_

10. us _i_

11. ur _ora_

12. y _ies_

The following medical words have *plural* endings. Write in the *singular* for each term listed:

13. vertebrae _Verteba_

14. thoraces _thoax_

15. lumina _lumen_

16. crises _crisis_

17. ovaries _ovary_

18. arteries _artery_

19. diverticula _diverticulum_

20. nuclei _____

21. meninges _____

22. diagnoses _____

23. spermatozoa _____

24. femora _____

25. appendices _____

26. ova _____

27. thrombi _____

■ BUILDING MEDICAL TERMS

Build a medical term that means:

1. A hollow space within the body _____

2. Stretched open beyond normal dimensions _____

3. A natural opening through a bone _____

4. The opening within an artery _____

5. Opening from the colon to the outside of the body made by surgery _____

6. A small chamber in the brain _____

7. An unplugged tube _____

8. The hollow space that extends from vulva to cervix _____

9. The tube extending from mouth to anus _____

10. A gap or cleft that allows a part of the alimentary canal to protrude through the diaphragm _____

_____

■ DEFINITIONS

Define these body parts used in Chapter 4:

1. femur _____

2. meninx _____

3. thorax _____

4. bursa _____

5. phalanx _____

6. artery _____

7. foramen _____

8. ovary _____

9. appendix _____

10. spermatozoan _____

11. erythrocyte _____

12. diverticuli _____

13. os _____

14. introitus _____

CHAPTER 5

Numbers, Positions, and Directions

OBJECTIVES

After completing this chapter and the exercises, the student should be able to:

1. Identify the location of any given body part.
2. Use appropriate prefixes to describe the direction of any movement and part of the body.
3. Give the meaning of prefixes that denote number and define given examples.
4. Identify commonly used prefixes that describe locations.
5. Describe body positions that indicate placement of a patient for a procedure or treatment.
6. Define the three major systems of weight and measurement used most often in medicine.
7. Convert Celsius to Fahrenheit or Fahrenheit to Celsius as needed.
8. Recognize commonly used symbols and/or abbreviations.
9. Define given word elements and transition to another system if required.

LESSON ONE   MATERIALS TO BE LEARNED

PART 1: PREFIXES—NUMBERS

Prefixes that denote number tell you if something is one-half, one, two, three, or more; if it is single or multiple; and if it involves one side, two sides, or more. Table 5–1 contains definitions and examples of some of the commonly used prefixes for numbers.

41

Table 5–1 Prefixes for Numbers

Prefix	Definition	Word Example	Pronunciation	Definition
uni- (mono-)	one	unilateral	u'-ni-<u>lat</u>-er-al	affecting only one side
bi- (diplo-)	two (double), twice	bilateral	bi-<u>lat</u>-er-al	having two sides; pertaining to both sides
		bicuspid	bi-<u>kus</u>-pid	having two points or cusps, e.g., bicuspid (mitral) valve; a bicuspid (premolar) tooth
gemin-	double, pair	gemini	<u>jim</u>-in'-eh	twins
tri-	three	tricuspid	tri-<u>kus</u>-pid	having three points or cusps, as a valve of the heart; the valve that guards the opening between the right atrium and right ventricle
		triceps	<u>tri</u>-seps	a muscle of the upper arm having three heads
quadri-	four	quadriplegic	kwod'-ri-<u>ple</u>-jic	paralysis of all four limbs
tetra-	four	tetrasomic	tet-rah-some-ik	having four chromosomes where there should be only two
quint-	five	quintipara	kwin-<u>tip</u>-ah-rah	a woman who has had five pregnancies which resulted in viable offspring (Para V)
sexti-	six	sextuplet	<u>sexs</u>-tu-plit	any one of six offspring produced at the same birth
septi-	seven	septuplet	<u>sep</u>-tu-plit	one of seven offspring produced at one birth
octa- (octo-)	eight	octahedron	ok-ta-<u>he</u>-dron	an eight-sided solid figure
nona-	nine	nonan	<u>no</u>-nan	having symptoms that increase or reappear every ninth day; malarial symptoms are an example
deca-	ten	decagram	<u>dek</u>-a-gram	a weight of 10 grams
multi-	many (more than one)	multicellular	mul'-ti-<u>sel</u>-u-lar	composed of many cells

Prefix	Definition	Word Example	Pronunciation	Definition
primi-	first	primigravida	pri-mi-<u>grav</u>-i-dah	a woman pregnant for the first time
semi-	half (partially)	semicircular	sem'i-<u>ser</u>-ku-lar	shaped like a half circle
hemi-	half, also one-sided	hemianopsia	hem'e-ah-<u>nop</u>-se-ah	defective vision or blindness in half of the visual field
ambi-	both or both sides	ambidextrous	am'bi-<u>deks</u>-trus	able to use either hand with equal dexterity
		ambivalence	am-<u>biv</u>-ah-lens	simultaneous existence of conflicting emotional attitudes toward a goal, object, or person
null-	none	nullipara	null-eh-pair-ah	a woman with no childen
pan-	all	pancytopenia	pan-site-oh-peen'-ee-ah	decreased number of all blood cells

PART 2: PREFIXES—POSITIONS AND DIRECTIONS

Prefixes that indicate directions describe a location. They tell you whether the location is above, below, inside, in the middle, around, near, between, or outside a body structure. Table 5–2 contains definitions and examples of commonly used prefixes that describe locations.

Table 5–2 Prefixes for Positions and Directions

Prefix	Definition	Word Example	Pronunciation	Definition
ab-	away from	abduction	ab-<u>duk</u>-shun	to draw away from; the state of being abducted
ad-	toward	adduction	ah-<u>duk</u>-shun	to draw toward a center or median line
circum-	around	circumcision	ser'kum-<u>sizh</u>-un	surgical removal of all or part of the foreskin, or prepuce, of the penis
contra-	opposition, against	contraindicated	kon'tra-<u>in</u>-di-ka-ted	any condition that renders a particular line of treatment improper or undesirable

Prefix	Definition	Word Example	Pronunciation	Definition
de-	down, away from	decay	deh-kay′	waste away (from normal)
ecto-, exo-	outside	ectopic	ek-<u>top</u>-ik	located away from normal position; arising or produced at an abnormal site or in a tissue where it is not normally found
		exogenous	ek-<u>soj</u>-e-nus	originating outside or caused by factors outside the organism
		exocrine	<u>ek</u>-so-krin	secreting externally via a duct; denoting such a gland or its secretion
endo-	within	endocrine	<u>en</u>-do-krin	pertaining to internal secretions; hormonal
		endogenous	en-<u>doj</u>-e-nus	produced within or caused by factors within the organism
epi-	upon, over	epigastric	ep′i-<u>gas</u>-tric	the upper and middle region of the abdomen
extra-	outside	extrauterine	ek′-strah-<u>u</u>-ter-in	situated or occurring outside the uterus
infra- (sub)	below, under	infrasternal	in′frah-<u>ster</u>-nal	beneath the sternum
intra-	inside	intracellular	in-tra-<u>sel</u>-u-lar	inside a cell
ipsi- (iso)	same (equal)	ipsilateral	ip′si-<u>lat</u>-er-al	situated on or affecting the same side
ir-	into, toward	irrigate	ir′-reh-gate	wash into
meso-	middle, pertaining to mesentery	mesoderm	<u>mez</u>-o-derm	the middle of the three primary germ layers of the embryo
meta- (supra)	after, beyond, over; change or transformation; following in a series	metastasis	me-<u>tas</u>-tah-sis	the transfer of disease from one organ or part to another not directly connected with it

Prefix	Definition	Word Example	Pronunciation	Definition
meta- (supra)		metabolism	me-<u>tab</u>-o-lizm	the sum of the physical and chemical processes by which living organized substance is built up and maintained and by which large molecules are transformed into energy
		metamorphosis	met'ah-<u>mor</u>-fo-sis	change of structure or shape; transition from one developmental stage to another
para-	near, beside	paramedical	par'ah-<u>med</u>-i-kal	having some connection with or relation to the science or practice of medicine
		paranormal	par'ah-<u>nor</u>-mal	near-normal function
peri-	around, surrounding	periodontal	per'e-<u>o</u>-don-tal	around a tooth
		pericardium	per'i-<u>kar</u>-de-um	pertaining to the fibrous sac enclosing the heart and the roots of the great vessels
retro-	behind, backward	retroperitoneal	ret'ro-<u>per</u>-i-to-<u>ne</u>-al	behind the peritoneum
sub-	under, near	submerged	sub-<u>mer</u>-j-ĕd	under the surface
trans-	across, through	transverse	trans'<u>verz</u>	positioned across
		transvaginal	trans'<u>vaj</u>-i-nal	through the vagina

PART 3: TERMS—DIRECTIONS AND POSITIONS

Table 5–3 contains both prefixes and suffixes, many of which you learned in the preceding chapters and some of which will be new. Both prefixes and suffixes are needed to describe body positions that indicate placement of a patient for procedures and/or treatments. Some words, such as Sims and Trendelenberg positions, are understood terms that denote the correct position without elaboration.

Table 5–3 Terms for Directions and Positions

Term	Pronunciation	Definition
anterior	an-<u>ter</u>-e-or	situated at or directed toward the front; opposite of posterior
posterior	pos-<u>ter</u>-e-or	directed toward or situated at the back; opposite of anterior
cephalic	se-<u>fal</u>-ik	pertaining to the head, or the head end of the body
caudal	<u>kaw</u>-dal	situated toward the tail (coccygeal area)
decubitus	de-<u>ku</u>-bi-tus	the act of lying down; the position assumed in lying down
eversion	e-<u>ver</u>-zhun	a turning inside out; a turning outward
extension	ek-<u>sten</u>-zhun	the movement bringing the members of a limb into or toward a straight condition
flexion	<u>flek</u>-zhun	the act of bending or the condition of being bent
Fowler's	<u>fow</u>-lerz	the head of the patient's bed is raised 18–20 inches above level
internal	in-<u>ter</u>-nal	situated or occurring within or on the inside
external	eks-<u>ter</u>-nal	situated or occurring on the outside
knee-chest	<u>ne</u> chest	the patient rests on his or her knees and chest. The head is turned to one side, and the arms are extended on the bed, the elbows flexed and resting so that they partially bear the weight of the patient
lateral	<u>lat</u>-er-al	midline of the body; pertaining to the side
bilateral	bi-<u>lat</u>-er-al	having two sides; pertaining to both sides
lithotomy	li-<u>thot</u>-o-me	position in which the patient lies on his or her back, legs flexed on the thighs, thighs flexed on the abdomen and abducted
medial	<u>me</u>-de-al	situated toward the midline
oblique	o-<u>blek</u>	slanting; incline
peripheral	pe-<u>rif</u>-er-al	an outward structure or surface; the portion of a system outside the central region
proximal	<u>prok</u>-si-mal	toward the center or median line; the point of attachment or origin

Term	Pronunciation	Definition
distal	<u>dis</u>-tal	remote; farther from any point of reference
quadrant	<u>kwod</u>-rant	one of four corresponding parts, or quarters, as of the surface of the abdomen or the field of vision
recumbent	re-<u>cum</u>-bent	lying down
rotation	ro-<u>ta</u>-shun	the process of turning around an axis
Sims'	simz	the patient lies on his or her left side and chest, the right knee and thigh drawn up, the left arm along the back
sinistro	<u>sin</u>-is-tro	left; left side
dextro	<u>dek</u>-stro	right; right side
superior	soo-<u>per</u>-e-or	situated above, or directed upward
inferior	in-<u>fer</u>-e-or	situated below, or directed downward
supine	<u>soo</u>-pīn	lying with the face upward or on the dorsal surface
supination	soo'-pi-<u>na</u>-shun	the act of placing or lying on the back
prone	prōn	lying face downward or on the ventral surface
pronation	prō-<u>na</u>-shun	the act of assuming the prone position
trans	trans	through; across; beyond
Trendelenburg's	tren-<u>del</u>-en-bergz	the patient is supine on a surface inclined 45 degrees, the head lower than the legs
upright	<u>up</u>-rit	perpendicular; vertical; erect in carriage or posture

UNITS OF WEIGHT AND MEASUREMENT

This section contains weights and measures used most often in medicine. The transition between apothecary, avoirdupois, and metric is sometimes confusing to the beginning student. For the convenience of the learner, the units and equivalents are provided here, along with some symbols frequently encountered.*

Table 5–4 Units of Weight and Measurement

Unit	Abbreviation(s)	Definition
Apothecaries' weight (ah-<u>poth</u>-e-ka'-rez)		System used for measuring and weighing drugs and solutions, precious metals, and precious stones. Fractions are used to designate portions of a unit. Small Roman numerals are used to designate amounts. Example: iss = one and one-half
grains	gr	
minims	m	
drams	dr	
ounces	oz	
pounds	lb	
	(12 oz = 1 lb)	
Avoirdupois weight (aver-du-<u>poiz</u>)		The system of measuring and weighing used in English-speaking countries for all commodities except drugs, precious stones, and precious metals.
drops	gtt	
teaspoon	tsp	
tablespoon	T	
ounces	oz	
pound	lb	
	(16 oz = 1 lb)	
Metric system (<u>met</u>-rik)		A system of weighing and measuring based on the meter and having all units based on the power of 10.
Word elements:		
tera (10^{12})	T	monster: one trillion times the size of a unit
giga (10^{9})	G	one billion times the size of a unit

---

* *Note:* Some textbooks in science and engineering use ML, others use both mL and ml. This book uses both abbreviations.

Unit	Abbreviation(s)	Definition
mega (10^6)	M	one million times the size of a unit
kilo (10^3)	k	one thousand times the size of a unit
hecto (10^2)	h	one hundred times the size of a unit
deka (10)	dk	ten times the size of a unit
Unit is one:		
deci(10^{-1})	d	1/10 of a unit
centi (10^{-2})	c	1/100 of a unit
milli (10^{-3})	m	1/1000 of a unit
micro (10^{-6})	µ	1/1,000,000 of a unit
nano (10^{-9})	n	1/1,000,000,000 of a unit
pico (10^{-12})	p	1/1,000,000,000,000 of a unit
Metric weight		
microgram	µg or mcg	1000 mcg = 1 milligram (mg)
milligram	mg	1000 mg = 1 gram (g or gm)
centigram	cg	100 cg = 1 g
decigram	dg	10 dg = 1 g
gram	g or gm	1 g = 1 g
dekagram	dkg	1 dkg = 10 g
hectogram	hg	1 hg = 100 g
kilogram	kg	1 kg = 1000 g
Metric length		
millimeter	mm	1000 mm = 1 meter (m)
centimeter	cm	100 cm = 1 m
decimeter	dm	10 dm = 1 m
meter	m	1 m = 1 m
dekameter	dkm	10 m = 1 dkm
hectometer	hm	100 m = 1 hm
kilometer	km	1000 m = 1 km
Metric volume		
cubic centimeter	cc	1 cc = 1 ml (milliliter)
milliliter	ml or mL	1000 ml = 1 L (liter)

Unit	Abbreviation(s)	Definition
centiliter	cl	100 cl = 1 L
deciliter	dl	10 dl = 1 L
liter	l or L	1 L = 1 L
dekaliter	dkl	10 L = 1 dkl
hectoliter	hl	100 L = 1 hl
kiloliter	kl	1000 L = 1 kl
Equivalents (equal to)	=	Conversions from apothecary and avoirdupois to metric
weight	μg/mg	1000 μg = 1 mg
	mg/g	1000 mg = 1 g
	g/kg	1000 g = 1 kg
	kg/lb	1 kg = 2.2 lb
length	cm/in	2.5 cm = 1 in
volume	ml/cc/L	1000 ml = 1000 cc = 1 L
energy		
joule	J	1 J = 0.24 c
calorie	c	1 c = 4.18 J
Temperature	°T	the degree (°) of sensible heat or cold expressed in terms of a specific scale
Celsius (or centigrade)	°C	scale at which the boiling point of water (H_2O) is 100° and the freezing point of H_2O is 0°
Fahrenheit	°F	scale at which the boiling point of H_2O is 212° and the freezing point of H_2O is 32°
conversion		to change from one scale or system to another
temperature		to convert Celsius to Fahrenheit, multiply by 9, divide by 5, and add 32: $°F = (°C \times 9/5) + 32$ to convert Fahrenheit to Celsius, subtract 32, multiply by 5, and divide by 9: $°C = (°F - 32) \times 5/9$

Weights and Measures

Table 5–5

U.S. System to Metric		Metric to U.S. System	
U.S. Measure	Metric Measure	Metric Measure	U.S. Measure
Length		*Length*	
1 in	25.0 mm	1 mm	0.04 in
1 ft	0.3 m	1 m	3.3 ft
Mass		*Mass*	
1 gr (grain)	64.8 mg	1 mg	0.015 g
1 oz	28.35 g	1 gr (grain)	0.035 oz
1 lb	0.45 kg	1 kg	2.2 lb
Volume		*Volume*	
1 cu in	16.0 cm^3	1 cm^3	0.06 in^3
1 tsp	5.0 ml	1 ml	0.2 tsp
1 T	15.0 ml	1 ml	0.07 T
1 fl oz	30.0 ml	1 ml	0.03 oz
1 c	0.24 L	1 L	4.2 c
1 pt	0.47 L	1 L	2.1 pt
1 qt (liq)	0.95 L	1 L	1.1 qt
1 gal	0.004 m^3	1 m^3	264.0 gal
Energy		*Energy*	
1 cal (c)	4.18 J	1 J	0.24 cal (c)

Common Weights and Measures

Table 5–6

Measure	Equivalent	Measure	Equivalent
3 tsp	1 T	1 fl oz	30 g
2 T	1 oz	1/2 c	120 g
4 T	1/4 c	1 c	240 g
8 T	1/2 c	1 lb	454 g
16 T	1 c		

Measure	Equivalent	Measure	Equivalent
		1 g	1 ml
2 c	1 pt	1 tsp	5 ml
4 c	1 qt	1 T	15 ml
4 qt	1 gal	1 fl oz	30 ml
		1 c	240 ml
1 tsp	5 g	1 pt	480 ml
1 T	15 g	1 qt	960 ml
1 oz	28.35 g	1 L	1000 ml

FREQUENTLY USED SYMBOLS

This unit contains the symbols most frequently used in medical fields of practice. A symbol is a graphic portrayal of words, phrases, or sentences.

Table 5–7

Symbol	Meaning	Symbol	Meaning
♂, □	male	$\bar{c}$	with
♀, ○	female	$\bar{s}$	without
*	birth	↓	decreased, depressed
†	death	↑	increased, elevated
$\bar{a}$	before	ϴ	absent
$\bar{p}$	after	∨	systolic blood pressure
∧	diastolic blood pressure	℥	dram
℞	take (prescription)	ℨ	fluidram
°T	degree (temperature)	±	indefinite (yes and no)
∞	infinity	#	number; weight; gauge

Symbol	Meaning	Symbol	Meaning
′	foot	/	per
″	inch	Ⓛ	left
:	ratio (is to)	Ⓡ	right (also registered trademark)
+	plus; positive; present	≥	greater than or equal to
−	minus, negative; absent	≤	less than or equal to
℥	ounce	@	at
f℥	fluid ounce	%	percent
μg	microgram		

LESSON TWO   **PROGRESS CHECK**

■ COMPARE AND CONTRAST

Explain the *differences* in the following prefixes:

   Example: ab/ad
          ab: away from; **ad:** toward (center or median)

1. circum/contra _circum = around   contra = against_
2. ecto/endo _ecto = outside   endo = inside_
3. infra/ipsi _infra = below   ipsi = same_
4. para/per _para = near   per = about/around_
5. uni/bi/tri _uni = one   bi = two   tri = three_
6. prima/multi _prima = first   multi = many_
7. semi/hemi _semi = half   hemi = one sided_
8. ambi/quadri _ambi = both   quadri = four_

9. meso/meta _Meso = Middle   meta = after/beyond_

10. retro/trans _retro = behind/   trans = across (through)_
, backward

■ IDENTIFY THE LOCATION

Identify these locations by writing in the correct medical term:

1. Toward the front _anterior_

2. Situated at the back _posterior_

3. Toward the head _cephalic_

4. Toward the tail _caudal_

5. Lying-down position _supine/prone_

6. Turned inside out _eversion_

7. Straightening a limb _extension_

8. Slanting/inclined _oblique_

9. Middle of the body _medial_

10. Part of the body that is attached to another part _adjacent_

■ MATCHING: POSITIONS

Match the position at the left to its correct direction:

m	1. Fowler's	a.	one of four parts
O	2. flexion	b.	lying on left side and chest; right knee and thigh up, left arm to back
N	3. lithotomy	c.	to the left; left side
J	4. peripheral	d.	on top; above
A	5. quadrant	e.	lying face up
L	6. recumbent	f.	lying face down
B	7. Sims'	g.	through; across; beyond
C	8. sinistro	h.	lying with head lower than legs
K	9. dextro	i.	bottom; below
D	10. superior	j.	outside; outward
I	11. inferior	k.	right side; to the right
E	12. supine	l.	lying down
F	13. prone	m.	head and knees elevated
H	14. Trendelenburg's	n.	back position with legs bent or flexed and thighs abducted
G	15. trans	o.	bending; being bent

■ DEFINE THE TERM

Define the following terms:

1. apothecaries' _system for weighing + measuring drugs, precious metals, solutions, + precious stones_
2. avoirdupois _English system of wts + measurements except for drugs, stones, + metals_
3. metric _system of wts + m based on meter + multiples of 10_
4. tera _master_
5. micro _small_
6. temperature _degree of cold/heat based on specific scale_
7. Celsius _temp scale - water boils at 100° + freezes at 0°_
8. Fahrenheit _temp scale - H₂O boils at 212° + freezes at 32°_
9. conversion _Δ from one scale/system to another_
10. equivalent _conversions that are equal_

■ MATCHING: METRIC UNITS

Match the units at the right to their metric weight on the left:

D **1.** ten times the size of the unit   **a.** milli

C **2.** one thousand times the size of the unit   **b.** pico

G **3.** one hundred times the size of the unit   **c.** kilo

E **4.** one tenth of a unit   **d.** deka

F **5.** one hundredth of a unit   **e.** deci

A **6.** one thousandth of a unit   **f.** centi

B **7.** one trillionth of a unit   **g.** hecto

■ SHORT ANSWER

1. A milligram equals _1000_ micrograms.
2. A gram equals _1000_ milligrams.
3. A gram equals _100_ centigrams.
4. A gram equals _10_ decigrams.
5. A hectogram equals _100_ grams.
6. A kilogram equals _1000_ grams.
7. One meter equals _1000_ millimeters.

8. One cubic centimeter equals __1__ milliliter(s).

9. One kilogram equals __2.2__ pounds.

10. One inch equals __2.5__ centimeters.

11. One liter equals __1000__ milliliters or __1000__ cubic centimeters.

12. To convert Celsius to Fahrenheit, multiply by __9__ divide by __5__, and add __32__.

13. To convert Fahrenheit to Celsius, subtract __32__, multiply by __9__, and divide by __5__.

14. One calorie equals __4.18__ joules (J).

15. __3__ teaspoon(s) equal(s) 1 tablespoon.

16. One fluid ounce equals __30__ milliliters.

17. One cup equals __240__ milliliters.

18. One liter equals __4.2__ cups.

■ FILL-IN

Write the term for the following abbreviations and/or symbols:

1. mg __milligram__

2. μg __microgram__

3. kg __kilogram__

4. gtt __drops__

5. ʒ __dram__

6. ℥ __ounce__

7. G __giga__

8. L __liter__

9. J __joule__

10. T __tera__

11. °C __degrees Celsius__

12. g __gram__

13. ↑ __evaporated / high__

14. ℞ __take, prescription__

15. s̄ __without__

16. c̄ __with__

17. ∞ __infinity__

18. $\bar{a}$ _before_

19. $\bar{p}$ _after_

20. ♀, ○ _Male_

CHAPTER 6	# Medical and Health Professions

LESSON ONE — MATERIALS TO BE LEARNED

SCIENTIFIC STUDIES

Table 6–1

Root	Suffix	Word Example	Pronunciation	Definition
audi/o	-logy	audiology	aw'de-<u>ol</u>-o-je	the science concerned with the sense of hearing, especially the evaluation and measurement of impaired hearing and the rehabilitation of those with impaired hearing
bacteri/o		bacteriology	bak-te're-<u>ol</u>-o-je	scientific study of bacteria
bi/o		biology	bi-<u>ol</u>-o-je	scientific study of living organisms
cardi/o		cardiology	kar'de-<u>ol</u>-o-je	study of the heart and its functions
dermat/o		dermatology	der'mah-<u>tol</u>-o-je	the medical specialty concerned with the diagnosis and treatment of skin diseases
endocrin/o		endocrinology	en'do-krin-<u>nol</u>-o-je	study of the endocrine system

Root	Suffix	Word Example	Pronunciation	Definition
gastr/oenter/o	-logy	gastroenterology	gas'tro-en'ter-<u>ol</u>-o-je	study of the stomach and intestine and their diseases
gynec/o		gynecology	gi'ne-<u>kol</u>-o-je	the branch of medicine dealing with diseases of the genital tract in women
hemat/o		hematology	he'mah-<u>tol</u>-o-je	the science dealing with the morphology of blood and blood-forming tissues and with their physiology and pathology
neur/o		neurology	nu-<u>rol</u>-o-je	the branch of medical science that deals with the nervous system, both normal and diseased
onc/o		oncology	ong-<u>kol</u>-o-je	the sum of knowledge regarding tumors; the study of tumors
ophthalm/o		ophthalmology	of'thal-<u>mol</u>-o-je	the branch of medicine dealing with the eye
path/o		pathology	pah-<u>thol</u>-o-je	the branch of medicine treating the essential nature of disease, especially changes in body tissues and organs that cause or are caused by disease
physi/o		physiology	fiz'e-<u>ol</u>-o-je	the science that treats the functions of the living organism and its parts, and the physical and chemical factors and processes involved
proct/o		proctology	prok-<u>tol</u>-o-je	the branch of medicine concerned with disorders of the rectum and anus
		psychology	si-<u>kol</u>-o-je	the science dealing with the mind and mental processes, especially in relation to human and animal behavior
radi/o		radiology	ra'de-<u>ol</u>-o-je	the branch of medical science dealing with the use of x-rays, radioactive substances, and other forms of radiant energy in the diagnosis and treatment of disease

Root	Suffix	Word Example	Pronunciation	Definition
ur/o	-logy	urology	u-<u>rol</u>-o-je	the branch of medicine dealing with the urinary system in the female and the genitourinary system in the male
phys	-iatry	physiatry	<u>fiz</u>-e-ah-tree	the branch of medicine that deals with the physical restoration, rehabilitation, and maintenance of the body structures
psych		psychiatry	si-<u>ki</u>-ah-tree	the branch of medicine that deals with the study, treatment, and prevention of mental illness

SPECIALTIES AND SPECIALISTS

Physicians and Medical Specialties

Table 6–2

Root	Suffix	Word Example	Pronunciation	Definition
-esthesia	-ologist	anesthesiologist	an′es-the′ze-<u>ol</u>-o-jist	a physician who specializes in anesthesiology. An anesthesiologist administers anesthetics, of which there are two types: *general* anesthetics, which produce sleep, and *regional* anesthetics, which render a specific area insensible to pain
cardi/o		cardiologist	kar′de-<u>ol</u>-o-jist	a physician skilled in the diagnosis and treatment of heart disease
derm/o (dermat/o)		dermatologist	der′mah-<u>tol</u>-o-jist	a physician who specializes in the treatment of infections, growths, and injuries related to the skin

Root	Suffix	Word Example	Pronunciation	Definition
endocrin/o	-ologist	endocrinologist	en'do-kri-<u>nol</u>-o-jist	a physician skilled in the diagnosis and treatment of disorders of the glands of internal secretion
gastr/oenter/o		gastroenterologist	gas-tro-en'ter-<u>ol</u>-o-jist	a physician who specializes in the study of the stomach and intestines and their diseases
geriatric	-ician	geriatrician	jer'e-a-<u>trish</u>-an	a physician who specializes in the diagnosis and treatment of the diseases of the aging and elderly
gynec/o		gynecologist	gi'ne-<u>kol</u>-o-jist	a physician who specializes in the diseases of the genital tract in women
hemat/o		hematologist	he'mah-<u>tol</u>-o-jist	a physician who specializes in the science of blood and blood-forming tissues
intern		internist	in-<u>ter</u>-nist	a physician who specializes in internal organs of the body and their function
neur/o		neurologist	nu-<u>rol</u>-o-jist	a physician who specializes in the science of the central nervous system
obstetric		obstetrician	ob'ste-<u>trish</u>-an	a physician who specializes in pregnancy, labor, and the puerperium
onc/o		oncologist	ong-<u>kol</u>-o-jist	a physician who specializes in the study of tumors

Root	Suffix	Word Example	Pronunciation	Definition
ophthalm/o		ophthalmologist	of'thal-<u>mol</u>-o-jist	a physician who specializes in diagnosing and prescribing treatment for defects, injuries, and diseases of the eye
orth/o		orthopedist	<u>or</u>-tho-pe'dist	a surgeon who specializes in the preservation and restoration of the function of the skeletal system, its articulation, and associated structures
ot/orhin/olaryng/o		otorhinolaryngologist	o'to-ri'no-lar-ing-<u>gol</u>-o-jist	a physician who specializes in the diseases of the ear, nose, and throat
path/o		pathologist	pah-<u>thol</u>-o-jist	a physician who specializes in diagnosing changes in body tissues and organs that cause or are caused by disease
pediatric		pediatrician	pe'de-ah-<u>trish</u>-an	a physician who specializes in the diagnosis and treatment of children's diseases
phys		physiatrist	fiz'-i-<u>a</u>-trist	a physician who specializes in prescribing and providing physical therapy and rehabilitation for patients requiring it
phys	-ician	physician	fi-<u>zish</u>-an	one who studies body function; an authorized practitioner of medicine

Root	Suffix	Word Example	Pronunciation	Definition
practice	-itioner	practitioner (family practice: M.D.)	prak-<u>tish</u>-a-ner	a physician who is schooled in six basic areas: internal medicine, obstetrics and gynecology, surgery, psychiatry, pediatrics, and community medicine. The practitioner can treat the whole family and coordinate specialty care if necessary
proct/o		proctologist	prok-<u>tol</u>-o-jist	a physician who specializes in the diagnosis and treatment of diseases of the rectum and anus
psych	-iatrist	psychiatrist	si-<u>ki</u>-a-trist	a physician who specializes in the diagnosis and treatment of mental disorders
radi/o	-ologist	radiologist	ra'de-<u>ol</u>-o-jist	a physician who specializes in the interpretation of x-rays and other radioactive substances used for diagnostic purposes
		General Practitioner (Doctor of Osteopathy: D.O.)		a physician who also specializes in surgical and physical manipulation for correcting body functions: the D.O. treats the patient as a holistic entity
		Preventive Medicine (practitioner)		a specialty that includes occupational medicine, public health, and general preventive medicine

Root	Suffix	Word Example	Pronunciation	Definition
		Emergency Medicine (practitioner)		relatively new specialty in emergency room care that treats acute illness and crisis situations

Other Health Professions

Table 6–3

Specialty	Title	Pronunciation	Definition
Chiropractic (ki'ro-prak-tik)	Chiropractor (D.C.)	ki'ro-<u>prak</u>-tor	a person trained in the manipulation of the vertebral column
Dentistry (den-tis-tre)	Dentist (D.D.S./D.M.D.)	<u>den</u>-tist	a physician who is concerned with the teeth and associated structures
Subspecialties	endodontist	en'do-<u>don</u>-tist	a dentist who specializes in conditions of the tooth pulp and root and the periapical tissues
	oral surgeon		a dentist who specializes in surgery of the mouth
	orthodontist	or'tho-<u>don</u>-tist	a dentist who specializes in the treatment of irregularities of the teeth, malocclusion, and associated facial problems
	pedodontist	pe'do-<u>don</u>-tist	a dentist who treats children's teeth
	periodontist	per'e-o-<u>don</u>-tist	a dentist who treats diseases of the gums
	prosthodontist	pros'tho-<u>don</u>-tist	a dentist who constructs artificial appliances designed to restore and maintain oral function
Related fields	Dental hygienist	<u>den</u>-tal hi'<u>je</u>-nist	a dental specialist (not an M.D.) whose primary concern is maintenance of dental health and prevention of oral disease
	Dental assistant		a person who assists the dentist at chairside

Specialty	Title	Pronunciation	Definition
	Dental technician		a person specially trained to prepare prosthetics, such as dentures, crowns, bridges, and partials
Dietetics	Registered Dietitian (R.D., M.S., Ph.D.)	reg-is-ter-ed di'e-tish-an	a specialist schooled in the use of proper diet for the promotion of health, prevention of disease, and therapy for the treatment of disease
	Dietetic Technician (D.T.R.)		a person with an associate of science degree trained to work under the guidance of a dietitian. Can plan menus and/or nutritional care for patients
Foot care	Podiatrist (D.M.P.)	po-di-ah-trist	a specialist who deals with the study and care of the foot
Medical assisting	Medical Assistant		a person trained to assist physicians in examining and treating patients, routine laboratory testing, and assigned clerical duties
Medical library	Medical Librarian (M.L.A.)		a professional person skilled in providing large volumes of current information to professional staff and personnel in medicine, dentistry, nursing, pharmacy, and other allied health professions
Medical records	Medical Record Administrator		a person skilled in managing an information system that meets medical, ethical, and legal requirements, compiling statisticsn and directing and controlling medical record staff
	Accredited Record Technician (ART)		a person who organizes, handles, and evaluates patient medical records
Medical technology	Medical Technologist or Clinical Laboratory Scientist (A.S.C.P.)		a person skilled in performing tests in a laboratory to identify and track disease

Specialty	Title	Pronunciation	Definition
Nursing	Registered Nurse (R.N.) or Advanced Practice Nurse (A.P.N.)		a specialist, licensed to work directly with patients, administering treatments as ordered by the physician
	Nurse Midwife (R.N. or A.P.N.)	mid-wif	a professional nurse with additional training who specializes in the care of women throughout pregnancy, delivery, and the postpartum period
	Nurse Practitioner (R.N. or A.P.N.)		a registered nurse who has completed required additional training and certification. A nurse practitioner, with physician referral, is able to offer patients personal attention and follow-up care
	Public Health Nurse (P.H.N.)		a registered nurse concerned with the prevention of illness and care of the sick in a community setting rather than a health care facility
Nursing, practical	Licensed Practical Nurse/ Licensed Vocational Nurse (L.P.N./L.V.N.)		a person who has completed a 1-year program in a state-recognized school and has taken and passed the state licensing test; works under the supervision of an R.N.
	Nursing Assistant (C.N.A.)		a person trained to help the R.N. and L.P.N. in a clinical situation
Physician assistant	Physician Assistant (P.A.)		a professional person trained in some medical procedures (not a physician) who performs limited duties under physician guidance
Occupational therapy	Occupational Therapist (O.T.R.)		a professional person schooled in the rehabilitation of fine motor skills who coordinates patient activities
Optometry	Optometrist (O.D.)	op-tom-e-trist	a professional person trained to examine the eyes and prescribe corrective lenses when there are irregularities in vision

Specialty	Title	Pronunciation	Definition
Pharmacy	Pharmacist (R.Ph.) (Pharm.D.)	<u>far</u>-mah-sist	one who is licensed to prepare, sell, or dispense drugs, compounds, and prescriptions
Physical therapy	Physical Therapist (R.P.T.)		a professional person skilled in the techniques of physical therapy and qualified to administer treatment prescribed by a physician or referred by a physician
Psychology	Psychologist (Ph.D.) (M.S.)	si-<u>kol</u>-o-jist	a person with advanced degrees who specializes in the treatment of disturbed mental processes and abnormal behavior. Does not prescribe drugs
Radiology	Radiology Technologist (R.R.T.)		one who specializes in the use of x-rays and radioactive isotopes in the diagnosis and treatment of disease and who works under the supervision of a radiologist
Respiratory therapy	Respiratory Therapist (A.R.R.T.)		one who holds at least an associate degree in respiratory therapy and who assists patients to improve impaired respiratory functions under a physician's direction
Social work	Health Care Social Worker (M.S.W./Ph.D.)		a professional person skilled in helping patients and their families handle personal problems that result from long-term illness or disability
	Psychiatric Social Worker (M.S.W./Ph.D.) (A.C.S.W.)		a professional person skilled in maintaining contact between patients with mental illness, their psychiatrist, families, and return to community life
Veterinary medicine	Veterinarian (D.V.M.)	vet'er-i-<u>na</u>-re-an	a doctor trained and authorized to practice veterinary medicine and perform surgery on animals. May also do research

Space limitations prohibit a complete presentation on known health professionals recognized by state and federal health authorities. Instead, Table 6–4 lists other health professions not covered in Lesson 1.

Table 6–4

Additional Health Professions	
Animal Technicians	Nuclear Medicine Technologists
Art Therapists	Occupational Therapy Assistants
Athletic Trainers	Opticians, Paraoptometrics
Biological Photographers	Orientation and Mobility Instructors for the Blind
Community Health Educators	Paramedics
Corrective Therapists	Pharmacy Assistants
Dance Therapists	Physical Therapy Assistants and Aides
Dietetic Assistants and Aides	Psychiatric/Mental Health Technicians
Educational Therapists	Radiation Therapists
EEG Technologists and Technicians	Radiology Technicians
EKG Technicians	Recreational Therapists
EMTs	Rehabilitation Teachers
Health Care Administrators	Respiratory Technicians
Health Sciences Library Technicians	Sanitarians
Horticulture Therapists	School Health Educators
Manual Arts Therapists	Social Service Assistants
Medical Illustrators	Speech-Language Pathologists/Audiologists
Medical Secretaries	Surgical Technicians
Medical Transcriptionists	Teachers of the Visually Handicapped
Music Therapists	Writers—Medical, Science, and Technical

LESSON TWO   PROGRESS CHECK

■ MULTIPLE CHOICE: SCIENTIFIC STUDIES

Circle the letter of the correct answer:

1. The science concerned with the evaluation and measurement of hearing is

    a. neurology
    b. biology
    c. anesthesiology
    d. audiology

2. The scientific study of living organisms is

    a. bacteriology
    b. biology
    c. pathology
    d. hematology

3. The study of conditions of the blood and blood-forming organs is called

    a. endocrinology
    b. cardiology
    c. hematology
    d. bacteriology

4. Oncology is the study of

    a. tumors
    b. kidneys
    c. diseases
    d. eyes

5. The science that specializes in diseases of the stomach and intestines is

    a. gynecology
    b. enterology
    c. gastroenterology
    d. radiology

6. The branch of medicine dealing with the mind and its diseases is

    a. neurology
    b. physiatry
    c. proctology
    d. psychiatry

7. The branch of medicine dealing with disorders of the rectum and anus is

    a. neurology
    b. physiatry
    c. proctology
    d. psychiatry

■ MATCHING

Match the specialist with the field of practice:

1.	anesthesiologist	**a.**	children's diseases
2.	dermatologist	**b.**	diseases of the elderly
3.	gastroenterologist	**c.**	interpretation of diagnostic x-ray studies
4.	internist	**d.**	skin diseases
5.	gynecologist	**e.**	diseases of stomach and intestines
6.	otorhinolaryngologist	**f.**	diseases of female genital tract
7.	ophthalmologist	**g.**	diseases of the ear, nose, and throat
8.	radiologist	**h.**	administration of therapeutic measures for pain insensibility
9.	geriatrician	**i.**	diseases and functions of body organs
10.	pediatrician	**j.**	diseases of the eye

■ SHORT ANSWER

Describe these *specialties* related to the medical profession and *name* the specialist, including his or her title:

1. Dentistry _____

2. Dietetics _____

3. Podiatry _____

4. Midwifery _____

5. Practical Nursing _____

6. Psychology _____

7. Pharmacy _____

8. Nursing _____

9. Veterinary Medicine _____

■ COMPLETION

1. The specialist who performs surgery on the mouth is called a(n)_____

2. The specialist who treats diseases of the gums is called a(n) _____

3. A specialist whose primary concern is prevention of oral disease is a(n)_____

4. A person who assists in the nutritional care of patients in a health care facility is a(n) _____

5. A person who treats problems and maintains the health of the foot is a(n)_____

6. A professional person who performs specialized tests in a laboratory is a(n) _____

7. A professional person who helps to restore and
   rehabilitate a patient to physical use of body parts is a(n) _____

8. The specialist who treats behavior and
   mental disturbances with communication therapies is a(n) _____

9. The specialist who dispenses medications is a(n) _____

10. The specialist who examines the eyes and prescribes corrective lenses is a(n) _____

■ MULTIPLE CHOICE: PROFESSIONS

For the following professions, circle *all* the answers that apply:

1. A nurse may be

   (a) licensed   (b) certified   (c) registered   (d) a Ph.D.

2. A physician may be

   (a) M.D.   (b) D.D.S.   (c) certified   (d) licensed

3. A dentist may be

   (a) M.D.   (b) D.D.S.   (c) licensed   (d) certified

4. A chiropractor must be

   (a) licensed   (b) certified   (c) M.D.   (d) registered

■ ABBREVIATIONS

List the appropriate letters (abbreviations) for the following professional titles:

1. Occupational Therapist _____

2. Physical Therapist _____

3. Public Health Nurse _____

4. Registered Dietitian _____

5. Vocational Nurse _____

6. Professional Nurse _____

7. Medical Technician _____ or _____

8. Radiology Technician _____

9. Dentist _____

10. Veterinarian _____

11. Optometrist _____

12. Ophthalmologist _____

13. Psychologist _____

14. Psychiatrist _____

15. Pharmacist _____

16. Respiratory Therapist _____

17. Osteopathy Practitioner _____

18. Family Practitioner _____

■ DESCRIBE THE SPECIALTY

Describe the specialty of the following practitioners:

1. Anesthesiologist _____

2. Endocrinologist _____

3. Hematologist _____

4. Radiologist _____

5. Pathologist _____

6. Bacteriologist _____

7. Biologist _____

8. Geriatrician _____

9. Pediatrician _____

10. Podiatrist _____

11. Dietitian _____

12. Obstetrician _____

Abbreviations

CHAPTER 7 Medical Abbreviations

LESSON ONE   MATERIALS TO BE LEARNED

The following information will help you in your study of medical abbreviations:

1. There are numerous medical abbreviations. Only samples are given in this chapter.
2. The necessity to learn certain medical abbreviations is directly related to a student's health career plan. For example, laboratory abbreviations and terms are essential for students planning to be Clinical Laboratory Technologists.
3. Physicians' handwriting, especially abbreviations, is difficult to read.
4. Purchase a medical abbreviations book recommended by your instructor.

ABBREVIATIONS FOR SERVICES OR UNITS IN A HEALTHCARE FACILITY

Table 7–1

Abbreviation	Definition
A & D	Admitting and Discharge
CS	Central Service (or Supply)
OR	Operating Room (surgery); MOR, Minor Surgery
RR	Recovery Room

Abbreviation	Definition
PT & OT	Physical Therapy and Occupational Therapy (may be under PM & R, Physical Medicine and Rehabilitation)
X-ray	Radiology
Lab	Medical Laboratory
MR	Medical Records
Peds	Pediatrics
Med-Surg	Ward for medical and surgical patients (may be combined or separate)
OB	Obstetrics (includes labor and delivery rooms, postpartum ward, and newborn nursery for healthy babies)
ICN or NICU	Intensive Care Nursery, or Newborn Intensive Care Unit, for premature or unhealthy babies
OPD	Out-Patient Department
ER	Emergency Room; ED, Emergency Department
ENT	Ear, Nose, and Throat
GU	Genitourinary
NP	Neuropsychiatric
SS	Social Service
CCU or ICU	Coronary Care Unit or Intensive Care Unit
DOU	Definitive Observation Unit (less than intensive care, but more than "floor" care)
Dietary (FS)	Food Service/Dietary Department
Housekeeping	Janitorial Service
Pharmacy	Drugstore
Morgue	Unit for autopsies/holding the deceased
Pathology (Path)	Laboratory for study of diseased tissues, including blood

ABBREVIATIONS FOR FREQUENCIES

Table 7–2

Abbreviation	Definition
q	every
qd	once a day
qod	every other day
q___h	every ___ hours (insert hours)
bid	twice a day
tid	three times a day
qid	four times a day
hs	at bedtime (hour of sleep)
ac	before meals
pc	after meals
prn	when needed
ad lib	as desired
stat	immediately

ABBREVIATIONS FOR UNITS OF MEASURE

Table 7–3

Abbreviation	Definition	Abbreviation	Definition
tabs.	tablets, pills	mEq	milliequivalent
g or gm	grams	U	units
gr.	grains	gtts	drops
cc	cubic centimeters	oz	ounces
mL or ml	milliliters	dr.	drams
L	liter (1000 cc or ml)		

ABBREVIATIONS FOR MEANS OF ADMINISTERING SUBSTANCES INTO THE BODY

Table 7–4

Abbreviation	Definition
PO	by mouth (*per os*)
IV	intravenously (into a vein; usually a peripheral vein)
IM	intramuscularly (into a muscle)
H	hypodermically (with a needle)
subcu, subq	subcutaneously (through the skin, into the fatty tissue)
subling	sublingually (under the tongue)
R	rectally (by rectum)
parenteral	a solution given intravenously
enteral	tube feeding (into stomach or small intestine)
D_5W	5% glucose in distilled water; use IV
caps.	capsules
supp	suppository
ss	one-half
mg	milligrams
N.S.	normal saline solution: isotonic solution
clysis	fluids given by needle, under skin (not in vein)
TKO	to keep open (vein)
KVO	keep vein open

ABBREVIATIONS FOR DIET ORDERS

Table 7–5

Abbreviation	Definition
NPO	nothing *per os* (nothing to eat or drink orally)
I & O	intake and output (measured)
Cl Liq	clear liquids only: ginger ale, tea, broth, Jell-O, 7-Up, coffee
F Liq	full liquid: addition of milk and milk products; liquid at body temperature
Lo Salt, Low Na, Salt Free	restricted in sodium: ordered by mg or g of sodium desired, i.e., 2 g Na, 500 mg Na
NAS	no added salt packet; usually 4–6 g Na (mild restriction)
reg	regular diet ("house" or "normal" sometimes used). A balanced diet without restrictions as to the type of food texture, seasoning, or preparation method
mech soft	mechanical soft; a regular diet with alteration in texture only. Sometimes called "edentulous"
med soft	medical soft; alterations in texture, preparation methods, and seasonings
bland	a medical soft diet further altered to omit acid-producing beverages and restrict seasonings. Altered feeding intervals
Lo res	low residue; alteration in texture and a limited food selection to yield little intestinal residue
high fiber	a regular diet with increased amounts of foods containing dietary fiber
FF or PF	force or push fluids; increasing the liquid intake by addition of extra fluids
int fdg or int nour	interval feeding; supplemental nourishment served between meals
DAT	diet as tolerated
dysphagia pureed	regular diet pureed to a smooth, homogeneous, and cohesive consistency like pudding
consistent or controlled carbohydrate (CCHO)	consistent amounts of carbohydrate at meals and snacks to regulate blood glucose levels primarily for diabetes
Lo Fat, Lo Chol	low saturated fat, low cholesterol. A "Healthy Diet" based on *The Dietary Guidelines for Americans*, 2005, to reduce the risk of heart disease

ABBREVIATIONS FOR ACTIVITY AND TOILETRY

Table 7–6

Abbreviation	Definition
CBR	complete bed rest; ABR (absolute bed rest)
dangle	sit at edge of bed, legs over side
ambulate	Walk
OOB	out of bed
BRP	bathroom privileges; may be up to bathroom only
commode	bedside toilet

ABBREVIATIONS FOR LABORATORY TESTS, X-RAY STUDIES, AND PULMONARY FUNCTION

Table 7–7

Abbreviation	Definition
AP and Lat	routine x-ray picture of chest (front to back and side view)
up	upright x-ray picture
decub	decubitus (lying) position
IVP	intravenous pyelogram (kidney)
BE	barium enema (colon)
2GI series	upper (barium swallow): x-ray of stomach/duodenum; lower (same as BE): x-ray of lower bowel/colon
GB series	gallbladder x-ray picture
MRI	magnetic resonance imaging; noninvasive procedure using a magnetic field that yields images for Dx
RAI, RAIU	radioactive iodine (uptake) for diagnosing thyroid function
SCAN	CT, CAT: computed tomography, computerized axial tomography
CBC	complete blood count
UA	urinalysis
VC	vital capacity (lungs)

ABBREVIATIONS FOR MISCELLANEOUS TERMS

Table 7–8

Abbreviation	Definition
qns	quantity not sufficient (lab requires a larger specimen). Also refers to insufficient food/liq intake
$\bar{c}$	with (con)
$\bar{s}$	without (sans)
dc	discontinue
TLC	tender loving care
stat	immediately
ASAP	as soon as possible
CPR	cardiopulmonary resusitation
EUA	examination under anesthesia
DOA	dead on arrival
OD	overdose; also means right eye (refer to context where used)
prep	prepare
V/S	vital signs
ECG, EKG	electrocardiogram
EEG	electroencephalogram
Dx	diagnosis
Tx	treatment
Rx	prescription
Sx	symptoms
Na^+	natrium: sodium (chemical symbol for)
K^+	potassium (chemical symbol for)
Ca^{++}	calcium (chemical symbol for)
P^{+++}	phosphorus (chemical symbol for)
Cl^-	chloride (chemical symbol for)

Abbreviation	Definition
I-	iodine (chemical symbol for)
Fe^{++}	iron (chemical symbol for)
Hg^{++}	mercury (chemical symbol for)

LESSON TWO   PROGRESS CHECK

■ IDENTIFY THE DEPARTMENT

As a new employee of the hospital, you are given a list of departments that you will tour. Identify these units, which are on your list:

1. A & D _____

2. CS _____

3. OR _____

4. PM & R _____

5. X-ray _____

6. Lab _____

7. OB _____

8. Peds _____

9. OPD _____

10. ER _____

11. SS _____

12. ICU _____

13. FS _____

■ IDENTIFY THE PRESCRIPTION

Medications are given in many different forms, and dosages, and at scheduled times. They are administered into the body in various ways. In the following questions, identify (a) the form, (b) the type of administration, (c) the scheduled time of the dose, and (d) the dosage amount:

1. 2 g PO tid _____

2. 60 mEq R supp hs _____

3. gtts vi subling $\overline{q}$4h _____

4. 2 L IV $\overline{q}$d _____

5. 30 U IM ac _____

6. 10 ml subcu prn _____

7. gr. ii in 10 cc n.s. clysis $\overline{q}$d _____

8. īiss mg $\overline{pc}$ PO _____

■ IDENTIFY THE DIET ORDER

Identify the following *diet orders* from their abbreviations:

Room	Name	Diet	
1. 123	Mr J	NPO	_____
2. 231	Mrs K	DAT	_____
3. 301	Ms B	CCHO	_____
4. 111	Mr H	2 g Na med soft	_____
5. 112	Mr P	mech soft	_____
6. 321	Mrs L	cl liq	_____
7. 222	Mr K	Reg Hi Fiber FF	_____
8. 232	Mrs R	f. liq $\overline{c}$ int. nour. 10–2–HS. I&O	_____

■ MATCHING

Match the abbreviation to its description:

1. AP and Lat   **a.** diagnostic for thyroid function

2. IVP   **b.** measuring lung capacity

3. BE   **c.** diagnostic for gastric diseases

4. GB series   **d.** kidney function test

5. upper GI   **e.** analysis of kidney excretion

6. UA   **f.** routine chest x-rays

7. VC   **g.** diagnostic for colon diseases

8. RAI   **h.** diagnostic for cholecystic diseases

■ SPELL OUT THE ABBREVIATION

In the following sentences, write in the complete words for the abbreviations given:

1. The nurse told the aide to *prep* the patient *pre-op*. _____

2. That man was *DOA*. _____

3. They took him $\bar{c}$ the others $\bar{s}$ doing *TPR*. _____

4. She required *CPR*. _____

5. *BP* was 110/80 *mm Hg*. _____

6. What I need is *TLC*. _____

7. *DC* the *IV ASAP*. _____

8. End products of respiration are CO_2 and H_2O. _____

9. The *Tx* was more painful than the *Sx*. _____

10. Her serum NA^+ was elevated, but the K^+ was low. _____

11. The *Dx* was Fe^{++} deficiency anemia. _____

CHAPTER 8 # Diagnostic and Laboratory Abbreviations

LESSON ONE MATERIALS TO BE LEARNED

DIAGNOSTIC ABBREVIATIONS

Table 8–1

Abbreviation	Definition
A & P	auscultation and percussion
ASHD	arteriosclerotic heart disease
CA	carcinoma (cancer)
CBS	chronic brain syndrome
CC	chief complaint
CHD	coronary heart disease; congenital heart disease
CHF	congestive heart failure
c/o	complains of
COPD/COLD	chronic obstructive pulmonary (lung) disease
CP	cerebral palsy
CVA	cerebrovascular accident (stroke)
CVD	cardiovascular disease

Abbreviation	Definition
DJD	degenerative joint disease (osteoarthritis)
Dx	diagnosis
FH	family history
FUO	fever of undetermined origin
GC	gonorrhea
HEENT	head, eyes, ears, nose, throat
Hx	history
(S)LE	(systemic) lupus erythematosus
m	murmur
MD	muscular dystrophy
MI	myocardial infarction
MS	multiple sclerosis
P & A	percussion and auscultation
PE	physical examination
PERRLA	pupils equal, round, react to light and accommodation (eyes)
PH	past history
PI	present illness
PID	pelvic inflammatory disease
RA	rheumatoid arthritis
R/O	rule out
Rx	recipe, take, prescription
SOB	short of breath
SR or ROS	systemic review or review of systems
Sx	symptoms
T & A	tonsillectomy and adenoidectomy

Abbreviation	Definition
TIA	transient ischemic attack
TPR	temperature, pulse, respiration
URI	upper respiratory infection
UTI	urinary tract infection

LABORATORY ABBREVIATIONS

Table 8–2

Abbreviation	Definition
AFB	acid-fast bacillus (tuberculosis organism)
C & S	culture and sensitivity
CATH	catheterize
CBC	complete blood count
Crit, Hct	hematocrit
diff	differential
ESR	erythrocyte sedimentation rate
FBS	fasting blood sugar
GTT	glucose tolerance test
Hb, Hgb	hemoglobin
RA	rheumatoid arthritis
RBC	red blood (cell) count (erythrocytes); red blood cells
STS	serologic test of syphilis
VDRL	venereal disease research laboratory
WBC	white blood (cell) count (leukocytes); white blood cells

A LIST OF COMMON DIAGNOSTIC AND
LABORATORY ABBREVIATIONS*

Table 8–3

Name of Test, Screening, Procedure, or Others	Explanatory Notes
cardio CRP™ (high-sensitivity C-reactive protein)	as stated in name
cervical biopsy	as stated in name
chlamydia tests	sexually transmitted diseases (STDs)
chloride (Cl)	blood/chemistry tests
cholesterol and triglycerides tests	blood/chemistry tests
chromosome analysis	as stated in name
CK (creatine kinase)	as stated in name
colon biopsy	as stated in name
colorectal cancer screen	as stated in name
complete blood count (CBC)	blood/chemistry tests
creatinine and creatinine clearance	blood/chemistry tests
C-reactive protein	as stated in name
cystic fibrosis test	screening
esophageal biopsy	as stated in name
fecal occult blood test	as stated in name
ferritin	blood/chemistry tests
folic acid	blood/chemistry tests
follicle-stimulating hormone (FSH)	as stated in name
glycohemoglobin (GHb)	as stated in name
gonorrhea test	sexually transmitted diseases (STDs)
Helicobacter pylori (*H. pylori*) tests	as stated in name
hemoglobin (part of CBC)	as stated in name
hepatitis B antigen and antibody tests	sexually transmitted diseases (STDs)
hepatitis C genotype	as stated in name

Name of Test, Screening, Procedure, or Others	Explanatory Notes
hepatitis C viral load	as stated in name
hepatitis C virus test	as stated in name
herpes test	sexually transmitted diseases (STDs)
HIV testing	sexually transmitted diseases (STDs)
HIV viral load	as stated in name
homocysteine	as stated in name
HPV test (human papillomavirus)	sexually transmitted diseases (STDs)
human chorionic gonadotropin (hCG)	blood/chemistry tests
iron tests	blood/chemistry tests
lactic dehydrogenase (LDH)	blood/chemistry tests
lead	as stated in name
luteinizing hormone (LH)	as stated in name
magnesium (Mg)	blood/chemistry tests

maternal serum screening
   alpha-fetoprotein (AFP) in blood
   estrogens
   human chorionic gonadotropin (hCG)
   maternal serum triple test
	blood/chemistry tests

osteoporosis/bone mineral density testing	as stated in name
ovarian cancer	as stated in name
Pap test	as stated in name
parathyroid hormone (bio-intact PTH)	as stated in name
partial thromboplastin time (PTT)	as stated in name

phosphorus
   phosphate in blood
   phosphate in urine
	blood/urine chemistry tests

potassium (K)	blood/chemistry tests
progesterone	as stated in name
prolactin	as stated in name

Name of Test, Screening, Procedure, or Others	Explanatory Notes
prostate biopsy	as stated in name
prostate-specific antigen (PSA)	as stated in name
prothrombin time (PT)	as stated in name
rheumatoid factor (RF)	as stated in name
rubella test	as stated in name
sedimentation rate	as stated in name
sickle cell testing	as stated in name
skin biopsy	as stated in name
sodium (Na)	blood/chemistry tests
stomach biopsy	as stated in name
syphilis tests	sexually transmitted diseases (STDs)
testosterone	as stated in name
thyroid hormone tests (T-3 total; T-3 uptake; T-4 total [thyroxine])	blood/chemistry tests
total serum protein and/or albumin	blood/chemistry tests
TSH	blood/chemistry tests

uric acid
    uric acid in blood
    uric acid in urine
	blood/chemistry tests

urine test	as stated in name
vitamin B_{12}	as stated in name

*This list is provided here for reference only. The instructor may choose examples for discussion or testing.

LESSON TWO PROGRESS CHECK

■ IDENTIFY THE DISEASE

Identify the following diseases or conditions from the diagnostic abbreviations given:

1. ASHD _____
2. CHD _____
3. CHF _____
4. CVD _____
5. CVA _____
6. CBS _____
7. COPD _____
8. MI _____
9. RA _____
10. TIA _____

■ SHORT ANSWER

To what *procedure* do the following abbreviations refer?

1. A & P _____
2. PERRLA _____
3. P & A _____
4. R/O _____
5. SR _____
6. T & A _____
7. PE _____
8. Rx _____
9. HEENT _____
10. Dx _____

■ MATCHING

Match the laboratory abbreviation to its descriptive term at the right:

1. Hct   **a.** test for abnormal blood sugar levels

2. C & S   **b.** test for blood sugar level before eating

3. ESR   **c.** test for volume of packed red cells

4. FBS   **d.** test for iron-containing red blood cells

5. GTT   **e.** count of both white and red cells

6. CBC   **f.** determination of rate of settling of red cells

7. AFB   **g.** test for tuberculosis organism

8. Hb   **h.** culture for organism sensitivity

9. EEG   **i.** bathroom privileges

10. qns   **j.** right eye

11. dc   **k.** examination under anesthesia

12. decubitus   **l.** out of bed

13. CAT   **m.** electroencephalogram

14. OD   **n.** computerized axial tomography

15. DOA   **o.** x-ray study taken in a lying position

16. OOB   **p.** inadequate quantity

17. BRP   **q.** discontinue

18. EUA   **r.** dead on arrival

■ DEFINE THE ABBREVIATION

Define the following abbreviations commonly used by medical personnel to speed up their charting in the patient's record:

1. CC _____

2. c/o _____

3. FH _____

4. FUO _____

5. Hx _____

6. SOB _____

7. URI _____

8. UTI _____

9. m _____

10. PI _____

11. Sx _____

12. PH _____

Review

CHAPTER 9 — Review of Word Parts of Units I, II, and III

OBJECTIVES

After completion of this chapter, the student should be able to:

1. Define the meaning of given word elements.
2. Define whole medical terms by applying knowledge gained from previous study.
3. Recognize the meaning of new terms by dividing them into their respective elements.

OVERVIEW

This review chapter is designed to assist you by pulling together the terminology to reinforce your learning.

These exercises are designed as learning tools. They give you the opportunity to write in your answers and test yourself. Check your answers carefully against the information contained in the previous three units. You may also use your medical dictionary. Check your spelling of the terms, as spelling is very important to the meaning of medical words.

If you have audio tapes with your text, listen to each term for the correct pronunciation and repeat the word out loud several times so you will be comfortable using it in conversation.

LESSON ONE | **MATERIALS TO BE LEARNED**

■ REVIEW A: SUFFIXES

Write the meaning of each suffix in the space provided:

Table 9–1

Suffix	Meaning
-algia	
-cele	
-dynia	
-ectasis	
-emia	
-gen	
-gram	
-graph	
-graphy	
-gravid	
-iasis	
-itis	
-logy	
-malacia	
-megaly	
-meter	
-metry	
-oid	
-oma	
-pathy	
-penia	
-phagia	
-phasia	
-phobia	
-plegia	

Suffix	Meaning
-ptosis	
-rrhage	
-rrhea	
-rrhexis	
-sclerosis	
-scopy	
-sis	
-spasm	
-stasis	

■ REVIEW B: PREFIXES

Write the meaning of each prefix in the space provided:

Table 9–2

Prefix	Meaning
a-, an-	
ab-	
ad-	
aero-	
aniso-	
bi-	
brady-	
de-	
di-	
dia-	
dif-, dis-	
dys-	
ec-, ecto-	
end-, endo-	
ep-, epi-	
eu-	
ex-, exo-	

Prefix	Meaning
extra-	
hemi-	
hemo-	
hetero-	
homo-	
hyper-	
hypo-	
in-	
iso-	
lip-	
mal-	
mega-	
megalo-	
meno-	
meta-	
noct-	
nyct-	
pan-	
para-	
per-	
peri-	
poly-	
post-	
pre-	
pro-	
pyo-	
pyro-	
re-	
super-	
supra-	
syn-	
tachy-	

■ REVIEW C: ROOT WORDS FOR BODY PARTS

Many of the words in this section have been introduced to you in previous chapters. They should serve as a small review of root words.

Cover each definition in the right column and try to define the term before looking at the answer by using previous knowledge of word parts. A short definition is okay. The answer column contains a more detailed definition, but your answer may contain just the essential meaning of the word at this time.

Table 9–3

Root Word	Meaning	Word Example	Pronunciation	Definition
carp/o	wrist	metacarpal	met'ah-<u>kar</u>-pal	the bones between the wrist and fingers
celi/o	abdomen			see lapar/o
cervic/o	neck	cervical	<u>serv</u>-i-cal	pertaining to the neck or to the cervix
		cervix (of uterus)	<u>ser</u>-viks	the narrow lower end (neck) of the uterus
chondr/o	cartilage	chondritis	kon-<u>dri</u>-tis	inflammation of a cartilage
colp/o	vagina	colpitis	kol-<u>pi</u>-tis	inflammation of the vagina; vaginitis
dent/o-odont	teeth	dentist	<u>den</u>-tist	a person who has received a degree in dentistry and is authorized to practice dentistry
		orthodontia	or-tho-<u>don</u>-ti-a	the branch of dentistry concerned with correcting and preventing irregularities of the teeth
esophag/o	esophagus	esophagitis	e-sof'ah-<u>ji</u>-tis	inflammation of the esophagus
lapar/o	abdominal wall	laparotomy	lap'ah-<u>rot</u>-o-me	incision through the flank or, more generally, through any part of the abdominal wall
laryng/o	larynx	laryngitis	lar'in-<u>ji</u>-tis	inflammation of the larynx
myring/o	eardrum			see tympan/o

Root Word	Meaning	Word Example	Pronunciation	Definition
onych/o	nail	paronychia	par'o-nik-e-ah	inflammation in the folds of the tissue around the fingernail
oophor/o	ovary	oophorectomy	o'of-o-rek-to-me	excision of one or both ovaries
ophthalm/o	eye	ophthalmologist	of'thal-mol-o-jist	a physician who specializes in diseases of the eyes
pancreat/o	pancreas	pancreatitis	pan'kre-ah-ti-tis	inflammation of the pancreas
pelv/i	pelvis	pelvimeter	pel-vim-e-ter	an instrument for measuring the pelvis
phleb/o	vein	phlebitis	fle-bi-tis	inflammation of a vein
pleur/o	pleura	pleurisy	ploor-i-se	inflammation of the pleura
pod/o	foot	podiatry	po-di-ah-tre	specialized field dealing with the treatment and care of the foot
psych/o	mind	psychiatrist	si-ki-ah-trist	a physician who specializes in treatment of the mind
pub/o	pubes (pubic bones)	suprapubic	soo'prah-pu-bik	above the pubes
rhin/o	nose	rhinoplasty	ri-no-plas'te	plastic surgery of the nose
salping/o	fallopian tube or eustachian tube	salpingitis	sal'pin-ji-tis	inflammation the auditory or uterine tube
soma	body	psychosomatic	si'ko-so-mat-ik	pertaining to the mind–body relationship; having bodily symptoms of psychic, emotional, or mental origin
splen/o	spleen	splenectomy	sple-nek-to-me	excision of the spleen
spondyl/o	vertebra	spondylitis	spon'di-li-tis	inflammation of the vertebrae
stomat/o	mouth	stomatitis	sto'mah-ti-tis	generalized inflammation of the oral mucosa
tars/o	ankle	metatarsal	met'ah-tar-sal	bones between the ankle and toes

Root Word	Meaning	Word Example	Pronunciation	Definition
thorac/o	thorax (chest)	thoracentesis	tho'rah-sen-te-sis	surgical puncture of the chest wall into the parietal cavity for aspiration of fluids
tympan/o	tympanum (eardrum or middle ear)	tympanotomy	tim'pah-not-o-me	incision of the tympanic membrane
myring/o	myringo (eardrum)	myringotomy	mir'ing-got-o-me	incision of the tympanic membrane; tympanotomy
ureter/o	ureter	ureteritis	u-re'-ter-i-tis	inflammation of a ureter
urethr/o	urethra	urethritis	u're-thri-tis	inflammation of the urethra
vas/o	vessel	cardiovascular	kar'de-o-vas-ku-lar	pertaining to the heart and blood vessels
ven/o	vein	intravenous	in'trah-ve-nus	within a vein

■ REVIEW D: DESCRIPTIVE WORD ELEMENTS

Table 9–4

Root Word	Meaning	Word Example	Pronunciation	Definition
ankyl/o	stiffening or fusion	ankylosis	ang'ki-lo-sis	immobility and consolidation of a joint from disease, injury, or surgical procedure
carcin/o	cancer (malignancy)	carcinomo	kar'si-no-mah	a malignant new growth made up of epithelial cells that may infiltrate surrounding tissues
cry/o	cold	cryosurgery	kri'o-ser-jer-e	the destruction of tissue by application of extreme cold
crypt/o	hidden (small hidden sac)	cryptorchidism	krip-tor-ki-dism	failure of one or both testes to descend into the scrotum

Root Word	Meaning	Word Example	Pronunciation	Definition
esthesia	feeling	anesthesia	an'es-<u>the</u>-ze-ah	loss of feeling or sensation, especially the loss of pain sensation induced to permit surgery
gravid/o	pregnant	primigravida	pri'mi-<u>grav</u>-i-dah	a woman pregnant for the first time, gravida I
lip/o	fat	lipoma	li-<u>po</u>-mah	a benign fatty tumor
lith/o	stone	cholelithiasis	ko'le-li-<u>thi</u>-ah-sis	the presence or formation of gallstones
necr/o	dead (decayed)	necrosis	ne-<u>kro</u>-sis	cell death: it may affect groups of cells or part of a structure or an organ
par-	to bear (children)	multipara	mul-<u>tip</u>-ah-rah	a woman who has had two or more pregnancies
path/o	disease state	osteopathy	os'te-<u>op</u>-ah-the	any disease of a bone
phag/o-phagia	eating, swallowing	dysphagia	dis-<u>fa</u>-je-ah	difficulty in swallowing
-phasia	speech	aphasia	ah-<u>fa</u>-zhe-ah	defect or loss of the power of expression by speech, writing, or signs or of comprehending spoken or written language, caused by injury or disease of the brain centers
phon/o	voice	aphonia	a-<u>fo</u>-ne-ah	loss of voice; inability to produce vocal sounds
schiz/o	split	schizophrenia	skit'so-<u>fre</u>-ne-ah	any of a group of severe emotional disorders characterized by withdrawal from reality, delusions, hallucinations, and bizarre behavior
scler/o	hardening	arteriosclerosis	ar-te're-o'skle-<u>ro</u>-sis	hardening and thickening of the walls of arterioles

Root Word	Meaning	Word Example	Pronunciation	Definition
sta	slowed, halted, controlled	hemostasis	he′mo-<u>sta</u>-sis	the arrest of bleeding, either by vasoconstriction and coagulation or by surgical means
therap	treatment	psychotherapy	si-ko-<u>ther</u>-ah-pe	treatment designed to produce a response by mental rather than physical effects
therm/o	heat	thermometer	ther-<u>mom</u>-e-ter	an instrument for determining temperatures
thromb/o	clot, lump	thrombosis	throm-<u>bo</u>-sis	the formation or presence of a thrombus (clot)
traumat/o	injury, wound, damage from an external source	traumatopenea	<u>traw</u>-ma-top-ne′ah	passage of air through a wound in the chest wall

■ REVIEW E: ADDITIONAL MEDICAL TERMS

Review E (additional medical terms) contains some words with which you will not be familiar. Test your ability to recognize the meaning of new medical terms by covering the definition column on the right side, dividing the word into its respective parts, and seeing if you can define it before you look at the answer.

Table 9–5

Word	Pronunciation	Definition
abdomen	<u>ab</u>-do′men	that part of the body lying between the thorax and the pelvis and containing the abdominal cavity and viscera
abdominal	ab-<u>dom</u>-i-nal	pertaining to the abdomen
abortion	ah-<u>bor</u>-shun	expulsion from the uterus of the products of conception before the fetus is viable
abscess	<u>ab</u>-ses	a localized collection of pus in a cavity formed by disintegration of tissues
acute	ah-<u>kut</u>	sharp; having severe symptoms and a short course
adhesion	ad-<u>he</u>-zhun	stuck together; abnormal joining of parts to one another

Word	Pronunciation	Definition
adnexa	ad-<u>nek</u>-sah	accessory structures of an organ: of the eye, including the eyelids and tear ducts; of the uterus, including the uterine tubes and ovaries
anomaly	ah-<u>nom</u>-ah-le	marked deviation from normal, especially as a result of congenital or hereditary defects
auscultation	aws'kul-<u>ta</u>-shun	listening for sounds within the body, chiefly to detect conditions of the thorax, abdominal viscera, or a pregnancy
autoclave	<u>aw</u>-to-klav	a self-locking apparatus for the sterilization of materials by steam under pressure
axilla (axillary)	ak-<u>sil</u>-ah	the armpit
biopsy	<u>bi</u>-op-se	removal and examination, usually microscopic, of tissue from the living body, performed to establish precise diagnosis
catgut	<u>kat</u>-gut	an absorbable, sterile strand obtained from collagen derived from healthy mammals, used to suture
catheter	<u>kath</u>-e-ter	a tubular, flexible instrument passed through body cavities for withdrawal of fluids from (or introduction of fluids into) a body cavity
cervical	<u>ser</u>-vi-kal	pertaining to the neck or to the cervix
chronic	<u>kron</u>-ik	persisting for a long time
coccyx	<u>kok</u>-siks	see tables of bones in Chapter 17. Triangular bone formed usually by fusion of last four vertebrae; the "tailbone"
congenital	kon-<u>jen</u>-i-tal	existing at the time of birth
defibrillator	de-fib'ri-<u>la</u>-tor	an apparatus used to produce defibrillation by application of brief electric shock to the heart directly or through electrodes placed on the chest wall
dilatation	dil'ah-<u>ta</u>-shun	the condition of being stretched open beyond normal dimensions
dilation	di-<u>la</u>-shun	the act of dilating or stretching
edema	e-<u>de</u>-mah	an abnormal accumulation of fluid in intercellular spaces of the body
embolus	<u>em</u>-bo-lus	a clot or other plug brought by the blood from another vessel and forced into a smaller one, thus obstructing the circulation
emesis	<u>em</u>-e-sis	the act of vomiting. Also used as a word termination, as in hematemesis

Word	Pronunciation	Definition
enema	<u>en</u>-e-mah	introduction of fluid into the rectum for evacuation of feces or as a means of introducing nutrient or medicinal substances, or the opaque material used in roentgenographic examination of the lower intestinal tract (BE)
exacerbation	eg-zas'er-<u>ba</u>-shun	increase in severity of a disease or any of its symptoms
excretion	eks-<u>kre</u>-shun	the act of eliminating waste
fascia	<u>fash</u>-e-ah	a sheet or band of fibrous tissue that lies deep to the skin or binds muscles and various body organs
febrile	<u>feb</u>-ril	pertaining to fever; feverish
fibrillation	fib'ri-<u>la</u>-shun	a small, local, involuntary, muscular contraction caused by activation of muscle cells or fibers
defibrillator	de-fib'ri-<u>la</u>-tor	an electronic apparatus used to produce defibrillation by application of brief electroshock to the heart, directly or through electrodes placed on the chest wall
hemorrhage	<u>hem</u>-o-rij	the escape of blood from the vessels; bleeding
icterus	<u>ik</u>-ter-us	jaundice
immunization	im'u-ni-<u>za</u>-shun	the process of providing immunity to disease processes
incontinence	in-<u>kon</u>-ti-nens	inability to control bowel and bladder functions
inflammation	in'flah-<u>ma</u>-shun	a protective tissue response to injury or destruction of tissues
ischemia	is-<u>ke</u>-me-ah	deficiency of blood in a part, caused by functional constriction or actual obstruction of a blood vessel
jaundice	<u>jawn</u>-dis	icterus; yellowness of the skin, sclerae, mucous membranes, and excretions
metastasis	me-<u>tas</u>-tah-sis	transfer of disease from one organ or body to another not directly connected with it
mucus	<u>mu</u>-kus	the free slime of the mucous membranes, composed of secretions of the glands, various salts, desquamated cells, and leukocytes
obese	o-<u>bes</u>	very fat; stout; corpulent
obesity	o-<u>bes</u>-i-te	an increase in body weight beyond the limitation of skeletal and physical requirements: the result of excessive accumulation of body fat
palpable	<u>pal</u>-pah-bul	felt by touching

Word	Pronunciation	Definition
paralysis	pah-<u>ral</u>-i-sis	loss or impairment of voluntary motor function
paralyzed	<u>par</u>-e-lizd	a condition of helplessness caused by inability to move; being ineffective or powerless
parietal	pah-<u>ri</u>-e-tal	pertaining to the walls of a cavity or located near the parietal bone
percussion	per-<u>kush</u>-un	the act of striking a part with short, sharp blows as an aid in diagnosing the condition of the underlying parts by the sound obtained
perineum	per'i-<u>ne</u>-um	the pelvic floor and associated structures occupying the pelvic outlet
peritoneum	per'i-to-<u>ne</u>-um	the serous membrane lining the walls of the abdominal and pelvic cavities and the contained viscera
pleura (pleural, adj.)	<u>pleu</u>-ra (<u>pleu</u>-ral)	serous membrane investing the lungs and lining the walls of the thoracic cavity
prolapse	<u>pro</u>-laps	the falling down, or downward displacement, of a part
prophylaxis	pro-fi-<u>lak</u>-sis	prevention of disease; preventive treatment
purulent	<u>pur</u>-roo-lent	containing or forming pus
remission	re-<u>mish</u>-un	having periods of abatement or of exacerbation
rheumatic	roo-<u>mat</u>-ik	a state of inflammation; inflammatory diseases
serous	<u>se</u>-rus	pertaining to or resembling serum
sputum	<u>spu</u>-tum	matter ejected from the trachea, bronchi, and lungs, through the mouth
suture	<u>su</u>-chur	a stitch or series of stitches made to secure the edges of a surgical or traumatic wound; used also as a verb to indicate application of such stitches
virus	<u>vi</u>-rus	a minute infectious agent that, with certain exceptions, cannot be seen by microscope and is able to reproduce only within a living host cell
viscera, viscus	<u>vis</u>-er-ah, <u>vis</u>-kus	any large interior organ in any of the four great body cavities, especially those in the abdomen
void (voided)	void	to urinate

LESSON TWO PROGRESS CHECK

■ COMPARE AND CONTRAST

In the following sets of words, explain the differences by contrasting the meaning of each word:

EXAMPLE: cry/o—crypt/o
cry/o means *cold,* but crypto is a term meaning *hidden*

1. lipo—litho _____

2. para—pathy _____

3. phagia—phasia—phonia _____

4. schizo—sclera _____

5. thrombo—thermo—trauma _____

6. abscess—adnexa _____

7. axilla—anomaly _____

8. cervical—coccyx _____

9. edema—embolus _____

10. emesis—enema _____

11. icterus—ischemia _____

12. palpable—parietal _____

13. prolapse—prophylaxis _____

14. suture—sputum _____

15. viscera—virus _____

■ BUILDING MEDICAL TERMS

Recall the rule for combining vowels, and the suffix for inflammation.
Build a medical word meaning *inflammation* of:

1. a cartilage _____

2. the vagina _____

3. the larynx _____

4. folds of tissue around a fingernail _____

5. the pancreas _____

6. a vein _____

7. a uterine tube_____

8. a eustachian tube_____

9. the pleura _____

10. the vertebrae _____

11. the mouth and oral mucosa _____

12. a ureter _____

13. a urethra_____

14. the esophagus _____

15. a nerve _____

Build a medical word that means:

16. Loss of the power of speech_____

17. Difficulty swallowing _____

18. A malignant new growth _____

19. Cell death _____

20. A fat _____

21. Thickening of the skin _____

22. Controlling the blood flow_____

23. Any injury _____

24. Severe but short duration _____

25. A congenital defect _____

26. Persisting for a long time _____

27. A clot or a plug in the bloodstream _____

28. Vomiting _____

29. Urinating _____

30. Abnormal fluid accumulation _____

31. "Tailbone" _____

32. Vertebrae in the neck _____

33. Eliminating waste _____

34. Increased severity of disease symptoms_____

35. Inability to control bowel and bladder function _____

36. A protective tissue response to injury or destruction_____

37. Deficiency of blood in a part _____

38. Escape of blood from vessels _____

39. Transfer of a disease from one part or organ to another not directly connected _____

40. Excessive accumulation of adipose tissue _____

41. Felt by touching _____

42. Preventive treatment _____

43. Matter ejected from lungs through the mouth _____

44. An infectious agent too small to be seen by an ordinary microscope_____

45. Securing the edges of a wound with stitches _____

■ FILL-IN

Fill in the blanks:

1. The bones between the wrist and fingers are the _____

2. An incision through part of the abdominal wall is a (an) _____

3. Excision of the ovaries is called a (an) _____ or a (an)

_____

4. The specialty dealing with care of the foot is called _____

5. Plastic surgery of the nose is _____

6. The bones between the ankle and the toes are the _____

7. Surgical puncture of the chest wall to aspirate fluid is known as a (an) _____

8. Failure of the testes to descend is called_____

9. A woman pregnant for the first time is a (an) _____

10. A woman who has had two or more pregnancies is a (an)_____

■ DEFINE THE TERM

Define the following terms:

1. abortion _____

2. auscultation _____

3. catgut _____

4. catheter _____

5. dilatation _____

6. embolus _____

7. exacerbation _____

8. fascia _____

9. metastasis _____

10. percussion _____

■ MATCHING

Match the body parts at the left to their medical terms on the right:

1.	mind	**a.**	cervical
2.	body	**b.**	ophthalm/o
3.	neck	**c.**	thorax
4.	wrist	**d.**	soma
5.	teeth	**e.**	psyche
6.	abdomen	**f.**	myring/o
7.	eye	**g.**	vas/o
8.	chest	**h.**	carpal
9.	eardrum	**i.**	celi/o
10.	blood vessel	**j.**	odont

■ SHORT ANSWER: ROOT WORDS

State the *root* word for the following body parts:

1. wrist _____

2. neck _____

3. teeth _____

4. esophagus _____

5. abdomen _____

6. fingernail _____

7. eye _____

8. pancreas _____

9. body _____

10. foot _____

11. pubic bone _____

12. nose _____

13. mouth _____

14. ankle _____

15. chest _____

■ SHORT ANSWER: BODY PARTS

State the *body part or organ* involved in the following conditions:

1. colpitis _____

2. phlebitis _____

3. pleurisy_____

4. spondylitis _____

5. stomatitis _____

UNIT V

Medical Terminology and Body Systems

CHAPTER 10 Body Organs and Parts

OBJECTIVES

After completing this chapter and the exercises, the student should be able to:

1. Identify the parts of a cell and the specialized functions of tissues
2. Identify the body systems
3. Describe the functions of the body systems and how they work together
4. Define the anatomical positions of the body and directional terms used to indicate them
5. List the body cavities and the organs contained within them
6. Identify nine body regions
7. Use appropriate medical terms when describing locations of various parts of the body

OVERVIEW

This chapter will focus on the way medical terms that you have previously learned relate to the body as a whole. In order to accurately understand and communicate data from medical reports, medical personnel use topographic anatomy. Topographic refers to the surface landmarks of the body. They are used as guides to the internal structures that lie beneath them, as well as the major regions of the body and their locations.

In order to describe the position of a structure or locate one structure in relation to another, medical professionals start with a position called the anatomical position. In this position, a person is standing erect, facing you, with hands at sides and palms forward, and feet and head pointed straight ahead. This is the position you will use to find the landmarks of the body. We will begin with a discussion of cells, the structural and functional unit of all living matter.

LESSON ONE   MATERIALS TO BE LEARNED

STRUCTURAL UNITS OF THE BODY

Table 10–1

Unit	Pronunciation	Definition
Cell	sel	minute protoplasmic masses making up organized tissue, consisting of the nucleus surrounded by cytoplasm enclosed in a cell or plasma membrane. Fundamental, structural, and functional unit of living organisms. Each cell performs functions necessary for its own life. Cells multiply by dividing. This is called mitosis
nucleus	<u>nu</u>-kle-us	cell nucleus; a spheroid body within a cell, consisting of a thin nuclear membrane and genes or chromosomes
chromosomes	kroh'-moh-sohms	thread-like structures in the cell nucleus that control growth, repair, and reproduction of the body
cytoplasm	<u>si</u>-to-plasm	the protoplasm of a cell exclusive of that of the nucleus (nucleoplasm)
cell membrane	sel <u>mem</u>-bran	a thin layer of tissue, serving as the wall of a cell. Selectively allows substances to pass in and out of the cell. Refuses passage to others
Tissue	<u>tish</u>-u	a group of similarly specialized cells that together perform certain special functions
epithelial tissue	ep'-i-<u>the</u>-le-al <u>tish</u>-u	the skin and lining surfaces that protect, absorb, and excrete
connective tissue	ko-<u>nek</u>-tiv <u>tish</u>-u	the fibrous tissues of the body; that which binds together and is the ground substance of the various parts and organs of the body; examples are bones, tendons, and so on
muscle tissue	<u>mus</u>-el <u>tish</u>-u	tissue that contracts; consists of striated (striped), cardiac, and smooth muscle
nerve tissue	nerv <u>tish</u>-u	a collection of nerve fibers that conduct impulses that control and coordinate body activities

Unit	Pronunciation	Definition
Organ	<u>or</u>-gan	tissues arranged together to perform a specific function. These internal structures are contained within the body cavities. Some examples include the heart, lungs, and organs of digestion, such as the liver and gallbladder, and the organs of reproduction
System	<u>sis</u>-tem	a set of body organs that works together for a common purpose
integumentary system	in-teg'u-<u>men</u>-ter-e <u>sis</u>-tem	skin serves as the external covering of the body. Accessory organs of this system are nails, hair, and oil and sweat glands
musculoskeletal system	mus'ku-lo-<u>skel</u>-e-tal <u>sis</u>-tem	skeleton and muscles: the 206 bones, the joints, cartilage, ligaments, and all of the muscles of the body
cardiovascular system	kar'de-o-<u>vas</u>-ku-lar <u>sis</u>-tem	heart and blood vessels; blood pumped and circulated through the body
gastrointestinal system	gas'tro-in-tes-ti-nal <u>sis</u>-tem	a long tube commonly called the GI tract: consists of mouth, esophagus, stomach, and intestines. Accessory organs are pancreas, liver, gallbladder, and salivary glands
respiratory system	re-spi-rah-to're <u>sis</u>-tem	nose, pharynx, larynx, trachea, bronchi, and lungs. Furnishes oxygen, removes carbon dioxide (respiration)
genitourinary system	jen'i-to-u-re-ner'e <u>sis</u>-tem	reproductive and urinary organs; also called urogenital system (GU or UG). The urinary organs are the kidneys, ureters, bladder, and urethra. The reproductive organs are the gonads and various external genitalia and internal organs
endocrine system	<u>en</u>-do-krin <u>sis</u>-tem	glands and other structures that make hormones and release them directly into the circulatory system; ductless glands
nervous system	<u>ner</u>-vus <u>sis</u>-tem	brain and spinal cord make up the central nervous system (CNS); the autonomic nervous system (ANS), or peripheral nervous system, consists of 12 pairs of cranial nerves and 31 pairs of spinal nerves

BODY CAVITIES AND PLANES

Refer to Figures 10–1, 10–2, and 10–3 when studying body cavities and planes.

The Body Cavities

The body has two main large cavities that contain the internal body organs—the *ventral* and *dorsal* cavities. Each of these cavities is further divided into smaller cavities that contain specific organs. Ventral refers to the front or belly portion of the body, and dorsal refers to the back portion of the body. Chapter 5 in your text contains the complete direction/position tables.

Table 10–2

Term	Pronunciation	Definition
Body cavities		hollow spaces containing body organs
pleural cavity	pleu'ral kav-i-te	the thoracic cavity containing the lungs, trachea, esophagus, and thymus gland
mediastinum	me'de-ah-sti-num	the mass of tissues and organs separating the sternum in front and the vertebral column behind, containing the heart and its large vessels
peritoneal cavity	per'i-to-ne-al kav-i-te	the space containing the stomach, intestines, liver, gallbladder, pancreas, spleen, reproductive organs, and urinary bladder
cranial cavity	kra-ne-al kav-i-te	space enclosed by skull bones, containing the brain
spinal cavity	spi-nal kav-i-te	cavity containing the spinal cord
diaphragm	di-ah-fram	dome-shaped muscle separating the abdominal and thoracic cavities
Body planes		imaginary lines that divide (used in anatomic diagrams)
sagittal	saj-i-tal	a sagittal plane divides the body into right and left portions
midsagittal	mid-saj-i-tal	a plane that vertically divides the body, or some part of it, into equal right and left portions (medial)
coronal	ko-ro-nal	also called frontal; a plane that divides the body into anterior and posterior sections (front and back)
transverse	trans-vers	a plane that divides the body into superior and inferior sections (top and bottom)

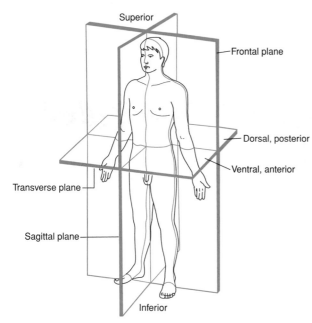

FIGURE 10–1 Body planes and directions

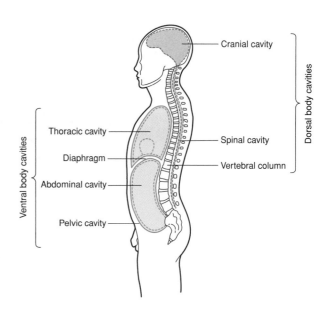

FIGURE 10–2 Sagittal section of the body, showing the dorsal and ventral body cavities

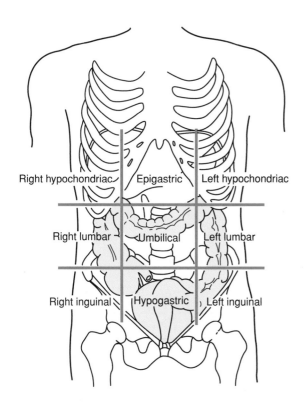

FIGURE 10–3 Abdominal regions

METABOLISM AND HOMEOSTASIS

There are two important terms in medicine that have general application.
They are described in Table 10–3.

Table 10–3

Term	Pronunciation	Definition
metabolism	me-<u>tab</u>-o-lizm	sum of the body's physical and chemical processes that convert food into elements for body growth, energy, building body parts (anabolism), and degrading body substances for recycling or excretion (catabolism)
homeostasis	ho'me-o-<u>sta</u>-sis	a steady state: the tendency of stability in the normal physiologic systems of the organism to maintain a balance optimal for survival. Body temperature, osmotic pressure, normal cell division rate, and nutrient supply to cells are a few examples

LESSON TWO   PROGRESS CHECK

■ SPELLING AND DEFINITION

Spell and *list* the parts of each of these body systems:

1. Serves as a covering:

    _____ system. Consists of _____

    _____

2. Pumps and circulates blood:

    _____ system. Consists of _____

    _____

3. Bones and muscles:

    _____ system. Consists of _____

    _____

4. A long tube for input of nutrients and excretion of solid wastes:

    _____ system. Consists of _____

    _____

5. Furnishes oxygen and removes carbon dioxide:

   _____ system. Consists of _____

   _____

6. Reproductive organs and liquid waste disposal:

   _____ system. Consists of _____

   _____

7. Makes hormones and releases them directly into the blood:

   _____ system. Consists of _____

   _____

8. Controls all thought and movement:

   _____ system. Consists of _____

   _____

■ FILL-IN

Fill in the blanks to make a complete, accurate sentence:

1. The _____ is the functional unit of all living organisms.

2. The function of the nucleus is to furnish _____ material.

3. Cell division is called _____ .

4. When cells divide they are really _____ .

5. The wall of the cell is called a (an) _____ .

6. When groups of cells have specialized functions they are called _____ .

7. The skin and lining surfaces that protect, absorb, and excrete are _____ .

8. The fibrous bonds that are the ground substance of various parts are called _____ .

9. Groups of cells that contract are _____ .

10. Those fibers that conduct impulses are _____ .

11. A body part that performs special functions is called a (an) _____ .

12. When a set of body parts works together for a common purpose it is called _____ .

13. The space that contains body organs is called a (an) _____ .

14. Imaginary lines that divide the human anatomy are called _____ .

15. The _____ separates the abdomen from the lungs.

■ DEFINITIONS

1. metabolism _____

_____

2. homeostasis _____

_____

■ SHORT ANSWER

Name the four types of specialized body tissues and one major function of each:

Specialized Tissue	*Function*
1. _____	_____
2. _____	_____
3. _____	_____
4. _____	_____

5. What is the function of a *cell membrane*? _____

6. Of what does a *cell nucleus* consist? _____

CHAPTER 11	Integumentary System

OBJECTIVES

Upon completion of this chapter, the student should be able to:

1. Identify the structures of the skin and accessory organs
2. List and describe the five functions of the skin
3. Identify and describe the lesions and pathological conditions that affect the integumentary system
4. Describe laboratory tests and clinical procedures used in diagnosing and treating skin disorders
5. Identify and define commonly used vocabulary terms that pertain to the skin

OVERVIEW

The skin and its accessory organs are called the *integumentary system*. The *integument* (skin) is a vital organ serving as a protective barrier that responds to internal and external stimuli and contributes to the maintenance of homeostasis. The integument forms the outer covering of the body. It consists of the skin and certain specialized tissues. Specialized tissues are hair, nails, *sebaceous* (oil) and *sudoriferous* (sweat) glands (Plate 16), and mammary glands.

The skin is the largest organ of the body, weighing about 9 lbs and covering approximately 18 square feet in the adult. It consists of two layers of tissue, the *epidermis* and *dermis,* and a layer of *subcutaneous* tissue. Embedded in these layers are various accessory appendages. Skin components are defined under Parts of the Skin in Lesson One of this chapter. A brief discussion of the components and functions of the integument follows.

The epidermis is the skin's outer layer. It contains no blood vessels and receives its nourishment from the dermis. The cells are packed closely together, being thickest on the palms of the hands and soles of the feet. The epidermis is firmly attached to the dermis, the deeper layer of skin that lies below it. In turn, the dermis is attached through subcutaneous tissue to underlying structures such as muscle and bone.

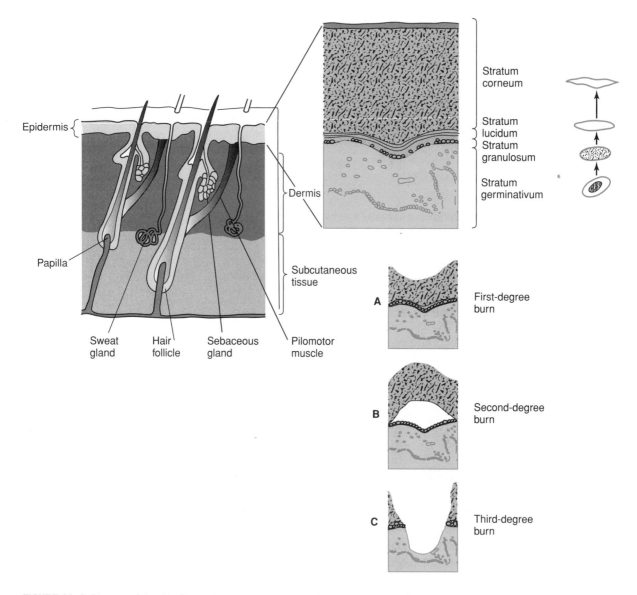

FIGURE 11–1 Diagram of the skin. The nucleated cell produced by the stratum germinativum dies (granulates) as it is forced outward to become the dead, scaly stratum corneum. The number of layers of the epidermis affected by the three types of skin burns is also shown. **A**, Only corneum cells are involved in first-degree burns. **B**, Damage to the upper three layers occurs in second-degree burns, forming a blister between layers 3 and 4. **C**, A third-degree burn involves all epidermal layers and, therefore, usually requires a skin graft to replace the stratum germinativum.

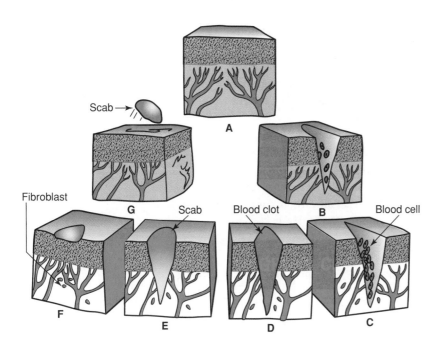

FIGURE 11–2 If normal skin **(A)** is injured deeply **(B)**, blood escapes from dermal blood vessels **(C)**, and a blood clot soon forms **(D)**. The blood clot and dried tissue fluid form a scab **(E)**, which protects the damaged region. Later, blood vessels send out branches, and fibroblasts migrate into the area **(F)**. The fibroblasts produce new connective tissue fibers, and when the skin is largely repaired, the scab sloughs off **(G)**.

The appendages of fingernails and toenails are found only in humans and other primates, and hair is characteristic only of mammals.

HAIR

A strand of hair is a tightly fused meshwork of horny cells filled with keratin. It has a root embedded in the hair follicle and a shaft, which is the visible part of hair. Each hair develops in the hair follicle as new growth forms from keratin located at the bottom of the follicle. Cutting the hair does not affect its rate of growth. Melanocytes located at the root of the hair follicle gives hair its color, and the color is dependent on the amount of melanin produced. As people age, melanocytes stop producing melanin and the hair turns gray or white.

NAILS

Fingernails and toenails are composed of hard keratin plates that cover the dorsal surface of the tip of each toe and finger. The horny cells are tightly packed and cemented together, and will continue to grow indefinitely unless cut or broken off. Fingernails can be replaced in 3–5 months; toenails grow more slowly, requiring 12–18 months to be completely replaced.

The visible part of the nail is the nail body. At the base of the nail body and around the sides is a fold of skin called a *cuticle*. The *lunula* is a half-moon crescent at the base of the nail plate. Underneath the cuticle, the nail body extends into the root of the nail. It is nourished by the nail bed, an epithelial layer lying just beneath it, which contains a supply of blood vessels and gives the nails their pinkish coloring. Alterations in the growth and appearance can give an indication of systemic disease. For example, a flattened or spoon-shaped nail plate can result from iron deficiency anemia.

Skin glands in humans include sebaceous glands, sudoriferous glands, and *mammary* glands, which are modified sweat glands. The glands of the ear canal that produce *cerumen* (ear wax) are also modified sweat glands, as are the specialized glands found in the *axilla* (armpit) and the *anogenital* area. A modified type of sweat gland, active only from puberty onward, is concentrated near the reproductive organs and in the armpits. These glands secrete an odorless sweat, but contain substances that are quickly decomposed by bacteria on the skin. The end products of this breakdown are responsible for human body odor. Mammary glands are another type of modified sweat gland. They only secrete milk after a female has given birth. See Figures 11–1 and 11–2 for a diagram of the skin and some injuries to the skin.

The skin performs five essential functions: protection, temperature regulation, communication, metabolism, and excretion.

1. Protection: The skin protects the body from microorganisms, fluid loss or gain, and other mechanical and chemical irritants. Melanin pigment provides some protection against the sun's ultraviolet rays.
2. Temperature regulation: The blood supply to the skin nourishes the skin and helps regulate body temperature. Sweat glands also assist in the maintenance and regulation of body temperature.
3. Communication: All stimuli from the environment are received through the skin by receptors that detect temperature, touch, pressure, and pain. Skin is the medium of facial expression (e.g., smiles, frowns, grimaces).
4. Metabolism: In the presence of sunlight (ultraviolet radiation), the synthesis of vitamin D, essential for bone growth and development, is initiated from a precursor molecule (7-dehydrocholesterol) found in the skin.
5. Excretion: Fatty substances, water, and salts (mainly the Na^+ ion) are eliminated from the skin.

The study of the skin is called *dermatology*, and the M.D. who specializes in the study of the diseases and disorders of the skin is called a *dermatologist*. Details of the integumentary system are provided in succeeding sections of the chapter.

LESSON ONE MATERIALS TO BE LEARNED

PARTS OF THE SKIN

Table 11–1

Part	Pronunciation	Definition
skin	skin	the outer covering of the body
epidermis (cuticle)	ep'i-<u>der</u>-mis (<u>ku</u>-ti-kul)	the outermost, nonvascular layer of the skin; composed of, from within outward, five layers: basal layer, prickle-cell layer, granular layer, clear layer, and horny layer
dermis corium	<u>der</u>-mis <u>ko</u>-re-um	layer of the skin deep in the epidermis, consisting of a dense bed of vascular connective tissue and containing the nerves of terminal organs or sensation, the hair roots, and sebaceous and sweat glands
hair, nails	hare, nales	appendages of the skin
subcutaneous	sub'ku-<u>ta</u>-ne-us	beneath the skin, containing adipose tissue, connective tissue, vessels, and nerves
breasts	brests	mammary glands; the front of the chest. In female mammals, the breast contains milk-secreting elements for nourishing the young

FUNCTIONS OF THE SKIN

Table 11–2

Process or Part	Pronunciation	Definition
protection	pro-<u>tek</u>-shun	from microorganisms, injuries, and excessive exposure to the ultraviolet rays of the sun
sensory organ (receptor)	<u>sen</u>-so-re (re-<u>cep</u>-tor)	for the body to feel pain, cold, heat, touch, and pressure
temperature regulator	<u>tem</u>-per-ah-tur <u>reg</u>-u-la'tor	insulation against heat and cold, e.g., perspiration for cooling
metabolism	me-<u>tab</u>-o-lizm	in the presence of sunlight, synthesize vitamin D from a precursor molecule found in the skin
waste elimination	wast e-lim-i-<u>na</u>-shun	eliminate body wastes in the form of perspiration

SURGICAL PROCESSES AND THE SKIN

Table 11–3

Process	Pronunciation	Definition
biopsy	<u>bi</u>-op-se	removal of tissue from body for examination
cautery	<u>kaw</u>-ter-e	tissue destruction by electricity
debridement	da-<u>bred</u>-maw	removal of contaminated or devitalized tissue from a traumatic or infected lesion
dermabrasion	der-mah-<u>bra</u>-shun	planing of the skin done by mechanical means, e.g., sandpaper or wire brushes
dermatome	<u>der</u>′mah-tom	an instrument for cutting thin skin slices for grafting
electrodesiccation	e-lek′tro-des′i-<u>ka</u>-shun	destruction of tissue by dehydration with high-frequency electric current
escharotomy	es-kah-<u>rot</u>-omy	removal of burn scar tissue
fulguration	ful′gu-<u>ra</u>-shun	destruction of living tissue by electric sparks
graft	graft	a tissue or organ for implantation or transplantation; a piece of skin transplanted to replace a lost portion of the skin; pigskin may be used as a temporary graft. A new type of synthetic collagen is now being used for permanent skin grafts
hyfracator	hi-fra-<u>cate</u>-or	a type of machine for destroying tissue (high-frequency eradicator)

SKIN GROWTHS

Table 11–4

Growth	Pronunciation	Definition
carcinoma	kahr-suh-<u>noh</u>-muh	a malignant new growth made up of epithelial cells tending to infiltrate surrounding tissues and give rise to metastases
keratosis	ker′ah-<u>to</u>-sis	any horny growth, such as a wart or callosity
nevus(-i)	ne′-vus	a mole or growth, e.g., birthmark; there are many types
steatoma	ste′ah-<u>to</u>-mah	lipoma; a fatty mass retained within a sebaceous gland; sebaceous cyst
verruca(-ae)	ve-<u>roo</u>-kah	a wart, caused by viruses. A plantar wart is one on the sole or plantar surface of the foot

BIOLOGIC AGENTS AND SKIN INFECTION

Table 11–5

Infection	Pronunciation	Definition
Bacteria		
acne vulgaris	<u>ak</u>-ne vul-<u>ga</u>-ris	an inflammatory disease of the skin with the formation of an eruption of papules or pustules; chronic acne, usually occurring in adolescence. May be caused by foods, stress, hereditary factors, hormones, drugs, and bacteria
carbuncle, furuncle	<u>kar</u>-bung-k'l, <u>fu</u>-rung-k'l	boils, abscesses, and pustular lesions
cellulitis	sel'u-<u>li</u>-tis	inflammation of the skin and subcutaneous tissue. May lead to ulceration and abscess
impetigo	im-pe-<u>ti</u>-go	a streptococcal or staphylococcal skin infection marked by vesicles or bullae that become pustular, rupture, and form yellow crusts, especially around the mouth and nose
Virus		
herpes genitalis	<u>her</u>-pez jen'i-<u>tal</u>-is	blister-type inflammatory highly contagious skin disease of the genitals. May harm an infant if the mother is infected at the time of delivery, causing damage to the child's nervous system. A prevalent STD (sexually transmitted disease)
herpes ophthalmicus	<u>her</u>-pez oph-<u>thal</u>-mi-cus	severe herpes zoster involving the ophthalmic nerve (eye)
herpes simplex	<u>her</u>-pez <u>sim</u>-plex	an acute viral disease, often on the borders of the lips or nares (cold sores) or on the genitals
herpes zoster	<u>her</u>-pez <u>zos</u>-ter	shingles: an acute, unilateral, self-limited inflammatory disease of a nerve, e.g., on one side of the pelvis
verruca	ve-<u>ru</u>-kah	a wart
Fungus		
tinea	<u>tin</u>-e-ah	ringworm; a name applied to many different superficial fungal infections of different parts of the body
tinea barbae	<u>tin</u>-e-ah <u>bar</u>-bae	infection of the bearded parts of the face by ringworm
tinea capitis	<u>tin</u>-e-ah <u>kap</u>-i-tis	infection of the scalp by ringworm
tinea corporis	<u>tin</u>-e-ah <u>cor</u>-por-is	infection of the body by ringworm

Infection	Pronunciation	Definition
tinea cruris	tin-e-ah cru-ris	infection of the groin by ringworm ("jock itch")
tinea pedis	tin-e-ah pe-dis	athlete's foot; a chronic superficial infection of the skin of the foot by ringworm
tinea unguium	tin-e-ah un-guium	infection of the fingernails by ringworm; the nails become opaque, white, thickened, and friable
Parasites		
pediculosis capitis	pe-dik'u-lo-sis kap-i-tis	lice (head)
pediculosis corporis	pe-dik'u-lo-sis cor-por-is	lice (body)
pediculosis pubis	pe-dik'u-lo-sis pu-bis	pubic lice or crabs
scabies	ska-bez	a mite, a small parasite; can burrow under the skin

ALLERGY AND THE SKIN

Table 11–6

Term	Pronunciation	Definition
eczema	ek-ze-ma	redness in skin, caused by some substance, e.g., food
neurodermatitis	nu'ro-der'mah-ti-tis	a dermatosis presumed to be caused by itching related to emotional causes or psychological factors
psoriasis	so-ri-ah-sis	a chronic, hereditary, recurrent dermatosis marked by discrete vivid red macules, papules, or plaques covered with silvery laminated scales

SKIN DISORDERS FROM SYSTEMIC DISEASES

Table 11–7

Disease	Pronunciation	Definition
diabetes mellitus	di'ah-be-tez mel-li-tus	a disorder in which blood sugar (glucose) levels are abnormally high because the body does not produce enough insulin
erysipelas	er'i-sip-e-las	a contagious disease of the skin and subcutaneous tissues caused by infection with streptococci organisms; redness and swelling of affected areas

Disease	Pronunciation	Definition
histoplasmosis	his'to-plaz-<u>mo</u>-sis	a systemic fungal disease caused by inhalation of dust contaminated by fungus
lupus erythematosus	<u>loo</u>-pus er-i-<u>them</u>-a-to-sus	a chronic superficial inflammation of the skin; the lesions typically form a butterfly pattern over the bridge of the nose and cheeks
rubella	roo-<u>bel</u>-ah	German measles; a mild viral infection marked by a pink macular rash
rubeola	roo-<u>be</u>-o-lah	a synonym of measles in English and of German measles in French and Spanish
syphilis	<u>sif</u>-i-lis	a venereal disease; cutaneous lesions; caused by infection from direct sexual contact
varicella	var'i-<u>sel</u>-ah	chickenpox; residues itch and later become scabs

SKIN TESTS

Table 11–8

Term	Pronunciation	Definition
coccidioidin	kok-sid'e-<u>oi</u>-din	a sterile preparation injected intracutaneously as a test for valley fever (respiratory fungus disease)
Mantoux or PPD	man-<u>too</u>	a test for tuberculosis (TB), a bacterial disease
Dick test	dik test	an intracutaneous test for susceptibility to scarlet fever
Schick test	shik test	an intracutaneous test for diphtheria
sweat test	swet test	a test for presence of cystic fibrosis

VOCABULARY TERMS AND THE SKIN

Table 11–9

Term	Pronunciation	Definition
actinic	ak-<u>tin</u>-ik	referring to ultraviolet rays of the sun
albinism	<u>al</u>-bi-nizm	no body pigment; white skin and hair

Term	Pronunciation	Definition
alopecia	al'o-<u>pe</u>-she-ah	baldness; hereditary or caused by chemotherapy
bulla(-ae)	<u>bul</u>-ah	large blisters, as in burns
burn	bern	thermal injury to tissues. First-degree burns show redness. Second-degree burns produce blisters and are partial-thickness burns. Third-degree burns are full-thickness burns and involve subcutaneous tissue and muscle
callus	<u>kal</u>-us	localized hyperplasia of the horny layer of the epidermis (skin) caused by pressure or friction
cicatrix	sik'ah-triks	a scar
cyst	sist	a closed epithelium-lined cavity or sac, normal or abnormal, usually containing liquid or semisolid material
dermatology	der'mah-<u>tol</u>-o-je	the medical specialty concerned with the diagnosis and treatment of skin diseases
ecchymosis	ek'i-<u>mo</u>-sis	bruise, caused by bleeding under the skin
erosion	e-<u>ro</u>-shun	eating or gnawing away, e.g., an early ulcer
eruption	e-<u>rup</u>-shun	breaking out; a rash
erythema	er'i-<u>the</u>-mah	redness of the skin
eschar	<u>es</u>-kar	a slough (hard crust) produced by a thermal burn
exanthem	eg-<u>zan</u>-them	an eruptive (rose-colored) disease or fever
excoriation	eks-ko're-<u>a</u>-shun	a superficial loss of skin, e.g., by scratching
exfoliation	eks-fo'le-<u>a</u>-shun	a falling off in scales or layers
fissure	<u>fish</u>-er	a narrow slit on the skin surface, e.g., anal fissure, athlete's foot lesion
gangrene	<u>gang</u>-gren	necrotic or dead tissue
hirsutism	<u>her</u>-soot-ism	abnormal hairiness, especially in women
keloid	<u>ke</u>-loid	a sharply elevated, progressively enlarging scar that does not fade with time
laceration	las'e-<u>ra</u>-shun	cut; tearing; a torn wound
lesion	<u>le</u>-zhun	any pathologic or traumatic discontinuity of tissue, e.g., a sore

Term	Pronunciation	Definition
macule	<u>mak</u>-ul	a spot, or thickening, e.g., freckle, flat mole. Area is not raised above the surface
nodule	<u>nod</u>-ul	a small node that is solid and can be detected by touch; a rounded prominence, e.g., a boss
nummular	<u>num</u>-u-lar	coin-sized and coin-shaped
papulae	<u>pap</u>-ul	a small, circumscribed, solid elevated lesion of the skin, e.g., wart, acne, mole
paronychia	par'o-<u>nik</u>-e-ah	inflammation of the folds of tissue around the fingernail
plaque	plak	any patch or flat area; used to describe the silvery scales of psoriasis
pruritus	proo-<u>ri</u>-tus	itching
pustule	<u>pus</u>-tul	a small, elevated, pus-containing lesion of the skin
scales, crusts	scalz, krust	an outer layer formed by drying of a bodily exudate or secretion; flaking type of lesion, e.g., psoriasis, fungus
scar, cicatrix	skahr sik'ah-triks	a mark remaining after the healing of a wound or other morbid process
superfluous hair	soo-<u>pur</u>-floo-es har	excessive hair on the face of women
tumor	<u>too</u>-mor	swelling; may be benign or malignant; also called a neoplasm
ulcer	<u>ul</u>-cer	a local destruction of tissue from sloughing of necrotic inflammatory tissue, e.g., varicose ulcer, decubitus ulcer
urticaria	er'ti-<u>ka</u>-re-ah	hives; transient elevated patches (wheals)
vesicle	<u>ves</u>-i-k'l	a small blister containing liquid
vitiligo	vit'i-<u>li</u>-go	loss of pigment; white, patchy areas
wheal	hwel	a localized area of swelling on the body surface, e.g., produced by a skin test reaction

LESSON TWO   PROGRESS CHECK

■ **SPELLING AND DEFINITION**

Circle the correct spelling for the following terms and then define the term:

1. **(a)** epidermis   **(b)** epidermosis   **(c)** epedermis   **(d)** epodermasis

   Definition: _____

2. **(a)** subcutenous   **(b)** subcortenus   **(c)** subcutenous   **(d)** subcutaneous

   Definition: _____

3. **(a)** biopse   **(b)** biopsy   **(c)** biospy   **(d)** bispoy

   Definition: _____

4. **(a)** debraidment   **(b)** debrisment   **(c)** debridement   **(d)** derbrement

   Definition: _____

5. **(a)** escharotomy   **(b)** scarotomy   **(c)** eschrotomy   **(d)** secharotomy

   Definition: _____

6. **(a)** keratinous   **(b)** keratosis   **(c)** karatosis   **(d)** karathosis

   Definition: _____

7. **(a)** steatanoma   **(b)** steteanoma   **(c)** steatoma   **(d)** stetusoma

   Definition: _____

8. **(a)** verracula   **(b)** verookah   **(c)** veracola   **(d)** verruca

   Definition: _____

9. **(a)** impitigo   **(b)** impetigo   **(c)** impecito   **(d)** imtipego

   Definition: _____

10. **(a)** pediculosis   **(b)** pedicleiosis   **(c)** pedicullosis   **(d)** pediculasis

    Definition: _____

11. **(a)** exema   **(b)** exczema   **(c)** eczema   **(d)** ekzema

    Definition: _____

12. **(a)** posorasis   **(b)** psoriasis   **(c)** posorosis   **(d)** poriaahis

    Definition: _____

13. (a) erisepilas (b) erysipolus (c) erisipilas (d) erysipelas

    Definition: _____

14. (a) varicella (b) variccela (c) variccella (d) varecella

    Definition: _____

15. (a) actomic (b) actinic (c) actinus (d) actonus

    Definition: _____

■ WRITE-IN

Write in the medical terms for the following definitions:

1. _____ white skin and hair

2. _____ baldness

3. _____ medical specialty that deals with skin diseases

4. _____ redness of the skin

5. _____ a hard crust produced by a thermal burn

6. _____ coin-sized or coin-shaped

7. _____ small circumscribed solid elevated skin lesion

8. _____ transient elevated patches (wheals)

9. _____ small pus-containing lesion

10. _____ mark remaining after wound healing

■ MATCHING: SKIN TERMS

Match the following terms to their definitions:

1. ecchymosis   a. scales or layers

2. erosion   b. scratching off (of the skin)

3. eruption   c. a rose-colored disease or fever

4. erythema   d. hard crust

5. eschar   e. redness

6. exanthema   f. breaking out

7. excoriation   g. eating or gnawing

8. exfoliation   h. a bruise

■ DEFINITIONS

Describe the uses of the following tests:

1. Mantoux _____

2. Dick _____

3. Schick _____

4. sweat _____

5. coccidioidin _____

6. histoplasmosis _____

■ MATCHING: SKIN DISEASES

Match the terms on the left with their definitions on the right:

1. urticaria   a. excessive

2. vesicle   b. patch

3. vitiligo   c. venereal disease

4. syphilis   d. hives

5. gangrene   e. loss of pigment

6. plaque   f. dead tissue

7. superfluous   g. small blister

8. callus   h. a sac containing liquid

9. cyst   i. hyperplasia of the epidermis

■ LIST THE FUNCTIONS

List the five major functions of the skin:

1. _____

2. _____

3. _____

4. _____

5. _____

■ WORD PUZZLE ON THE INTEGUMENTARY SYSTEM

Find the 46 words about the integumentary system by reading up, down, forward, backward, or diagonally. When the 46 words have been circled, the remaining letters will spell INTEGUMENTARY SYSTEM.

```
M  E  T  S  Y  S  Y  R  A  T  N  E  M  U  G  E  T  N  I  C
A  C  C  E  S  S  O  R  Y  O  R  G  A  N  S  R  A  C  S  O
E  I  N  B  A  S  A  L  C  E  L  L  T  F  A  H  S  U  E  N
L  M  U  I  L  E  H  T  I  P  E  S  W  E  A  T  B  T  B  N
C  K  E  R  A  T  I  N  I  Z  A  T  I  O  N  C  A  D  A  E
S  E  S  T  R  A  W  S  U  O  E  N  A  T  U  C  M  N  C  C
U  P  E  H  S  K  I  N  G  S  T  R  A  T  U  M  E  I  E  T
M  I  E  M  U  T  D  U  D  E  R  M  A  L  M  E  H  M  O  I
I  D  V  A  N  N  E  C  C  R  I  N  E  T  A  N  T  A  U  V
L  E  I  R  L  E  R  N  T  O  E  N  A  I  L  S  Y  T  S  E
I  R  T  K  I  M  M  A  L  O  P  E  C  I  A  T  R  I  A  T
P  M  C  E  G  G  I  R  U  P  A  P  I  L  L  A  E  V  Y  I
R  I  E  L  H  I  S  S  U  D  O  R  I  F  E  R  O  U  S  S
O  S  T  O  T  P  L  S  E  T  Y  C  O  N  A  L  E  M  Q  S
T  S  O  I  S  A  P  O  C  R  I  N  E  G  L  A  N  D  U  U
C  E  R  D  Y  Y  N  O  I  T  A  R  O  P  A  V  E  S  A  E
E  L  P  E  U  S  S  I  T  E  S  O  P  I  D  A  T  E  M  E
R  O  R  D  E  R  M  A  T  I  T  I  S  E  R  O  P  M  O  N
R  M  E  L  A  N  I  N  L  I  A  N  R  E  G  N  I  F  U  C
A  H  A  I  R  E  N  I  R  C  O  L  A  H  M  U  B  E  S  A
```

WORDS TO LOOK FOR IN WORD PUZZLE

1. accessory organs
2. acne
3. adipose tissue
4. alopecia
5. apocrine gland
6. arrector pili muscle
7. basal cell
8. birthmark
9. connective tissue
10. cutaneous
11. dermal
12. dermatitis
13. dermis
14. eccrine
15. epidermis
16. epithelium
17. erythema
18. evaporation
19. fingernail
20. hair
21. halocrine
22. integumentary system
23. keloid
24. keratinization
25. melanin
26. melanocytes
27. moles
28. papilla
29. pigment
30. pores
31. protective
32. scars
33. sebaceous
34. sebum
35. shaft
36. skin
37. squamous
38. stratum
39. subcutaneous layer
40. sudoriferous
41. sunlight
42. sweat
43. tan
44. toenails
45. vitamin D
46. warts
INTEGUMENTARY SYSTEM

CHAPTER 12 Digestive System

OBJECTIVES

1. Identify the organs of the digestive system.
2. Describe the location and label the structures of the digestive system.
3. List the function(s) of each organ and accessory organ in the digestive system.
4. Identify and define clinical disorders affecting the system.
5. Define and explain medical words pertaining to tests and procedures used in the diagnosis and treatment of digestive system disorders.

OVERVIEW

The digestive system, also called the gastrointestinal (GI) system or alimentary tract, contains the organs involved in the ingestion and processing of food. Its general description is that of a long muscular tube extending from mouth to anus and the accessory organs, which include the teeth, tongue, salivary glands, liver, gallbladder, and pancreas. The physician who specializes in diagnosis and treatment of disorders of the stomach and intestines is called a *gastroenterologist*.

The primary function of the GI system is to provide the body with food, water, and electrolytes by digesting nutrients to prepare them for absorption. The following processes are involved in this function:

1. Ingestion: Taking food into the mouth.
2. Mechanical: Grinding or mincing food with the teeth and mixing with saliva from the salivary glands.
3. Peristalsis: Involuntary waves of smooth muscle contraction that move materials through the GI tract.
4. Digestion: Chemical breakdown of large molecules into small ones so that absorption can occur.

5. Absorption: The movement of end products of digestion from the lumen of the digestive tract into the blood and lymph circulation so that they can be used by body cells.

6. Egestion (defecation): Elimination of undigested wastes and bacteria from the tract as feces.

The major and accessory organs are defined in Lesson One; the structures are seen throughout this chapter. Color plates of the entire system illustrate the positions of the various organs (Plates 12 and 14). A brief discussion of the function of the major parts and accessory organs follows:

The upper digestive tract consists of the oral cavity, pharynx, esophagus, and stomach. The lower digestive tract is the small and large intestines. Accessory organs of the digestive system are the salivary glands, liver, pancreas, and gallbladder.

The digestive tract begins with the oral cavity (also known as *buccal cavity*). The major parts of the cavity are the lips, cheeks, hard palate, soft palate, and tongue.

The lips surround the opening of the cavity, and the cheeks, which are continuous with the lips and lined with mucous membrane, form the walls of the oval-shaped cavity. See Figure 12–1.

The hard palate forms the anterior portion of the roof of the mouth, and the muscular soft palate lies posterior to it. The hard palate, or roof of the mouth, is supported by bone. It has irregular ridges in its mucous membrane lining called *rugae*. The soft palate is composed of skeletal muscle and connective tissue. Hanging from the soft palate is a small soft tissue called a *uvula*. This structure aids in producing sound and speech.

The tongue is a solid, strong, flexible structure covered with mucous membrane. It extends across the floor of the oral cavity and strong, flexible, skeletal muscles attach it to the lower joint bone (*mandible*). It is the principal organ of taste and also assists in chewing by moving the food around (*mastication*) and swallowing (*deglutition*).

Across the surface of the tongue are small, rough elevations known as *papillae*. They contain taste buds that detect sweet, sour, salty, and bitter tastes of food (or liquid) as they move across the tongue.

The tongue aids the digestive process by mixing food with saliva and shaping it into a small mass (called a *bolus*), and moving it toward the throat (*pharynx*) to be swallowed. The release of saliva is triggered by the smell, taste, and sometimes even the thought of food.

Salivary glands are exocrine glands, of which there are three pairs—the *parotids*, *submandibulars*, and *sublinguals*—and they secrete most of the saliva produced each day. Saliva is a watery secretion released by the salivary glands containing some mucus and digestive enzyme.

The gums are made of fleshy tissue and surround the sockets of the teeth. Every individual has two sets of teeth during their lifetime. The first set, known as "baby teeth," are primary or *deciduous* teeth. There are 20 teeth in this set, 10 in each jawbone, and the baby will begin to cut them at about 6 month of age. The second set of teeth, the permanent teeth, begin to appear around age 6, replacing the deciduous teeth. There are 32 permanent teeth, 16 in each jaw bone. The last of these teeth, the third molar, or wisdom teeth, usually starts erupting at about age 17.

The shape of the tooth determines its name. The incisors have a chisel shape with sharp edges for biting, canine or cuspid teeth have a single cusp (point) used for grasping and tearing, and the bicuspids or premolars and the molars have flat surfaces with multiple cusps for crushing and grinding.

1. *Esophagus*—transports food from pharynx (throat) to *stomach* by peristalsis. Contains no digestive enzymes.

2. *Stomach*—primarily for food storage. Activity in the stomach results in formation of *chyme* and propels it into the *duodenum*. It secretes pepsin, hydrochloric acid, mucus, and intrinsic factor. The *gastric juices* initiate digestion of protein and fat.

3. *Small intestine*—completes digestion that started in the mouth and stomach by its intestinal enzymes, pancreatic enzymes, and bile from the liver. Also absorbs products of digestion. Peristalsis moves undigested residue to the large intestine.

4. *Pancreas*—the large, elongated gland located behind the greater curvature of the stomach. It contains both endocrine and exocrine glands. The endocrine cells, called islets of Langerhans, secrete the hormones insulin and glucagon. Exocrine glands secrete digestive enzymes, which allow them to digest protein, carbohydrate, and fat.

5. The *liver* is an important organ that plays a major role in many body functions, as follows:

   a. Produces bile to emulsify fats.
   b. Stores glycogen to maintain blood sugar levels.
   c. Forms urea from excess amino acids and nitrogenous wastes.
   d. Synthesizes fats from carbohydrate and protein.
   e. Synthesizes cholesterol and lipoproteins from fats.
   f. Synthesizes plasma proteins and blood clotting factors.
   g. Stores minerals and fat-soluble vitamins.
   h. Detoxifies drugs and toxins; inactivates hormones.
   i. Produces heat.
   j. Stores blood.

6. *Gallbladder*—concentrates and stores bile.

7. *Large intestine*—performs the following functions:

   a. Absorbs 80–90% of water and electrolytes and reduces chyme to a semisolid mass.
   b. Produces no digestive enzymes or hormones.
   c. Bacteria present in the colon produce vitamin K, riboflavin, and thiamin.
   d. Excretes waste and feces.

The abdominal cavity and all its organs, including the organs of the GI system, are lined by a membrane called the *peritoneum*. The portion surrounding the abdominal organs is called the *visceral peritoneum* and that which lines the abdominal cavity is the *parietal peritoneum*.

LESSON ONE   MATERIALS TO BE LEARNED

The digestive system involves the processes of ingestion, digestion, absorption, and elimination of food and food products. The most essential medical terms related to this system are described below and should be studied in conjunction with Figures 12-1 through 12-6.

The digestive system is a large organ system, which includes the accessory organs. It has myriad functions. In such a complex system, there will be many clinical disorders and diseases, some of which will require surgery. In order to properly diagnose and treat these conditions, specific medical tests are used. Great accuracy in pinpointing the exact location of the problem is essential.

To provide a simple method of learning the major terms related to this system, this lesson is divided into six segments: the organ and accessory organs (and processes), selective clinical disorders, surgery terms, medical tests, identification of divisions and quadrants of the abdomen, and some general terminology related to the system.

MAJOR AND ACCESSORY ORGANS

Table 12–1

Major and Accessory Organ	Pronunciation	Definition
mouth	mowth	oral cavity forming the beginning of the digestive system
teeth	teeth	structures of the jaws for biting and masticating food
tongue	tung	chief organ of taste; aids in mastication, swallowing, and speech
salivary glands	<u>sal</u>-i-ver-e glands	pertaining to the saliva; glands in the mouth that secrete saliva
pharynx	<u>far</u>-ingks	the throat; the membranous cavity behind the nasal cavities and mouth and before the larynx
esophagus	e-<u>sof</u>-ah-gus	membranous passage extending from the pharynx to the stomach

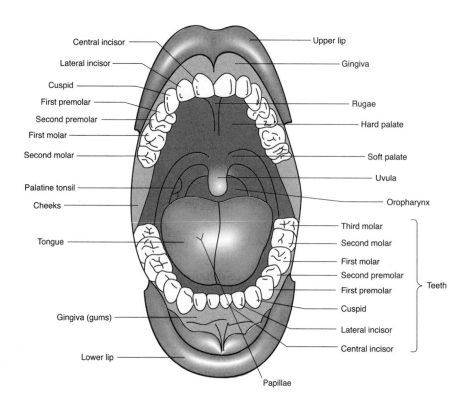

FIGURE 12–1 Oral cavity.

Major and Accessory Organ	Pronunciation	Definition
stomach	<u>stum</u>-ak	the musculomembranous expansion of the digestive tract between the esophagus and duodenum, consisting of a cardiac part, a fundus, a body, and a pyloric part
duodenum	du-o-<u>de</u>-num	the first portion of the small intestine
jejunum	je-<u>joo</u>-num	part of the small intestine from the duodenum to the ileum
ileum	<u>il</u>-e-um	last portion of the small intestine, from jejunum to cecum
pancreas	<u>pan</u>-kre-as	a large, elongated gland situated transversely behind the stomach. Externally, it secretes digestive enzymes into the common duct. Internally, its beta cells secrete insulin and glucagon. The alpha, beta, and delta cells of the pancreas form aggregates, called islets of Langerhans
liver	<u>liv</u>-er	the large, dark red gland in the upper part of the abdomen on the right side, just beneath the diaphragm. Its functions include storage and filtration of blood, secretion of bile, conversion of sugars into glycogen, and many other metabolic activities (see overview)

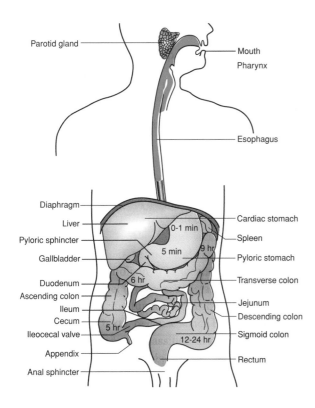

FIGURE 12–2 Human digestive tract. Times indicated along the tract represent how long it takes food to pass through each area during the process of digestion.

Major and Accessory Organ	Pronunciation	Definition
gallbladder	gall-blader	the pear-shaped reservoir for bile, behind the liver; stores and concentrates bile
cecum	se-kum	the first part of the large intestine, a dilated pouch
ascending colon	a-sen-ding ko-lon	portion of the colon from the cecum to the hepatic flexure
transverse colon	trans-vers ko-lon	portion of the large intestine passing transversely across the upper part of the abdomen, between the hepatic and splenic flexure
descending colon	di-send-ing ko-lon	portion of the colon from the splenic flexure to the sigmoid colon
sigmoid colon	sig-moid ko-lon	portion of the large intestine between descending colon and rectum
rectum	rek-tum	the last portion of the large intestine
anus	a-nus	opening of the rectum on the body surface

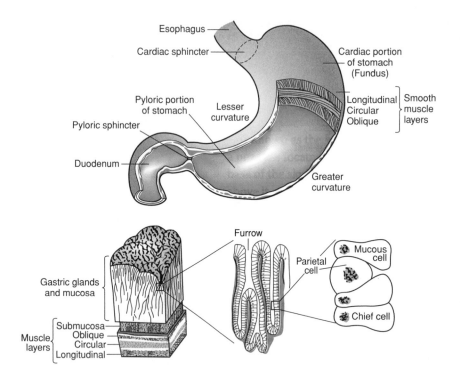

FIGURE 12–3 External and internal anatomy of the stomach.

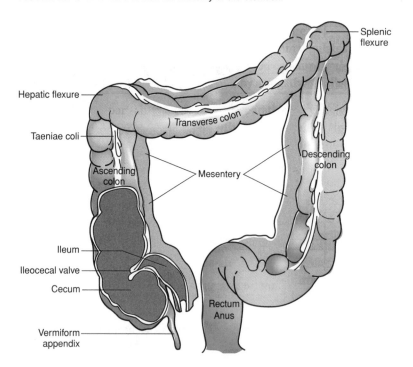

FIGURE 12–4 Large intestine. Each segment is named according to the direction it travels or according to its shape.

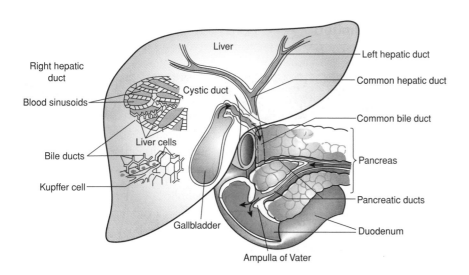

FIGURE 12–5 Liver and its interrelationship with the gallbladder, pancreas, and duodenum. A section has been removed from the liver and the area enlarged to show the arrangement of liver cells, bile ducts, Kupffer cells, and blood sinusoids to one another. Arrows indicate the direction of flow of bile from the gallbladder and liver and of digestive juices from the pancreas into the duodenum.

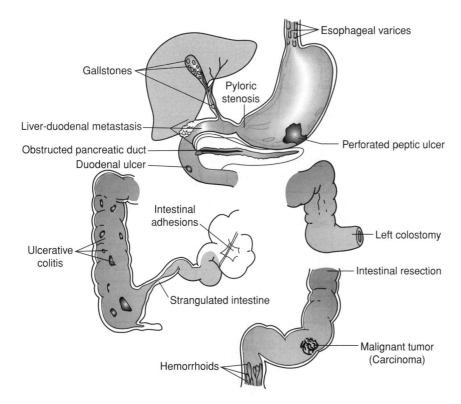

FIGURE 12–6 Pathologies of the alimentary tract.

CLINICAL DISORDERS

Table 12–2

Clinical Disorder	Pronunciation	Definition
adhesion	ad-<u>he</u>-zhun	union of two surfaces normally separate; also, any fibrous gland that connects them. Surgery within the abdomen may result in adhesions from scar tissue
alcoholism	<u>al</u>-ko-hol′ism	excessive consumption of alcoholic beverages, interfering with personal health and economy; an addiction. Although this disease affects the entire body, the liver is the organ most involved
anorexia nervosa	an′o-<u>rek</u>-se-ah ner-<u>vo</u>-sa	lack or loss of appetite for food; a psycho-physiologic condition characterized by symptoms of undernutrition
appendicitis	ah-pen′di-<u>si</u>-tis	inflammation of the appendix, which may rupture
borborygmus	bor-boh-rig′-mus	audible abdominal sound produced by hyperactive intestinal peristalsis. They are rumbling, gurgling, and tinkling noises heard when listening with a stethoscope
botulism	<u>boch</u>-oo-lizm	an extremely severe type of food poisoning caused by a neurotoxin (botulin) produced by *Clostridium botulinum* in improperly canned or preserved foods; can be fatal
carcinoma	kar′si-<u>no</u>-ma	a malignant tumor
celiac disease	<u>ce</u>-li-ac diz-ez	damage to the lining of the small intestine caused by the inability to digest gluten found in wheat, resulting in malabsorption of nutrients and malnutrition, if untreated
cholelithiasis	ko′le-li-<u>thi</u>-ah-sis	gallstones, hardened cholesterol stones formed from bile crystallization
cirrhosis	si-<u>ro</u>-sis	interstitial inflammation of an organ, particularly the liver; loss of normal architecture, with fibrosis and nodular regeneration
cleft lip/palate	cleft lip/<u>pal</u>-at	congenital fissure or split of the lip (cleft lip) or roof of the mouth (cleft palate)
colitis	ko-<u>li</u>-tis	inflammation of the colon, ulcerative or spastic
cryptitis	krip-<u>ti</u>-tis	inflammation of a crypt, especially the anal crypt
diverticulitis	di′ver-tik′u-<u>li</u>-tis	inflammation of the diverticula, the pouches that form in the walls of the large intestine

Clinical Disorder	Pronunciation	Definition
dysentery	<u>dis</u>-en-ter'e	inflammation of the intestine, especially the colon, with abdominal pain, diarrhea, and blood and mucus in stools; most commonly associated with bacterial or parasitic infection
emaciation	ee-may-she-ay'-shun	excessive leanness caused by disease or lack of nutrition
emesis	em'-eh-sis	material expelled from the stomach during vomiting; vomitus
esophageal atresia	e-sof'ah-<u>je</u>-al ah-<u>tre</u>-zhe-ah	congenital absence of the opening between esophagus and stomach
esophageal varices	e-sof'ah-<u>je</u>-al <u>var</u>-i-sez	enlarged, incompetent veins in the distal esophagus, usually caused by portal hypertension in liver cirrhosis
esophagitis	e-sof'ah-<u>ji</u>-tis	inflammation of the esophagus
femoral	<u>fem</u>-o-ral (pertaining to the groin)	hernia into the femoral canal
flexure	<u>flek</u>-sher	a bend or fold; as the hepatic flexure of the colon (near the liver)
gastric ulcers	<u>gas</u>-trik <u>ul</u>-serz	peptic or duodenal tissue inflammation of the stomach or intestinal linings, with pain and sometimes bleeding from perforation
gastritis	gas-<u>tri</u>-tis	inflammation of the stomach lining; a common stomach disorder
gastroenteritis	<u>gas</u>-tro-en'ter-i-tis	inflammation of the stomach and intestine caused by ingested harmful bacterial toxin, with acute nausea and vomiting, cramps, and diarrhea
gastroesophageal reflux disease (GERD)	gas-tro-e-soph-a-<u>ge</u>-al re-fluks diz-ez'	flow of gastric acid contents back up into the esophagus causing heartburn and, if chronic, esophagitis
glossitis	glo-<u>si</u>-tis	inflammation of the tongue
hepatitis	hep'ah-<u>ti</u>-tis	inflammation of the liver; may be type A, type B, or type C; types D and E have now also been identified
hernia	<u>her</u>-ne-ah	protrusion of a portion of an organ or tissue through an abnormal opening; there are many types
hiatal	hi-<u>a</u>-tal	protrusion of any structure through the esophageal hiatus of the diaphragm

Clinical Disorder	Pronunciation	Definition
Hirschsprung's disease	hirsh'-sprungz diz-ez'	congenital megacolon due to absence of autonomic ganglia in a segment of smooth muscle that normally stimulates peristalsis
impaction (fecal)	im-pak-shun (fek-al)	condition of being impacted. A collection of hardened feces in the rectum or sigmoid colon
inguinal	ing-gwi-nal (pertaining to the groin)	hernia into the inguinal canal; may be direct or indirect
intussusception	in'tuh-suh-sep-shun	prolapse of a part of the intestine into the lumen of an immediately adjacent part
irritable bowel syndrome (IBS) or spastic colon	eer-uh-tuh-bul bah-wul sin-drohm spas'-tic coh'-lon	increased motility of the small or large intestine causing nausea, pain, anorexia, and trapping of gas throughout the intestinal tract
melena	mell'-eh-nah	abnormal black, tarry stool containing digested blood
nausea and vomiting (N & V)	naw-ze-ah and vom-it-ing	common symptoms in many GI disorders
obesity	o-bes-i-te	Body Mass Index (BMI) of ≥30 using the formula: weight (kg) ÷ height squared (m²)
oral leukoplakia	or'-al loo-koh-play'-kee-ah	precancerous lesion in the mouth
pancreatitis	pan'kre-ah-ti-tis	inflammation of the pancreas
peritonitis	per'i-to-ni-tis	inflammation of the peritoneal cavity; may be due to chemical irritation or bacterial invasion
phenylketonuria (PKU)	fen-il-ke'to-nu-re-ah	a congenital inability to metabolize phenylalanine, a component of protein; may lead to retardation
polyposis	pol'i-po-sis	the formation of numerous polyps (growth hanging from a thin stalk)
pyloric stenosis	pi-lor-ik ste-no-sis	an obstruction of the pyloric orifice of the stomach, congenital or acquired
rectocele	rek-to-sel	hernia of the rectum through the vaginal floor
sialolith	si-al-o-lith	salivary duct stone
ulcers	ul-serz	a local defect of the surface of an organ or tissue

Clinical Disorder	Pronunciation	Definition
umbilical	um-<u>bil</u>-i-kal (pertaining to the umbilicus)	protrusion of the abdominal contents through the abdominal wall at the umbilicus

SURGERY

Table 12–3

Surgical Procedure	Pronunciation	Definition
anastomosis	ah-nas'to-<u>mo</u>-sis	surgical formation of a connection between two parts; ileorectal anastomosis connects the ileum and rectum after removal of the colon
appendectomy	ap'en-<u>dek</u>-to-me	excision of the appendix
biopsy	<u>bi</u>-op-se	removal of tissue for microscopic diagnosis
bypass	<u>bi</u>-pas	a shunt, e.g., a surgically created pathway
cheiloplasty	<u>ki</u>-lo-plas'te	surgical repair of a lip defect
cholecystectomy	ko'le-sis-<u>tek</u>-to-me	excision of the gallbladder
choledochoduodenostomy	ko-led'o-ko-du' o-de-<u>nos</u>-to-me	surgical formation of an opening into the duodenum that connects it with the common bile duct
colostomy	ko-<u>los</u>-to-me	surgical creation of an opening (stoma) between the colon and the body surface
gastrectomy	gas-<u>trek</u>-to-me	excision of the stomach, may be partial or subtotal
herniorrhaphy	her'ne-<u>or</u>-ah-fe	surgical creation of an opening into the ileum with a stoma on the abdominal wall
ileostomy	il'e-<u>os</u>-to-me	surgical creation of an opening into the ileum with a stoma on the abdominal wall
laparotomy	lap'ah-<u>rot</u>-o-me	incision through any part of the abdominal wall
portacaval shunt	por'tah-<u>ka</u>-val shunt	connecting the portal vein and inferior vena cava to bypass a cirrhotic liver

Surgical Procedure	Pronunciation	Definition
stomach stapling (gastric bypass)	<u>stum</u>-ak <u>sta</u>-pling	part of the stomach stapled to permit passage of a small amount of food, used to treat gross obesity
vagotomy	va-<u>got</u>-o-me	cutting the vagus nerve to reduce stomach stimulation, used to treat an ulcer

MEDICAL TESTS

Table 12–4

Medical Test	Pronunciation	Definition
barium swallow	bah'-ree-um swalo	also called upper GI series; the oral administration of a radiopaque contrast medium to view the esophagus by x-ray, while swallowing, to detect abnormalities
biopsy	<u>bi</u>-op-se	removal and examination, usually microscopic, of tissue from the living body, performed for diagnosis
blood tests or laboratory tests	blud tests	chemical analyses of various substances in the blood to make diagnoses. Some tests evaluate electrolytes, albumin and bilirubin levels, blood urea nitrogen (BUN), cholesterol, total protein, and serum glutamic–oxaloacetic transaminase (SGOT)
cholangiography	ko-lan'je-<u>og</u>-rah-fe	x-ray examination of the bile ducts, using a radiopaque dye as a contrast medium
colonoscopy	ko-lon-<u>os</u>-ko-pe	endoscopic examination of the colon, either transabdominally during laparotomy, or transanally by means of a colonoscope
digital examination	<u>dig</u>-i-tal eg-zam'i-na-shun	insertion of the gloved finger into the rectum or vagina
esophagogastroduodenoscopy (EGD)	e-sof'ah-go-gas'tro-du'o-de-<u>nos</u>-ko-pe	using endoscopes to examine esophagus, stomach, and duodenum

Medical Test	Pronunciation	Definition
flat plate of abdomen	flat plate <u>ab</u>-do-men	an x-ray film of the abdomen
fluoroscopy	floo-or-oh'-skop-ee	radiological technique to examine the function of an organ
gastrointestinal series (GIs)	gas'tro-in-<u>tes</u>-t-nal series	an examination of the upper gastrointestinal tract using barium as the contrast medium for a series of x-ray films; also called a barium meal
gastroscopy	gas-<u>tros</u>-ko-pe	inspection of the stomach's interior with a gastroscope
magnetic resonance imaging (MRI)	mag-neh'-tic rez'-oh-nans im'ij-ing	noninvasive scanning to visualize fluid, and soft and bone tissue; very precise and accurate
proctoscopy	prok-<u>tos</u>-ko-pe	inspection of the sigmoid and rectum with a proctoscope
scan	skan	an image produced using a moving detector or a sweeping beam of radiation, as in scintiscanning, B-mode ultrasonography, scanography, or CAT (computerized axial tomography)
serum glutamic oxalacetic transaminase (SGOT)	see-rum gloo-tam'-ik oks-al-ah-see-tic trans-am'-in-ays	an enzyme in high concentration in liver cells; high amounts in the blood indicate disease of liver cells
stool sample or specimen		a small stool sample for laboratory study, e.g., occult blood, parasites
ultrasonography	ul'trah-son-<u>og</u>-rah-fe	using ultrasound to obtain a visual record of any organ

ABDOMINAL REFERENCE TERMS

Table 12–5

Area	Right	Left	Middle
quadrant (kwod-rant)	right upper quadrant (RUQ) right lower quadrant (RLQ)	left upper quadrant (LUQ) left lower quadrant (LLQ)	

RUQ LUQ Quadrants RLQ LLQ	RH E LH RL U LL RI S or H LI

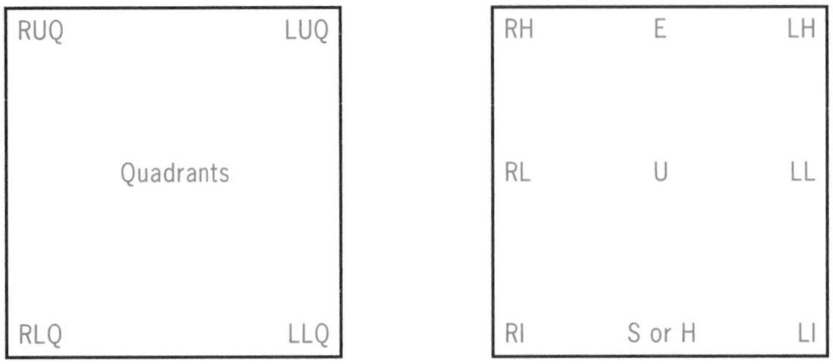

FIGURE 12–7 Quadrants and divisions of the abdomen.

Area	Right	Left	Middle
divisions (nine)	right hypochondrium (hi'po-<u>kon</u>-dre-um) (RH)	left hypochondrium (LH)	epigastric (ep'i-<u>gas</u>-trik) (E)
	right lumbar (<u>lum</u>-bar) (RL)	left lumbar (LL)	umbilical (um-<u>bil</u>-i-kal) (U)
	right inguinal (<u>ing</u>-gwi-nal) or iliac (il-e-ak) (RI)	left inguinal or iliac (LI)	suprapubic (S)

DIGESTIVE PROCESSES

Table 12–6

Substance or Process	Pronunciation	Definition
absorption	ab-<u>sorp</u>-shun	the uptake from the intestine of fluids, solutes, proteins, fats, and other nutrients into the intestinal wall cells, blood, lymph, or body fluids
anabolism	a-<u>nab</u>-o-lizm	building up using nutrients (proteins) for growth and development

Substance or Process	Pronunciation	Definition
catabolism	kah-<u>tab</u>-o-lizm	burning nutrients: breakdown in presence of oxygen
deciduous	de-<u>sid</u>-u-us	primary (baby) teeth replaced by permanent
deglutition	de'-glu-<u>ti</u>-shun	the act of swallowing
digestion	di-<u>jes</u>-chun	the act of converting food and fluids into chemical substances that can be absorbed and assimilated
elimination	e-lim-i-<u>na</u>-shun	excreting solid waste (feces)
epiglottis	epi-<u>glot</u>-is	thin leaf-shaped structure posterior to root of tongue
excretion	ek-<u>skre</u>-shun	excreting body solid and liquid waste (feces and urine)
incisors	in-size'-orz	front teeth used for biting, tearing
ingestion	in-<u>jes</u>-chun	taking food, liquids, drugs, etc., by mouth
mandible	<u>man</u>-di-ble	lower jaw
mastication	mas-ti-<u>kay</u>-shun	chewing
maxilla	mak-<u>sil</u>-a	upper jaw
molars	<u>moh</u>-lar	crushing and grinding teeth
palate	<u>pal</u>-at	roof of the mouth
papillae	pah-<u>pill</u>-ay	small rough elevations on tongue and roof of mouth; contain taste buds
periodontal disease	pair-ee-oh-don'tal diz-ez'	group of inflammatory gum disorders
peristalsis	peri-<u>stal</u>-sis	muscular movement of food and liquid through the GI tract
trachea	<u>tray</u>-kea	wide, short tube, commonly called the windpipe. Starts below larynx and enters thoracic cavity
uvula	yoo-vyoo-lah	small cone-shaped tissue hanging from soft palate of the mouth

MISCELLANEOUS TERMS

Table 12–7

Term	Pronunciation	Definition
achalasia	ak-al-lay′-zee-ah	decreased mobility of the lower two-thirds of the esophagus, along with constriction of the muscle between the esophagus and stomach, the lower esophageal sphincter (LES)
anasarca	an′ah-<u>sar</u>-kah	generalized massive edema
ascites	ah-<u>si</u>-tes	abnormal accumulation of (edematous) fluid within the peritoneal cavity
buccal	<u>buk</u>-al	pertaining to the cheek
cachexia	kah-<u>kek</u>-se-ah	severe malnutrition and wasting, emaciation
dental caries	den′tal cair′eez	tooth decay formed from microorganisms maintained in the mouth
enema	<u>en</u>-e-mah	introduction of fluid into the rectum to promote evacuation of feces or to administer nutrient or medicinal substances
enteropathy	en′ter-<u>op</u>-ah-the	a disease of the intestine
enzyme	<u>en</u>-zim	a protein produced in a cell capable of facilitating a specific biologic or chemical reaction. Enzymes perform this function without being destroyed or altered
fistula	<u>fis</u>-tu-lah	an abnormal passage between two internal organs, or leading to the body surface
gamma globulins	<u>gam</u>-ah <u>glob</u>-u-linz	substances containing antibodies; they provide passive immunity in some people against certain infectious diseases
gavage	gah-v<u>ahzh</u>	forced feeding, especially through a tube passed into the stomach; common for premature infants, the unconscious, and the critically ill
glossal	<u>glos</u>-al	pertaining to the tongue
hyperalimentation	hi′per-al′i-men-<u>ta</u>-shun	an intravenous feeding program similar to total perenteral nutrition
lavage	lah-<u>vahzh</u>	washing out an organ, e.g., the stomach or bowel
lingual	<u>ling</u>-gwal	pertaining to the tongue; sublingual means "under the tongue"

Term	Pronunciation	Definition
nasogastric (ng)	na'zo-<u>gas</u>-trik	a soft flexible tube introduced through the nose into the stomach for gavage, lavage, or suction
NPO (nothing per os)		no food or fluid by mouth or other body orifice (os means any body orifice)
parotid	pah-<u>rot</u>-id	near the ear
peritoneum	per'i'-to-<u>ne</u>-um	membrane lining abdominal walls and pelvis, cavities, and investing the contained viscera, the peritoneal cavity (see Plate 12)
stoma	<u>sto</u>-mah	"mouth"; an artificially created opening (e.g., in colostomy) on the surface of the abdomen
thrush	thrush	fungal infection of the mouth caused by *Candida albicans* resulting in painful creamy white raised patches of the tongue and oral mucosa
total parenteral nutrition	pah-<u>ren</u>-ter-al nu-<u>trish</u>-un	intensive intravenous feeding most often introduced through a subclavian vein
viscera	<u>vis</u>-er-ah	a large interior organ in a body cavity, especially the abdomen
volvulus	vol'vyoo-lus	loop of bowel twisting on itself resulting in bowel obstruction

LESSON TWO   PROGRESS CHECK

The following tests permit you to assess your progress in learning medical terms that pertain to the gastrointestinal system.

■ WRITE-IN

For each digestive disease or disorder described, write in the correct term.

1. Abnormal fibers that bind one organ to another_____ .

2. A severe type of food poisoning caused by anaerobic bacteria _____ .

3. A malignant tumor anywhere in the body _____ .

4. The term for stones in the gallbladder _____ .

5. Inflammation of the colon _____ .

6. Pouches in the sigmoid colon _____ .

7. An inflamed area with tissue destruction in the gastric mucosa _____ .

8. Inflammation of the stomach or intestines _____ .

9. Inflammation of the tongue _____ .

10. Protrusion of a part out of its natural place _____ .

11. Telescoping of the intestine into itself _____ .

12. A hernia that causes a bowel obstruction _____ .

13. Inflammation of the liver _____ .

14. The most common symptoms of GI disorders _____ .

15. Having a Body Mass Index (BMI) of ≥30 _____ .

16. Inflammation of the pancreas _____ .

17. Inflammation of the peritoneal membrane _____ .

18. A disease of infancy in which the outlet of the stomach is too narrow
    for food to pass through _____ .

19. Foamy, bulky, foul-smelling stool high in fat content _____

20. Replacement of liver cells by fibrous tissue _____ .

■ MATCHING

Match the parts of the digestive tract listed at the left with their respective functions listed on the right:

1. tongue
2. pharynx
3. parotid, submaxillary, sublingual
4. esophagus
5. gallbladder
6. liver
7. pancreas
8. ileum
9. gastric mucosa
10. gastric secretions

a. produces saliva
b. breaks up food for digestion
c. aids in swallowing
d. produces insulin and enzymes
e. stores bile
f. stores fat-soluble vitamins; manufactures bile
g. a tube that directs food to the next organ
h. carries food to the esophagus
i. digests and absorbs food
j. prevents acid from consuming the stomach

■ DEFINITIONS

Give a definition for each of the following terms:

1. small intestine _____

2. gastroenterologist _____

3. digestion _____

4. absorption _____

5. alimentary canal _____

6. peristalsis _____

7. mucus _____

8. duodenum _____

9. pyloric sphincter _____

10. ampulla of Vater _____

11. mesentery _____

12. hemorrhoids _____

13. peritoneum _____

14. colon _____

15. cecum _____

16. caries _____

17. bicuspid _____

18. ridges on the mucous membrane _____

■ WORD POOL: STRUCTURE OF THE DIGESTIVE TRACT

Select appropriate terms from the word pool below to complete these sentences:

1. The first part of the digestive system is called the _____ .

2. The chief organ of digestion is the _____ .

3. The first part of the small intestine is called the _____ .

4. The first part of the large intestine is called the _____ .

5. Three accessory organs are _____ .

6. Primary (baby) teeth replaced by permanent teeth are _____ .

7. The lower part of the large intestine is called the _____ .

8. The last part of the alimentary canal is the _____ .

9. A structure whose common name is the apron is the _____ .

10. The three divisions of the small intestine are the _____ .

11. A term meaning roof of the mouth is the _____ .

12. A group of inflammatory gum disorders is called _____ .

WORD POOL

Anus, ascending, bicuspid, cecum descending, deciduous, duodenum, gallbladder, greater omentum, ileum, jejunum, liver, mouth or oral cavity, pancreas, periodontal disease, rectosigmoid, rectum, small intestine, transverse, palate

■ MATCHING: SURGICAL PROCEDURES

Match the procedure on the left to its description on the right:

1. anastomosis   **a.** creation of a new opening into the abdomen

2. cholecystectomy   **b.** exploratory incision into the abdomen

3. colostomy   **c.** a bypass of an obstruction

4. gastrectomy   **d.** closing off of part of the stomach to permit passage of only small amounts of food

5. herniorrhaphy   **e.** surgical repair of a hernia

6. ileostomy   **f.** excision of the gallbladder

7. laparotomy   **g.** joining two parts together (intestine: ducts) when a portion has been removed

8. stapling   **h.** creating a stoma on the surface of the abdomen for excretion of waste

9. shunt   **i.** cutting the vagus nerve to reduce acid secretions

10. vagotomy   **j.** subtotal removal of the stomach

■ WORD PUZZLE ON THE DIGESTIVE SYSTEM

There are 51 words about the digestive system contained in this puzzle. Find them by reading forward, backward, up, down, or diagonally. When the 51 listed words have been located, the remaining letters (from left to right) will spell DIGESTIVE SYSTEM.

```
A  N  U  S  L  A  N  A  C  Y  R  A  T  N  E  M  I  L  A  F
I  L  E  U  M  A  E  N  H  B  D  I  S  E  P  N  D  G  A  P
X  A  S  D  S  M  S  A  Y  I  E  E  V  E  T  E  D  T  Y  A
I  S  R  I  T  Y  O  L  M  L  C  L  R  R  C  E  S  L  R  N
D  C  E  O  O  L  C  C  E  E  A  I  I  S  D  O  D  A  C
N  E  V  M  M  A  U  A  F  V  S  N  D  C  I  R  P  I  L  R
E  N  S  G  A  S  L  N  L  T  S  U  E  C  I  R  A  T  L  E
P  D  N  I  C  E  G  A  A  I  O  N  A  C  E  Y  L  O  I  A
P  I  A  S  H  O  C  L  C  U  D  C  S  D  C  R  A  R  X  T
A  N  R  S  R  E  S  F  S  I  I  P  D  N  E  E  T  A  A  I
M  G  T  A  C  I  A  U  N  R  H  A  G  I  C  T  E  P  M  C
R  C  L  O  S  C  G  G  O  I  L  N  A  M  U  N  U  J  E  J
O  O  E  T  T  A  C  L  N  B  M  C  S  A  M  E  R  P  I  U
F  L  V  O  H  O  H  C  L  U  G  R  T  T  U  S  E  H  E  I
I  O  R  P  L  C  T  L  N  S  U  E  R  I  C  E  C  A  N  C
M  N  O  O  O  E  A  E  V  Y  T  A  I  V  O  M  T  R  I  E
R  S  N  R  R  G  D  I  L  I  P  S  C  S  S  T  U  Y  S  D
E  F  D  O  S  O  L  I  V  E  R  E  T  S  A  T  M  N  P  I
V  Y  H  O  U  L  A  B  S  O  R  P  T  I  O  N  M  X  E  C
H  C  L  D  I  G  E  S  T  I  V  E  S  Y  S  T  E  M  P  A
```

WORDS TO LOOK FOR IN THE WORD PUZZLE

1. absorption	14. digestive system	27. intrinsic factor	40. pepsin
2. acid	15. duodenum	28. jejunum	41. peristalsis
3. alimentary canal	16. esophagus	29. lips	42. pharynx
4. amylase	17. fats	30. liver	43. pyloric sphincter
5. anal canal	18. feces	31. maxillary	44. rectum
6. anus	19. gallbladder	32. mesentery	45. sigmoid
7. ascending colon	20. gastric	33. mucosa	46. stomach
8. bile	21. glucose	34. oral	47. taste
9. cecum	22. gut	35. os	48. transverse
10. CHO	23. HCl	36. palate	49. vermiform appendix
11. chyme	24. hydrochloric acid	37. pancreas	50. villi
12. deciduous	25. ileocecal valve	38. pancreatic juice	51. vitamin
13. descending colon	26. ileum	39. parotid	**DIGESTIVE SYSTEM**

CHAPTER 13 Respiratory System

OBJECTIVES

1. Identify the organs of the respiratory system.
2. Describe the location and label the structures of the respiratory system.
3. List the functions of the respiratory system.
4. Identify and define clinical disorders affecting the respiratory system.
5. List and explain laboratory tests and medical procedures used to diagnose disorders of the respiratory system.

OVERVIEW

The respiratory system consists of a series of tubes that transport air into and out of the lungs. Its function is to supply oxygen (O_2) to the body cells and to transport carbon dioxide (CO_2) produced by the body cells into the atmosphere. The respiratory organs also have important functions for normal speech, acid-base balance, hormonal regulation of blood pressure, and defense against foreign material. The respiratory system also allows humans to perceive odors and to filter and moisten air.

Respiration involves the following processes:

1. Pulmonary ventilation (breathing).
2. External respiration (diffusion of O_2 and CO_2 between air in the lungs and the capillaries).
3. Internal respiration (diffusion of CO_2 and O_2 between blood and tissue cells).
4. Cellular respiration (use of O_2 by the body cells in production of energy and release of CO_2 and H_2O).

The respiratory tract is divided into the upper respiratory tract, consisting of the *nose, pharynx,* and *larynx,* and the lower respiratory tract, the *trachea, bronchi,* and *lungs.* These structures are defined and illustrated in Lesson One.

(Also see Plate 13.) A brief discussion of their respective functions follows:

1. *Nose* (nostrils or nares)—the external portion of the respiratory tract filters small particles, warms and humidifies incoming air, and receives odors. It is the primary organ for the sense of smell.

2. *Pharynx* (throat)—a 5-in. muscular tube that extends from the base of the skull to the esophagus. It is the airway that connects the mouth and nose to the larynx. Although it is a single organ, it is divided into three sections, the *nasopharynx, oropharynx*, and *laryngopharynx*. The nasopharynx is behind the nose and serves to equalize pressure on both sides of the tympanic membrane (eardrum). The oropharynx, behind the mouth, is a muscular soft palate containing the uvula and palatine tonsils. The laryngopharynx surrounds the opening of the esophagus, which is the gateway to the rest of the respiratory system. The pharynx is the common passageway for both air and food. To prevent food from entering the respiratory tract, a small flap called the *epiglottis* covers the opening of the larynx during the act of swallowing.

3. *Larynx* (voice box)—connects the pharynx with the trachea. It is a short tube shaped like a triangular box and is supported by nine cartilages, three paired and three unpaired. It contains the vocal cords and supporting tissue that make vocal sounds possible.

4. *Trachea* (windpipe)—a 10- to 12-cm-long tube, the trachea extends into the chest and serves as a passageway for air into the bronchi. It lies in front of the esophagus. It is kept permanently open by 16 to 20 C-shaped cartilaginous rings.

5. *Bronchi*—the trachea branches into two tubes called the bronchi (the bronchial tree). Each bronchus enters a lung. The right primary (main) bronchus is shorter than the left because the arch of the aorta displaces the lower trachea to the right. Foreign objects falling into the trachea are more likely to lodge in the right bronchus. Each bronchus subdivides into progressively smaller branches called *bronchioles*, which terminate in the *alveoli* (air space).

6. *Lungs*—pyramid-shaped, spongy, air-filled organs, which are molded into the thoracic cavity that contains them. The right lung has three lobes, the left has two. In the lungs, alveoli are surrounded by a network of tiny blood vessels called capillaries: O_2 from the lungs passes into these capillaries for distribution to the cells, and CO_2 from the blood cells passes into the lungs for removal (by exhalation). When O_2 is absorbed into the blood it attaches to *hemoglobin* and is released as needed.

The pleura are the serous membrane coverings that enclose each lung. The *parietal* pleura lines the *thoracic* (chest) cavity (rib cage, diaphragm, and mediastinum). The *visceral* pleura covers the lung and is continuous at the root of the lung, where it joins with the parietal pleura. The parietal and visceral pleura lie close together; between them is a thin film of lubricating fluid that prevents friction when the two slide against each other during respiration.

THE RESPIRATORY SYSTEM

The overview described the structure, function, and supporting systems of the respiratory system. The respiratory system involves the exchange of oxygen and carbon dioxide. We inhale oxygen (O_2) and exhale carbon dioxide (CO_2). This process is also known as *respiration (inspiration and expiration)*. To facilitate your learning of myriad medical terms within the respiratory system, we have divided them into tables. Lesson One identifies the body parts, and Table 13–2 names and defines common respiratory diseases and disorders. Table 13–3 provides terms pertaining to the tests and diagnostic and/or surgical aspects of treatment, as well as terminology needed for an understanding of the respiratory system. Refer to Figures 13-1 through 13-4 as needed.

RESPIRATORY BODY PARTS

Table 13–1

Body Part	Pronunciation	Definition
Organ		
nasal cavity	na-zal kav-i-te	nose, nares, cavity separated by septum
pharynx	far-ingks	throat, cavity behind the nasal cavities and mouth
larynx	lar-inks	voice organ, containing the vocal cords
trachea	tra-ke-ah	windpipe
lung	lung	two cone-shaped spongy organs consisting of alveoli, blood vessels, nerves, and elastic tissue. Each is enveloped in a double-folded membrane called the pleura
parietal pleura	par-ry'-e-tal ploo'-rah	the serous membrane that lines the thoracic (chest) cavity
visceral pleura	viss'-or-al ploo'-rah	membrane that covers the lungs. This membrane and the parietal membrane are close together. Between them is a thin film of lubricating fluid that prevents friction when they slide against each other
bronchus (pl., bronchi)	brong-kus (brong-ki)	one of the larger passages conveying air to (right or left principal lobe) and within the lungs

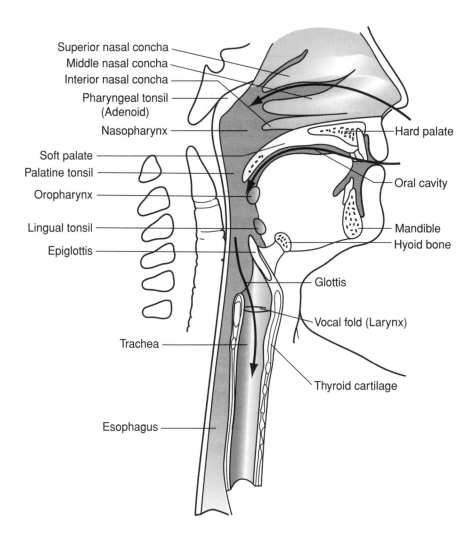

FIGURE 13–1 Sagittal section of the head and neck, showing the respiratory passage down to the bifurcation of the trachea.

Body Part	Pronunciation	Definition
bronchioles	brong-ke-olz	one of the subdivisions of the branched bronchial tree
alveolus (pl., alveoli)	al-ve-o-lus (al-ve-ol-i)	a small saclike dilation (outpocketing) of the alveolar ducts
diaphragm	dye'-ah-fram	muscular partition that separates the thoracic cavity from the abdominal cavity and aids in the process of breathing

COMMON DISORDERS OF THE RESPIRATORY SYSTEM

Table 13–2

Condition	Pronunciation	Definition
abscess (lung)	<u>ab</u>-ses	a localized collection of pus in a cavity formed by the disintegration of tissues
anthracosis	an-thrah-koh′-sis	accumulation of carbon deposits in the lung due to breathing smoke or coal dust, also known as black lung disease
ARDS		adult (acute) respiratory distress syndrome
asbestosis	as-beh-stoh′-sis	lung disease caused by inhaling asbestos particles. Associated with development of mesothelioma, a type of lung cancer
asphyxiation	as-fik′se-<u>a</u>-shun	suffocation
asthma	<u>az</u>-mah	spasm and narrowing of bronchi, leading to bronchial airway obstruction
atelectasis	at′e-<u>lek</u>-tah-sis	incomplete expansion of the lungs at birth, or collapse of the adult lung

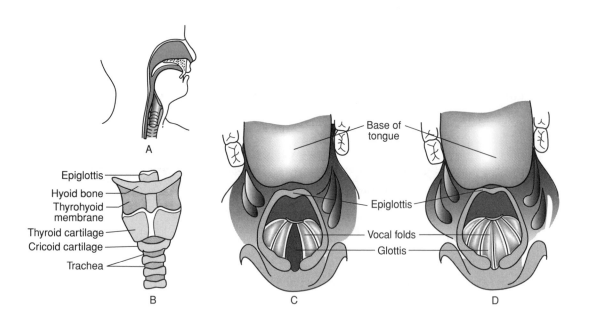

FIGURE 13–2 Larynx. **A**, In relation to the head and neck. **B**, Anterior aspect. **C**, Superior aspect with vocal folds open. **D**, Superior aspect with vocal folds closed.

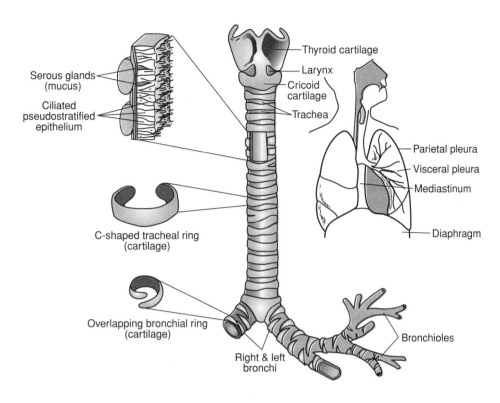

FIGURE 13–3 Human larynx, trachea, and bronchi, anterior aspect.

Condition	Pronunciation	Definition
bradypnea	brad-ip-nee'-ah	abnormally slow breathing
bronchiectasis	brong'ke-<u>ek</u>-tah-sis	chronic dilation of one or more bronchi
bronchitis	brong-<u>ki</u>-tis	inflammation of one or more bronchi
byssinosis	bis-ih-noh'-sis	lung disease resulting from inhaling cotton, flax, or hemp, also know as brown lung disease
carcinoma	kar'si-<u>no</u>-mah	a malignant new growth made up of epithelial cells tending to infiltrate surrounding tissues and to give rise to metastases
coccidioidomycosis	kok-sid'e-oi'-do-mi-<u>ko</u>-sis	a respiratory infection caused by spore inhalation of *Coccidioides immitis,* varying in severity from that of a common cold to symptoms resembling those of influenza; also called valley fever
COPD		chronic obstructive pulmonary (lung) disease, especially emphysema, chronic bronchitis, and asthma

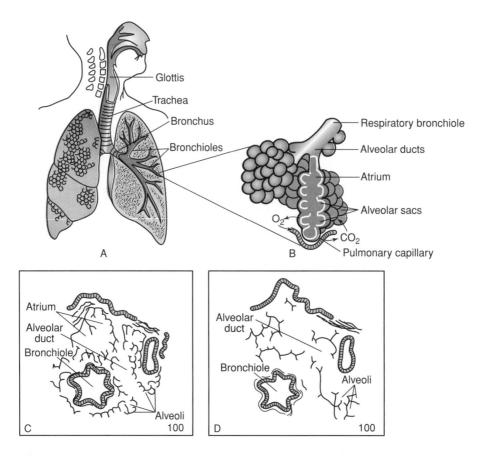

FIGURE 13–4 Internal structure of the lungs. **A**, Relationship of the lungs to the head and neck. **B**, External and internal appearance of a lung lobule, showing the atrium and alveolar sacs. **C**, Section of a lung, magnified 100 times. **D**, Section of a similar lung with emphysema. Note the decreased number of alveolar sacs and consequent diminishing in the gas exchange area of lung tissue.

Condition	Pronunciation	Definition
cor pulmonale	kor pul'mo-<u>nay</u>-lee	heart failure from pulmonary disease
coryza	ko-<u>ri</u>-zah	profuse discharge from the mucous membrane of the nose; the common cold
cough	koff	a forceful expiration preceded by a preliminary inhalation. Usually caused by irritation of the airways from dust, smoke, infection, or mucus. Can be described as croupy, rasping, harsh, hollow, loose, dry, productive, brassy, bubbly, or wracking
cystic fibrosis	<u>sis</u>-tik fi-<u>bro</u>-sis	generalized hereditary disorder of infants, children, and young adults associated with malfunctioning of the pancreas and frequent respiratory infections

Condition	Pronunciation	Definition
deviated septum	<u>de</u>-vi-ated <u>sep</u>-tum	defect in the wall between the nostrils that can cause partial or complete obstruction
diphtheria	dif-<u>the</u>-re-ah	an acute bacterial infection primarily affecting the membranes of the nose, throat, or larynx accompanied by fever and pain
effusion	e-<u>fu</u>-zhun	escape of a fluid; exudation or transudation
emphysema	em'fi-<u>se</u>-mah	a pathologic accumulation of air in tissues or organs
epistaxis	ep-ih-staks'-is	hemorrhage from the nose: nosebleed
expectoration	ex-pek-toh-ray'-shun	the act of spitting out saliva or coughing up material from the lungs
fibrosis	fi-<u>bro</u>-sis	formation of fibrous or scar tissue (in lungs) usually caused by previous infections
flail chest	flal chest	chest wall moves paradoxically with respiration, owing to multiple fractures of the ribs
"flu"	floo	popular name for influenza
hay fever	hay <u>fe</u>-ver	a hypersensitive state, e.g., allergy to pollen
hemothorax	he'mo'<u>tho</u>-raks	blood in the pleural thoracic cavity
hiatal hernia	hi-<u>a</u>-tal <u>her</u>-ne-ah	protrusion of part of the stomach into the chest through the esophageal hiatus defect of the diaphragm
hiccup	<u>hik</u>-up	sharp respiratory sound with spasm of the glottis and diaphragm
histoplasmosis	his'to-plaz-<u>mo</u>-sis	fungal infection of lungs, may be symptomatic or asymptomatic, resembling TB
hyaline	<u>hi</u>-ah-liln	glossy, translucent
hyaline membrane disease	<u>hi</u>-ah-lin mem-bran di-<u>zez</u>	lack of surfactant due to a layer of hyaline material lining the alveoli, alveolar ducts, and bronchioles. Leading cause of neonatal deaths
influenza	in'floo-<u>en</u>-zah	an acute viral infection of the respiratory tract; serious for the very young and old
laryngitis	lar'in-<u>ji</u>-tis	inflammation of the larynx
laryngotracheo-bronchitis	la-<u>rin</u>-go-tra-ke-o-brong-<u>ki</u>-tis	inflammation of the larynx, trachea, and bronchi

Condition	Pronunciation	Definition
lung abscess	lung ab'-sess	pus formed by the destruction of lung tissue and microorganisms by white blood cells that have gone to a localized area to fight infection
pertussis	per-<u>tus</u>-is	acute upper respiratory infectious disease caused by bacterium *Bordetella pertusis.* Commonly called whooping cough
pharyngitis	far'in-<u>ji</u>-tis	inflammation of the pharynx
pleural effusion	ploo'-ral eh-fyoo'-shun	accumulation of fluid in the pleural space, which compresses the underlying portion of the lung, resulting in dyspnea
pleurisy	<u>ploor</u>-i-se	inflammation of the pleura
pneumoconiosis	nu'mo-ko'ne-<u>o</u>-sis	any lung disease, e.g., anthracosis, silicosis, caused by permanent deposition of substantial amounts of particulate matter in the lungs
pneumothorax	new-moh-thoh'-racks	a collection of gas or air in the pleural cavity, resulting from a perforation through the chest wall or the visceral pleura
rhinitis rhinorrhea	ri-<u>ni</u>-tis ri'no-<u>re</u>-ah	inflammation of the nasal membrane; "runny nose"
SIDS	sidz	sudden infant death syndrome, or crib death; cause unknown. Associated failure of synapse of nerves to activate the diaphragm
sinusitis	si'nu'<u>si</u>-tis	inflammation of a sinus
sneeze	sneeze	spasmodic contraction of muscles causing air to be expelled forcefully through the nose and mouth
streptococcal throat	strep'to-<u>kok</u>-al	sore throat caused by the spore bacteria *Streptococcus*
tonsillitis	ton'si'<u>li</u>'tis	inflammation of the tonsils, especially the palatine tonsils
tuberculosis (TB)	too-ber'ku-<u>lo</u>-sis	an infectious disease, marked by tubercles and caseous necrosis in tissues of the lung
URI		upper respiratory infection, general term for colds or "flu"
valley fever		see coccidioidomycosis
wheezing	wheez-ing	a high-pitched, whistling sound from air movement through narrowed bronchioles during exhalation; symptom of asthma and COPD

Condition	Pronunciation	Definition
whooping cough	hoop-ing kof	a respiratory infection caused by *Bordetella pertussis*, marked by peculiar paroxysms of cough, ending in a prolonged crowing or whooping respiration

DIAGNOSTIC, SURGICAL, AND MEDICAL PROCEDURES, AND GENERAL TERMS

The signs and symptoms of respiratory diseases are unique to the system. They provide doctors, nurses, and patients with clues in terms of sight and sound. For example, wheezing (sound), a certain color of phlegm (sight), coughing (sound), sneezing (sight and sound), etc. These manifestations are all helpful in diagnosing the problem.

The medical terminology included in the following table on diagnostics should become part of your vocabulary.

Table 13–3

Term	Pronunciation	Definition
aerosol	a-er-o-sol′	a medication that can be sprayed from a container to relieve bronchial distress, especially asthma
anoxia	an-ok-se-ah	without oxygen
apnea	ap-ne-ah	temporary cessation of breathing; asphyxia
bifurcation	bi′fer-ka-shun	a division into two branches, e.g., bronchi
blood gases	blud gas-iz	oxygen, carbon dioxide, and other gases in the blood
bronchodilator	brong′ko-di-la-tor	an agent capable of dilating the bronchi
bronchoscope	brong-ko-skop	an instrument for inspecting the bronchi
bronchoscopy	brong-kos-ko-pe	lung examination using a bronchoscope
bronchospasm	brong-ko-spazm	spasmodic contraction of bronchi muscles, as in asthma
Cheyne-Stokes	Chan-Stokes	breathing characterized by waxing and waning of the depth of respiration: the patient breathes deeply a short time and then breathes slightly or stops altogether. The cycle repeats.

Term	Pronunciation	Definition
CO_2		carbon dioxide; an odorless, colorless gas resulting from oxidation of carbon, formed in the tissues and eliminated by the lungs
consolidation	kon-sol'i-<u>da</u>-shun	solidification of lung tissue, as in pneumonia
CPR		cardiopulmonary resuscitation; artificial means of providing circulation and breathing during cardiac and respiratory arrest
cyanosis	si-ah-<u>no</u>-sis	a bluish discoloration of skin and mucous membranes caused by insufficient oxygen in the blood
dysphonia	dis-<u>fo</u>-ne-ah	voice impairment; difficulty in speaking
dyspnea	<u>disp</u>-ne-ah	labored or difficult breathing
endotracheal (ET) tube	en'do-<u>tra</u>-ke-al	an airway catheter inserted in the trachea during surgery and for a temporary airway in emergency situations
expectorant	ek-<u>spek</u>-to-rant	an agent that promotes expectoration (loosening of secretions)
hemoptysis	he-<u>mop</u>-ti-sis	the spitting of blood or of blood-stained sputum (from the lungs)
hiatus	hi-<u>a</u>-tus	a gap (opening), especially in the diaphragm
hilus	<u>hi</u>-lus	part of lung where vessels, nerves, and bronchi enter
hypercapnia	hi'per-<u>kap</u>-ne-ah	an excess of carbon dioxide in the blood
hyperventilation	hi'per-ven'ti-<u>la</u>-shun	increased rate and/or depth of respiration, e.g., from anxiety
hyposensitization	hi'po-sen'si-ti-<u>za</u>-shun	the process of rendering hyposensitive, e.g., exposing a patient to an offending substance to reduce his or her sensitivity to the substance
hypoxia	hi-<u>pok</u>-see-ah	insufficient oxygen
IPPB		intermittent positive pressure breathing, used as treatment with ventilation
Kussmaul breathing	<u>koos</u>-mowl	gasping, labored breathing, also called air hunger
laryngectomy	lah-rin-<u>jek</u>-to-me	excision of the larynx

Term	Pronunciation	Definition
laryngoscopy	lar'ing-<u>gos</u>-ko-pe	visual examination of the interior larynx with an instrument called a laryngoscope
lavage of sinuses	lah-<u>vahzh</u> si-nus	the irrigation or washing out of sinuses
lobectomy	lo-<u>bek</u>-to-me	excision of a lobe of the lung
Mantoux (test)	man-<u>too</u>	TB skin test
O₂ (oxygen)	<u>ok</u>-si-jen	constitutes about 20% of atmospheric air; inhaled and carried in the blood
orthopnea	or'thop-<u>ne</u>-ah	difficult breathing, except in the upright position
oximetry	ox·im'e·try	measurement of the oxygen saturation of arterial blood
palpation	pal-pay-shun	application of hands and fingers to external surfaces to detect abnormalities
parenchyma (lung)	pah-<u>reng</u>-ki-mah	the essential elements or "working parts" of an organ, e.g., alveoli in the lung
peak expiratory flow rate	pek ex-pi'-ra-tory flo rat	measurement of how fast a person can exhale using a small handheld device to monitor treatment in asthma or COPD
percussion and auscultation (P & A)	per-<u>kush</u>-un aw'skul-<u>ta</u>-shun	striking the body (e.g., chest) with short, sharp blows of the fingers, and listening through a stethoscope for the sounds produced. Technique used by practitioners
perfusion	per-<u>fu</u>-zhun	the passage of a fluid through the vessels of a specific organ to supply nutrients and oxygen
pneumothorax	nu'mo-<u>tho</u>-raks	air or gas in the pleural space; from trauma or from deliberate introduction; may be spontaneous
postural drainage	<u>pos</u>-chur-al <u>dran</u>-ij	drainage by placing the patient's head downward so that the trachea will be inclined below the affected area and the secretions mobilized
PPD		purifed protein derivative (TB test)
productive cough	pro-<u>duk</u>-tiv kof	cough with spitting of material from the bronchi
pulmonary function	<u>pul</u>-mo-ner'e <u>fungk</u>-shun	tests to assess ventilatory status

Term	Pronunciation	Definition
rales, rhonchi	rahlz, rong-ki	an abnormal respiratory sound heard on auscultation, indicating some pathologic condition
rarefaction	rar'e-fak-shun	condition of being less dense, e.g., decreased density in x-ray films
residual air	re-zed-u-al	air remaining or left behind after expiration
respirator (ventilator)	res-pi-ra'tor (ven'ti-la-tor)	a device for giving artificial respiration or to assist in pulmonary ventilation
rhinoplasty	ri-no-plas'te	plastic surgery of the nose
scan (lung, pleura)	skan	an image or a "picture" produced using radioactive isotopes, e.g., B-mode ultrasonography
SMR		submucous resection, excision of a portion of the submucous membrane of the nose to correct a defect
SOB		shortness of breath
spirometer (spirometry)	spi-rom-e-ter (spi-rom-e-tre)	an instrument for measuring air taken into and expelled from the lungs; spirometry is the measurement of lung capacity
sputum	spu-tum	matter ejected from the trachea, bronchi, and lungs through the mouth
tachypena	tak'ip-ne-ah	very rapid respiration
thoracentesis	thor'rah-sen-te-sis	surgical puncture of the chest wall into the parietal cavity to remove fluid
tine test		TB test
tracheostomy	tra'ke-os-to-me	creation of an opening into the trachea through the neck, e.g., insertion of a tube to facilitate ventilation
tracheotomy	tra'ke-ot-o-me	incision of the trachea through the skin and muscles of the neck
ventilator	ven'ti-la-tor	an apparatus to assist in pulmonary ventilation; see also respirator
vital capacity	vi-tal kah-pas-i-te	amount of air that can be expelled from the lungs after deep inspiration (pulmonary function test)

Term	Pronunciation	Definition
wheeze	hweez	breathing with a raspy or whistling sound. Common symptom of asthma
x-ray examination		visual record made using x-rays, for diagnostic examination of the chest; may be AP (anteroposterior) or Lat (side) views

LESSON TWO   PROGRESS CHECK

■ MATCHING

Match the terms in the left-hand column to their definitions on the right.

J **1.** apnea
I **2.** dyspnea
E **3.** orthopnea
G **4.** tachypnea
A **5.** atelectasis
B **6.** bronchiectasis
H **7.** dysphagia
D **8.** emphysema
C **9.** asthma
F **10.** effusion

a. incomplete expansion or collapse of lung
b. chronic dilation of the lung
c. spasm and swelling in the airways
d. abnormal accumulation of air
e. difficulty breathing except when sitting up
f. escape of fluid
g. very rapid breathing
h. difficulty swallowing
i. difficult breathing
j. temporary cessation of breathing

■ MULTIPLE CHOICE

Circle the letter of the correct answer:

1. The pulmonary function test is used to
   a. diagnose abnormal lung tissue
   b. demonstrate abnormal pulmonary blood flow
   c. evaluate how a patient breathes
   d. measure obstructions to pulmonary function

2. When the chest wall is punctured with a needle to obtain fluid for diagnosis, the procedure is known as
   a. thoracentesis
   b. bronchoscopy
   c. pleural biopsy
   d. pulmonary angiogram

3. Coccidioidomycosis is
   a. a malignant lung tumor
   b. a disease caused by a fungus
   c. coughing up of blood
   d. a collection of fluid in the pleural cavity

4. Which of the following statements describes eupnea?
   a. shortness of breath
   b. lack of oxygen
   c. difficult breathing
   d. normal breathing

5. Heart failure caused by pulmonary disease is called
   a. coryza
   b. cor pulmonale
   c. COPD
   d. carcinoma

6. A deviated septum is a
   a. malfunctioning alveoli
   b. defect in the wall between nostrils
   c. broken nose
   d. pulmonary obstruction

7. Which of the following terms describes the coughing up of blood?
   a. expectorate
   b. hypoxia
   c. hemoptysis
   d. sputum

8. A hemothorax is a
   a. collection of blood in the chest
   b. collapsed lung
   c. creation of a new opening into the chest
   d. nosebleed

9. When part of the stomach protrudes through the diaphragm into the chest, the medical term is
   a. hyaline membrane disease
   b. hemothorax
   c. hiatal hernia
   d. histoplasmosis

10. The common name for pertussis is
   a. measles
   b. hay fever
   c. hiccups
   d. whooping cough

■ DEFINITIONS

Define the following terms:

1. pharynx _throat – cavity btwn nasal passages + mouth passageway for food, liquid + air_

2. larynx _voice box – contains vocal cords_

3. trachea _windpipe – long tube extending from trachea to chest_

4. alveoli _cluster of air sacs where walls exΔ O_2 + CO_2_

5. bronchi _main branches that convey air from trachea to lungs_

6. intercostal _btwn the ribs_

7. sinuses _(cavities) pockets in face + skull bones_

8. lungs _orgs of respiration where blood + air meet + mix_

9. diaphragm _main musc. of respiration, separates lungs from abdomen_

10. SIDS _crib death sudden infant death syndrome – dying of healthy baby during sleep cause = unknown_

11. COPD _chronic obstruction pulmonary disease chronic, progressively debilitating lung diseases_

12. pleurisy _inflammation of pleura (lining that encases lungs)_

13. cystic fibrosis _hereditary disorder present from birth associated w/ malfunct of pancrease + frequent resp. infects._

14. influenza _contagious inflamm. of upper respiratory tract_

15. emphysema _pus in body cavity_

16. ARDS _acute (adult) resp. distress syndrome – faulty gaseous exΔ leading to lung shock_

■ ABBREVIATIONS

Identify the following abbreviations:

1. URI _upper respiratory infection_

2. SOB _shortness of breath_

3. IPPB _intermittan positive pressure breathing_

4. SMR _submucous resection_

5. CBC _complete blood count_

6. TPR _temperature, pulse + respiration_

7. PPD _purified protein derivative (TB test)_

8. CPR _cardiopulmonary resuscitation_

9. ET tube _endotracheal tube_

10. A & P _auscultation + percussion_

■ NAMING

Name the following respiratory symptoms from their descriptions:

1. Excessive amount of carbon dioxide in the blood _hypercapnia_

2. Breathing is possible only in an upright position _orthopnea_

3. Difficult breathing _dyspnea_

4. Condition where there is a bluish discoloration of the skin _cyanosis_

5. Spitting up blood _hemoptysis_

6. Deficiency of oxygen _hypoxia_

7. Condition of pus in the pleural cavity _pyothorax/empyema_

8. High-pitched, harsh sound heard during inspiration _stridor_

9. Inability to make sounds _dysphonia_

10. Blood in the pleural cavity _hemothorax_

■ MATCHING

Match the following breath sounds on the left with their descriptions on the right.

F **1.** pleural rub   **a.** crackling sounds heard on auscultation, usually during inhalation

A **2.** rales   **b.** loud, coarse, rattling sounds heard on auscultation

B **3.** rhonchi   **c.** abnormally rapid breathing

E **4.** wheeze   **d.** labored or difficult breathing

D **5.** dyspnea   **e.** whistling sound heard without a stethoscope, usually during exhalation

C **6.** tachypnea   **f.** rubbing sound heard on auscultation

       g. abnormally slow breathing

       h. high-pitched sound made during inspiration

■ WORD PUZZLE ON THE RESPIRATORY SYSTEM

Find the 54 words related to the respiratory system by reading forward, backward, up, down, and diagonally. When the 54 listed words have been circled, the remaining letters spell the word AIR.

```
L  O  B  U  L  E  S  A  N  I  R  A  C  I  C  A  R  O  H  T
A  M  U  T  P  E  S  L  A  S  A  N  X  O  B  E  C  I  O  V
R  T  H  R  O  A  T  X  N  Y  R  A  H  P  S  T  I  D  A  L
Y  S  C  A  S  Y  R  A  N  O  M  L  U  P  A  S  S  A  G  E
N  I  N  S  P  I  R  A  T  I  O  N  I  N  H  A  L  E  A  B
X  N  O  I  T  A  R  I  P  S  E  R  C  I  L  I  A  B  S  R
E  E  R  U  S  S  E  R  P  L  A  I  T  R  A  P  T  R  E  O
D  S  H  A  L  L  O  W  C  T  R  A  C  H  E  A  I  O  X  N
I  A  E  R  A  T  E  I  O  E  V  R  E  S  E  R  V  N  C  C
X  H  E  T  A  R  B  R  L  S  U  L  O  E  V  L  A  C  H  H
O  C  S  A  A  O  Y  A  M  U  C  U  S  E  B  O  L  H  A  I
I  N  O  N  R  C  H  E  C  N  A  I  L  P  M  O  C  U  N  O
D  O  N  E  E  X  P  I  R  A  T  I  O  N  I  O  N  S  G  L
N  C  A  N  E  M  G  A  R  H  P  A  I  D  U  C  T  S  E  E
O  Y  T  I  L  I  B  I  S  N  E  T  S  I  D  T  U  B  E  S
B  E  E  R  T  L  A  I  H  C  N  O  R  B  O  X  Y  G  E  N
R  V  E  N  T  I  L  A  T  I  O  N  L  A  U  D  I  S  E  R
A  I  T  R  A  N  S  P  O  R  T  R  C  E  L  L  U  L  A  R
C  A  P  A  C  I  T  Y  T  I  V  A  C  L  A  R  U  E  L  P
G  N  U  L  S  U  R  F  A  C  T  A  N  T  B  R  E  A  T  H
```

WORDS TO LOOK FOR IN THE WORD PUZZLE

1. aerate	12. cilia	23. larynx	34. pleural cavity	45. tidal
2. aerobic	13. compliance	24. lobe	35. pulmonary	46. thoracic
3. alveolus	14. concha	25. lobules	36. pharynx	47. throat
4. breath	15. diaphragm	26. lung	37. rate	48. trachea
5. bronchial tree	16. distensibility	27. mucus	38. reserve	49. transport
6. bronchioles	17. ducts	28. nare	39. residual	50. tubes
7. bronchus	18. exhale	29. nasal septum	40. respiration	51. ventilation
8. capacity	19. expiration	30. nose	41. respiratory center	52. vital
9. carbon dioxide	20. gas exchange	31. oxygen	42. sacs	53. voice box
10. carina	21. inhale	32. partial pressure	43. shallow	54. ions
11. cellular	22. inspiration	33. passage	44. surfactant	AIR

CHAPTER 14   Cardiovascular System

OBJECTIVES

1. Identify the organs of the cardiovascular system.
2. Describe the location of the structures.
3. List the functions of the cardiovascular system.
4. Identify the structure and functions of the lymphatic system.
5. Name the five blood-forming organs associated with the circulatory system.
6. Identify and describe the types and functions of the blood vessels.
7. Identify and define selected clinical disorders affecting the cardiovascular system.
8. Explain medical tests and lab procedures used in the diagnosis of cardiovascular diseases/disorders.
9. Correctly spell and pronounce new medical terms.

OVERVIEW

The cardiovascular system is a subset of the circulatory system. It consists of the heart, blood vessels, and blood. The lymphatic system is also a part of the circulatory system, consisting of lymph vessels and lymph nodes within the larger vessels. Associated with the circulatory system are the blood-forming organs, that is, the spleen, liver, bone marrow, thymus gland, and lymph tissue (see Plates 6, 7, 8, and 10).

The heart is a four-chambered hollow organ that lies between the lungs in the middle of the *thoracic* cavity. Two-thirds of the heart lies left of the *midsternum*. It is about the size of the owner's fist. It is cone-shaped, the base directed toward the right shoulder and the apex pointed toward the left hip.

The heart is covered with a double-walled sac that encloses the heart and great blood vessels called the *pericardium*. It is attached to the *diaphragm*, the *sternum*, and the lung pleura. The tough outer layer of the pericardium protects the heart. The inner *serous* layer contains the visceral membrane (*epicardium*) that covers the heart surface and the parietal membrane that lines the inside of the pericardium. There is fluid in the space between these layers that lubricates the membrane and prevents friction.

There are four heart chambers, upper right and left *atria* and lower right and left *ventricles*. The ventricles are separated by the *interventricular* septum. The *tricuspid* valve lies between the right atrium and right ventricle. Blood flows back and forth through the valve and regulates blood pressure in the heart, sending blood into the right ventricle when the pressure is greater in the right atrium and preventing backflow of blood into the right atrium.

The blood vessels are a series of closed tubes that carry blood from the heart to the tissue and back to the heart. The three major types of vessels are *arteries*, *capillaries*, and *veins*.

Arteries carry blood from the heart. Elastic arteries are the largest arteries from the heart. Muscular arteries branch into medium-sized and small arteries that contain both muscular and elastic tissue. The smallest, the *arterioles*, deliver blood to capillary beds in the tissues.

Veins carry blood back to the atria of the heart. The venous system holds 75% of total blood volume and returns blood under low pressure. The venous system begins at the *capillary* beds and flows into larger *venules* and then into small, medium, and large veins.

The major arteries of systemic circulation are the *aorta*, the largest vessel in diameter in the body, and the branches from the aorta leading toward the head and neck, and descending into the trunk and lower extremities (see Plates 6, 7, and 8 for complete details).

An interesting feature of the circulatory system is fetal circulation, which is not discussed here. Details can be obtained from a standard textbook on the subject.

The circulatory system can be divided into three types of circulation: pulmonary (lung), systemic (whole body), and portal (intestine, liver, and spleen). Functions of the circulatory system are:

1. Transport—gases, hormones, minerals, enzymes, and other vital substances are carried in the blood to every cell in the body. All waste materials are carried by the blood to the lungs, skin, or kidneys for elimination from the body (*pulmonary circulation*).
2. Body temperature—the blood vessels maintain body temperature by dilating at the skin surface to dissipate heat or by constricting to retain heat.
3. Protection—the blood and lymphatic systems protect the body against injury and foreign invasion through the immune system. Blood clotting mechanisms protect against blood loss.
4. Buffering—blood proteins provide an acid-base buffer system to maintain optimum pH of the blood.

The parts of the heart are defined and illustrated in Lesson One of this chapter.

LESSON ONE   MATERIALS TO BE LEARNED

The human circulatory system consists of a pump (the heart) and a network of vessels that transport blood throughout the body. The workhorse of the circulatory system is the heart, propelling blood through approximately 60 miles of blood vessels in the body.

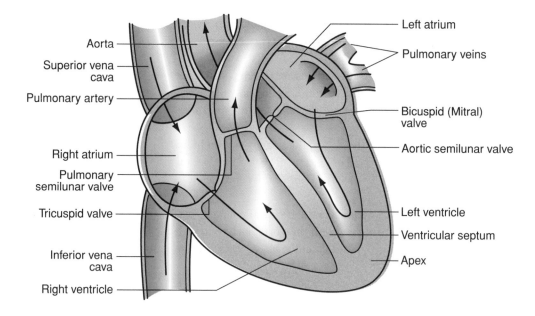

FIGURE 14–1 Diagram of the heart. Arrows indicate direction of blood flow.

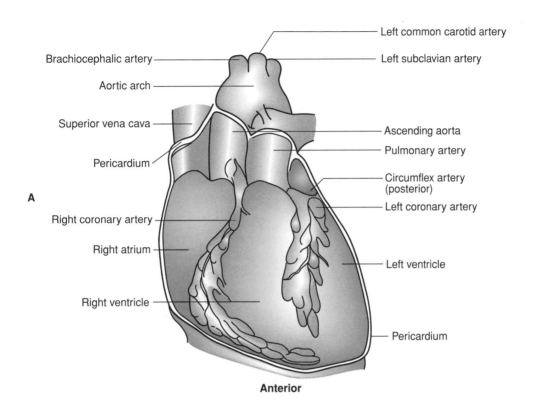

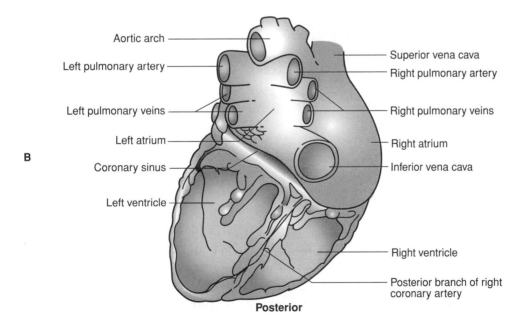

FIGURE 14–2 **A**, Anterior structure of the heart. **B**, Posterior structure of the heart.

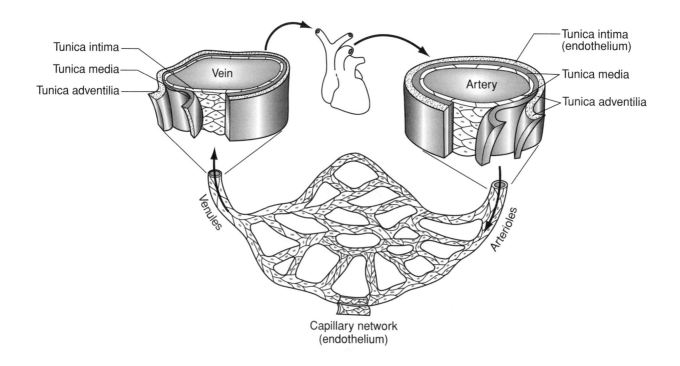

Tunica intima
Tunica media
Tunica adventilia

Vein

Tunica intima
(endothelium)

Tunica media

Tunica adventilia

Artery

Venules

Arterioles

Capillary network
(endothelium)

FIGURE 14–3 Blood vessels. Diagrammatic sketch showing the single-cell endothelium of all the vessels and the layered muscular coats of arteries and veins.

Lesson One explains the parts and functions of the heart and blood vessels and the terminology related to them. It also describes disorders/diseases affecting the system and some means of diagnosis and treatment of them. Blood pressure terminology, blood types, blood components, and other general and related terms are included.

The lymphatic system, which is an integral part of the circulatory system, is discussed in Lesson Two.

THE CARDIOVASCULAR SYSTEM

This information should be studied in conjunction with Figures 14–1, 14–2, 14–3, 14–4, and 14–5.

Parts of the Heart

The heart is a muscular, cone-shaped organ, about the size of a clenched fist, that pumps blood throughout the body and beats normally about 70 times per minute by coordinated nerve impulses and muscular contractions. The right side of the heart provides for oxygenation of blood (*pulmonary circulation*). The left side is responsible for transportation of blood to and from body cells (*systemic circulation*). The heart is enclosed in a fibroserous sac and is divided into four chambers.

Table 14–1

Parts of the Heart	Pronunciation	Definition
heart	hart	the organ of circulation of the blood
atrium (pl., atria)	a̱-tre-um a̱-tre-uh	one of the two (left and right) upper chambers of the heart; also known as the auricle. These upper chambers collect blood
ventricle	ven-tri-kul	one of the two (left and right) lower chambers of the heart. They pump blood from the heart
apex	a̱-peks	the pointed end (of the heart)
Valves	valvz	a membrane in a passage to prevent backward flow
tricuspid	tri-kus-pid	having three points or cusps, situated between the right atrium and the right ventricle
pulmonary semilunar	pul-mon-ner′e sem′i-lu-nar	pertaining to the lung and resembling a crescent valve; located between the right ventricle and the pulmonary artery
mitral	mi-tral	shaped like a miter, also called bicuspid valve; situated between the left atrium and the left ventricle
aortic	a-or-tic	located between the left ventricle and the aorta
septum	sep-tum	a dividing wall between the right and left sides of the heart
Muscle	muhs-uhl	
myocardium	mi′o-kar-de-um	middle, thickest layer of the heart wall, made of cardiac muscle
Membranes	mem-brânz	
pericardium	per′i-kar-de-um	the fibroserous sac enclosing the heart
endocardium	en′do-kar-de-um	lining membrane of the heart's cavities
epicardium	ep′i-kar-de-um	the visceral pericardium
Conduction system		
sinoatrial node or SA node	si′no-a̱-tre-al	atypical muscle fibers at the junction of the superior vena cava and right atrium. It originates the cardiac rhythm and is therefore called pacemaker of the heart
atrioventricular node	a′tre-o-ven-trik-u-lar nod	Purkinje fibers beneath the endocardium of the right atrium in the septum
bundle of His	bun-d′l of his	cardiac muscle fibers connecting the atria with the ventricles of the heart

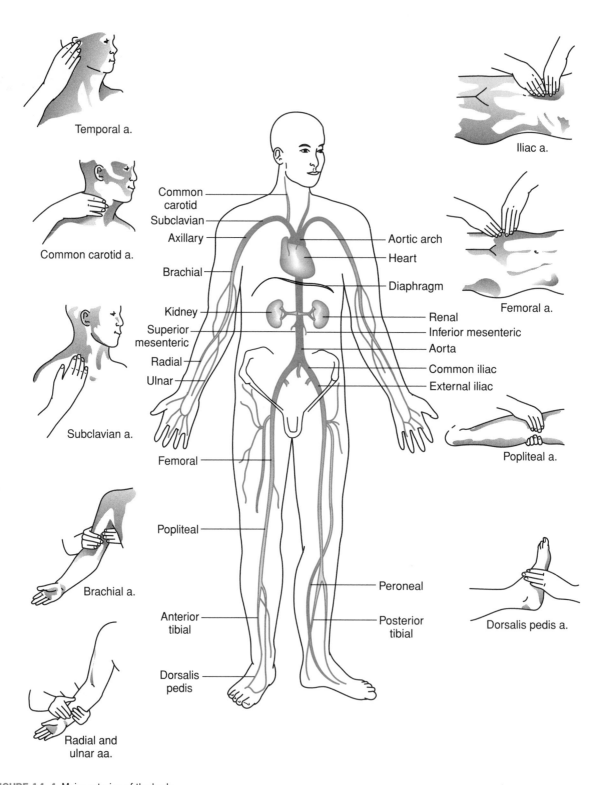

FIGURE 14–4 Major arteries of the body.

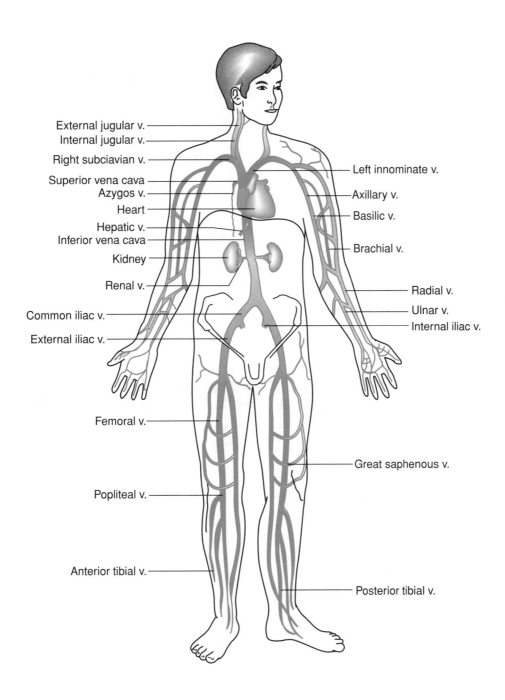

External jugular v.
Internal jugular v.
Right subciavian v.
Superior vena cava
Azygos v.
Heart
Hepatic v.
Inferior vena cava
Kidney
Renal v.
Common iliac v.
External iliac v.
Femoral v.
Popliteal v.
Anterior tibial v.

Left innominate v.
Axillary v.
Basilic v.
Brachial v.
Radial v.
Ulnar v.
Internal iliac v.
Great saphenous v.
Posterior tibial v.

FIGURE 14–5 Major veins of the body.

The Circulatory System

The circulatory system in the body transports oxygen and nutrients *to* and carbon dioxide and wastes *away from* the cells.

Table 14–2

Circulation	Pronunciation	Definition
Circulation	ser'ku-<u>la</u>-shun	movement in circuitous course; as the movement of blood through the heart and blood vessels
pulmonary	<u>pul</u>-mo-ner'e	movement of blood through the lungs and the pulmonary artery
systemic	sis-<u>tem</u>-ic	pertaining to movement of blood to the body as a whole
portal	<u>por</u>-tal	circulation of blood from the gastrointestinal tract and spleen through the portal vein to the liver

Types of Blood Vessels

Three types of vessels carry blood throughout the body. Each has a unique structure and function.

Table 14–3

Blood Vessels	Pronunciation	Definition
Artery	<u>ar</u>-ter-e	a vessel in which blood flows away from the heart, carrying oxygenated blood
aorta	a-<u>or</u>-tah	the great artery arising from the left ventricle; largest artery
coronary arteries	<u>kor</u>-o-ner'e <u>ar</u>-ter-es	arteries from the base of the aorta that supply the heart muscle with blood
Vein	vân	a vessel in which blood flows toward the heart, carrying blood with little oxygen
vena cava	<u>ve</u>-nah ca-vah	largest vein. *Inferior:* the venous trunk for the lower viscera. *Superior:* the venous trunk draining blood from head, neck, upper limbs, and thorax
Capillary	<u>kap</u>-i-ler'e	a minute, hairlike vessel connecting arterioles and venules

Blood Components

Table 14–4

Component	Pronunciation	Definition
Red blood cells (RBCs)	red blud	red blood cells or corpuscles, one of the formed elements in peripheral blood. They contain hemoglobin and transport oxygen. Also called erythrocytes
White blood cells (WBCs)	white blud	colorless blood corpuscles capable of amoeboid movement; protect the body against pathogenic microorganisms. There are five types of white blood cells. Also called leukocytes
granulocytes	<u>gran</u>-u-lo-sitz′	any cells containing granules, especially a granular leukocyte; formed in the bone marrow. There are three types: neutrophils, eosinophils, and basophils
neutrophils	<u>nu</u>-tro-filz	having a nucleus with three to five lobes and cytoplasm containing very fine granules. Neutrophils defend the body by ingesting invaders. Type I WBC
eosinophils	e′o-<u>sin</u>-o-filz	having a nucleus with two lobes and cytoplasm containing coarse, round granules. May be associated with allergy. Type-2 WBC
basophils	<u>ba</u>-so-filz	any structure cells staining readily with basic dyes; functions unknown. Type-3 WBC
agranulocytes	ah-<u>gran</u>-u-lo-sitz′	nongranular leukocytes, produced by the spleen and lymph nodes. There are two types
lymphocytes	<u>lim</u>-fo-sitz	participate in immunity; produced by the spleen and lymph nodes. Type-4 WBC
monocytes	<u>mon</u>-o-sitz	destroy foreign invaders in the body. Type-5 WBC
Other components		
fibrinogen	fi-<u>brin</u>-o-jen	promotes blood clotting
thrombocytes	<u>throm</u>-bo-sitz	blood platelets
plasma	<u>plas</u>-mah	the fluid portion of the blood or lymph, without the cells, amber-colored. When whole blood is undisturbed in a tube, clotting cells settle in the bottom, the clear plasma is on top
serum	<u>se</u>-rum	the clear portion of the blood separated from solid elements; plasma minus fibrinogen
platelet	<u>plât</u>-let	a disk-shaped structure in the blood, for blood coagulation; also called thrombocyte

Component	Pronunciation	Definition
reticulocytes	re-<u>tik</u>-u-lo'sitz	immature red blood cells, in the bone marrow
Landsteiner types	<u>land</u>-sti-ner	refers to the type of red blood cell: A, B, AB, and O
universal donor	<u>do</u>-ner	a person with group O blood; frequently used in emergency transfusion
universal recipient	re-<u>sip</u>-e-ent	able to receive blood of any type; group AB
type and crossmatch (x match)		determination of the compatibility of the blood of a donor and that of a recipient before transfusion by placing the donor's cells in the recipient's serum and the recipient's cells in the donor's serum; absence of agglutination, hemolysis, and cytotoxicity indicates compatibility
Rh factors		a genetically determined antigen, present on the surface of erythrocytes. There are at least eight variations. It is named for rhesus monkeys used in early experiments. One Rh factor present in blood means it is Rh positive; if no factor is found, the blood is Rh negative

Blood Pressure

Table 14–5

Term	Pronunciation	Definition
hypertension	hi'per-<u>ten</u>-shun	persistently high arterial blood pressure; causes may or may not be identifiable
sphygmomanometer	sfig'mo-mah-<u>nom</u>-e-ter	an instrument for measuring arterial blood pressure
systolic pressure	sis-<u>tol</u>-ic <u>presh</u>-ur	the contraction, or period of contraction, of the heart, especially of the ventricles. The top number in a blood pressure reading
diastolic pressure	di-ah-<u>stol</u>-ic <u>presh</u>-ur	the dilation, or the period of dilation of the heart, especially of the ventricles. The bottom number in a blood pressure reading
normal BP		an acceptable range for systolic pressure is ≤120, and for diastolic <80

Clinical Disorders Affecting the CV System

Table 14–6

Condition	Pronunciation	Definition
anemia	ah-<u>ne</u>-me-ah	reduction below normal of red blood cells, hemoglobin, or the volume of packed red cells in the blood; a symptom of various disorders
aneurysm	<u>an</u>-u-rizm	a sac formed by localized dilation of an artery or vein
angina pectoris	an-<u>ji</u>-nah <u>pek</u>-to-ris	pain in the chest, caused by decreased supply of oxygen to the heart muscle; can be precipitated by increased activity or stress
arrhythmia	ah-<u>rith</u>-me-ah	variation from the normal rhythm of the heartbeat
arteriosclerosis	ar-te're-o-skle-<u>ro</u>-sis	thickening and loss of elasticity of the arterial walls, slowing the flow of blood
asystole	a-<u>sis</u>-to-le	cardiac standstill; no heartbeat
atherosclerosis	ath'er-o-skle-<u>ro</u>-sis	a form of arteriosclerosis in which fats (e.g., cholesterol) are deposited on arterial walls
cardiac arrest	<u>kar</u>-de-ak ah-<u>rest</u>	cessation of heart function
coarctation	ko'ark-<u>ta</u>-shun	stricture or narrowing of a vessel
Congenital defects	kon-<u>jen</u>-i-tal <u>de</u>-fekts	defects present at birth
cyanosis	sigh'-ah-<u>no</u>-sis	dark, slightly bluish discoloration of the skin due to reduced hemoglobin in the blood
patent ductus arteriosus	<u>pa</u>-tent <u>duk</u>-tus ar-te-re-<u>o</u>-sus	birth defect; duct with an abnormal open lumen in the ductus arteriosus
tetralogy of Fallot	te-<u>tral</u>-o-je of Fah-<u>lo</u>	birth defect consisting of pulmonic stenosis, interventricular septal defect, hypertrophy of right ventricle, and transposition of the aorta
congestive heart failure (CHF)	kon-<u>jes</u>-tiv hart <u>fâl</u>-yer	defective blood pumping system, marked by breathlessness and abnormal retention of sodium and water
embolism	<u>em</u>-bo-lizm	the sudden blocking of an artery by an embolus
embolus	<u>em</u>-bo-lus	a foreign object (i.e., air, fat, tissue, or blood) brought by the blood and forced into a smaller vessel, thus obstructing the circulation

Condition	Pronunciation	Definition
endocarditis	en'do-kar-<u>di</u>-tis	exudative and proliferative inflammation of the endocardium
fibrillation	fi'bri-<u>la</u>-shun	a small, local, involuntary muscular contraction, caused by spontaneous activation of single muscle cells or muscle fibers
Heart attack		
coronary thrombosis	<u>kor</u>-o-ner-e throm-<u>bo</u>-sis	thrombosis of a coronary artery, often leading to myocardial infarction
infarction	<u>in</u>-fark-shun	a localized area of ischemic necrosis owing to occlusion of the arterial supply
myocardial infarction	<u>mi</u>-o-kar'de-al in-<u>fark</u>-shun	gross necrosis of the myocardium, caused by decreased blood supply to the area
occlusion	o-<u>kloo</u>-zhun	obstruction, a closing off of the coronary arteries, leading to a heart attack
heart block	hart blok	impairment of conduction in heart excitation; often applied specifically to arterioventricular heart block
heart murmur	hart <u>mer</u>-mer	an auscultatory sound (soft, blowing); a periodic sound of short duration of cardiac origin; may be due to an incompetent valve
hemophilia	he'mo-<u>fil</u>-e-ah	a hereditary hemorrhagic condition caused by lack of one or more clotting factors
Hodgkin's disease	<u>hoj</u>-kinz di-<u>zez</u>	painless progressive enlargement of lymph nodes, spleen, and lymphoid tissue; symptoms include anorexia, lassitude, weight loss, fever, itching, night sweats, and anemia
hypertension	hi'per-<u>ten</u> shun	persistently high arterial blood pressure; causes may or may not be identifiable
ischemia	is-<u>ke</u>-me-ah	deficiency of blood in a part; due to spasm of blood vessel, temporarily reducing blood flow
leukemia	loo-<u>ke</u>-me-ah	a malignant disease of the blood-forming organs, e.g., abnormal proliferation and development of leukocytes and related cells in blood and bone marrow
myocarditis	mi'o-kar-<u>di</u>-tis	inflammation of the myocardium
pericarditis	per'i-kar-<u>di</u>-tis	inflammation of the pericardium

Condition	Pronunciation	Definition
plaque	plak	a deposit of fatty material in the artery (atheroscloerosis)
rheumatic heart disease	roo-<u>mat</u>-ik	the most important manifestation and sequel to rheumatic fever, consisting chiefly of valvular deformities
stroke (cerebrovascular accident [CVA])	strôk	a sudden and acute vascular lesion of the brain caused by hemorrhage, embolism, thrombosis, or rupturing blood vessels
thrombophlebitis	throm'bo-fle-<u>bi</u>-tis	inflammation of a vein associated with thrombus formation
transient ischemic attack (TIA)	is-<u>kem</u>-ik ah-<u>tak</u>	brief interruption of circulation to a portion of the brain owing to vascular spasm, causing temporary loss of function. A precursor to CVA
varicose veins	<u>var</u>-i-kos vânz	a dilated, tortuous vein, usually in the leg, caused by a defective venous valve

Surgery, Lab, and Medical Tests

Table 14–7

Term	Pronunciation	Definition
angiography	an'je-<u>og</u>-rah-fe	x-ray technique using an injected contrast medium to visualize the heart and blood vessels
angioplasty	<u>an</u>-je-o-plas'te	surgical or percutaneous reconstruction of blood vessels
balloon angioplasty		insertion of a balloon to dilate a vessel (see PTCA)
anticoagulant	an'ti-ko-<u>ag</u>-u-lant	any substance that removes or prevents blood clotting
antihypertensive drug	an'ti-hi'per-<u>ten</u>-siv	a drug that reduces or eliminates high blood pressure
auscultation	aws'kul-<u>ta</u>-shun	the act of listening for sounds within the body chiefly to ascertain the condition of the thoracic or abdominal viscera; may be performed with the unaided ear or with a stethoscope
bradycardia	brad'e-<u>kar</u>-de-ah	slowness of the heartbeat, as evidenced by a pulse rate of <60
bypass	<u>bi</u>-pas	a surgically created route to circumvent the normal path

Term	Pronunciation	Definition
cardiac catheterization	<u>kar</u>-de-ak kath'e-ter-i-<u>za</u>-tion	a long, fine catheter is navigated through a peripheral blood vessel into the chambers of the heart using x-ray visualization as a guide
cardiac enzyme test	ca-dee-ak-en'-zym test	tests on drawn blood samples to determine if there is damage to the myocardial muscle
collateral circulation	ko-<u>lat</u>-er-al ser'ku-<u>la</u>-shun	circulation by secondary channels after obstruction of the principal channel supplying the heart
commissurotomy	kom'i-shur-<u>ot</u>-o-me	surgical incision of a defective heart valve to increase the size of the orifice; commonly done to separate adherent, thickened leaflets of a stenotic mitral valve
computed axial tomography (CAT scan or CT scan)	computed ak'-see-al toh-mog'rah-fee	diagnostic x-ray technique that uses ionizing radiation to produce cross-section images of the body. The x-ray feeds the images into a computer that produces cross-sectional pictures
coronary artery bypass graft	<u>kor</u>-o-ner-e <u>ar</u>-ter-e <u>bi</u>-pas	use of a leg vein or synthetic material to substitute for an occluded artery in the heart
digitalize	dij'i-tal-<u>iz</u>	to administer digitalis in a dosage schedule designed to produce and then maintain optimal heart contraction with nominal side effects
diuretic	di'u-<u>ret</u>-ik	an agent that promotes removal of excess interstitial fluid and results in increased urine secretion
Doppler	<u>dop</u>-ler	a device for measuring blood flow that transmits and reflects sound waves
dyscrasia	dis-<u>kra</u>-ze-ah	any abnormal condition of the blood
echocardiography	ek-oh-car-dee-og'-rah-fee	diagnostic procedure using ultrasound waves to study the structure and motion of the heart and to detect changes in some heart disorders
electrocardiogram	e-lek'tro-<u>kar</u>-de-o-gram'	the record produced by electrocardiography; abbreviated ECG or EKG
endarterectomy	en'dar-ter-<u>ek</u>-to-me	excision of thickened areas of the innermost coat of an artery to increase blood flow
exercise stress test		test widely used to assess cardiac function by means of subjecting the patient to controlled amounts of physical stress, such as the treadmill, pedaling a stationary bike, or climbing stairs

Term	Pronunciation	Definition
hemoglobin	he'mo-<u>glo</u>-bin	the oxygen-carrying pigment of the red blood cells; it contains iron and copper
heparin	<u>hep</u>-ah-rin	a substance that counteracts blood clotting, existing both as a natural substance in the blood and as a drug
Holter monitor	<u>hol</u>-tur	a portable device for monitoring blood pressure or heart/respiratory rate, e.g., ECG
low-salt diet		common term for a diet low in sodium content to reduce body-water level; correctly termed sodium-restricted diet
lumen	<u>loo</u>-men	the cavity or channel within a tube, e.g., a blood vessel
magnetic resonance imaging (MRI)	mag-neh'-tic rehz'oh-nans imaging	noninvasive procedure that uses strong magnetic fields and radiofrequency waves to produce images of soft tissue, heart, blood vessels, and brain. It can also show the heartbeat and blood flow. Used to detect possible tumors and other pericardial conditions
pacemaker	<u>pâs</u>-mâk-er	that which sets the pace at which a phenomenon occurs; often used alone to indicate the natural cardiac pacemaker or an artificial cardiac pacemaker
phlebotomy	fle-<u>bot</u>-o-me	incision of a vein
positron emission tomography (PET)	pawz'ih-tron ee-mish-un toh-mog'rah-fee	computerized x-ray technique using radioactive substances, which are given by injection, to measure blood flow and metabolic activity of the heart and blood vessels. The radiation emitted is measured by the PET camera
PTCA (percutaneous transluminal coronary angioplasty)	per'ku-<u>ta</u>-ne-us trans-<u>lum</u>-i-nul <u>kor</u>-o-ner-e <u>an</u>-je-o-plas'te	dilation of a blood vessel by means of a balloon catheter inserted through the skin and into the chosen vessel and then passed through the lumen of the vessel to the site of the lesion, where the balloon is inflated to flatten plaque against the artery wall
serum lipid test	see'-rum lip'-id test	tests on drawn blood samples to measure the amount of cholesterol, triglyceride and lipoprotein substances in the blood
sinus rhythm	<u>si</u>-nus rithm	the normal heart rhythm originating in the sinoatrial (SA) node
tachycardia	tak'e-<u>kar</u>-de-ah	abnormally rapid heart rate

Term	Pronunciation	Definition
thallium stress test	thal-ee-um stress test	thallium injections are given intravenously in conjunction with the stress test to determine if there are changes in coronary blood flow during exercise. Changes may be indicative of ischemia, severe coronary narrowing, or infarction
thrombolysis	throm·bo-li'-sis	injection of a drug to dissolve a blood clot and restore blood flow in the coronary artery to prevent heart damage during a heart attack
vasodilator	vas'o-di-<u>la</u>-tor	an agent that dilates blood vessels
vasopressor	vas'o-<u>pres</u>-or	an agent that constricts blood vessels
venipuncture	ven'i-<u>pungk</u>-chur	puncture of a vein with a needle to withdraw blood or infuse fluid

Abbreviations

These abbreviations are frequently used when diagnosing and/or charting cardiovascular disorders.

Table 14–8

Abbreviation	Definition
ALL	acute lymphocytic leukemia
AMI	acute myocardial infarction
AML	acute myeloblastic leukemia (myeloblast: a primitive bone marrow WBC)
ASD	arterial septal defect
ASHD	arteriosclerotic heart disease
BASO	basophil (type of WBC)
BBB	bundle branch block
BP	blood pressure
CABG	coronary artery bypass graft
CBC	complete blood count
CCU	coronary care unit
CHF	congestive heart failure
CO_2	carbon dioxide

Abbreviation	Definition
CPR	cardiopulmonary resuscitation
CVA	cerebrovascular accident
DOE	dyspnea on exertion
DVT	deep vein thrombosis
ECG, EKG	electrocardiogram
ECHO	echocardiogram
Eos	eosinophil (type of WBC)
HDL	high-density lipoprotein
LDL	low-density lipoprotein
Lymph	lymphocyte (type of WBC)
MI	myocardial infarction
Mono	monocyte (type of WBC); mono can also mean mononucleosis
MRI	magnetic resonance imaging
MVP	mitral valve prolapse
O_2	oxygen
PMI	point of maximal impulse (of heart on chest wall)
PMN	polymorphonuclear (leukocyte)
PTCA	percutaneous transluminal coronary angioplasty
PVC	premature ventricular contractions
RBC	red blood cell, red blood (cell) count
SA	sinoatrial
Segs	white blood cells with segmented nuclei
TIA	transient ischemic attack
VSD	ventricular septal defect
VT	ventricular tachycardia
WBC	white blood cell; white blood (cell) count

The lymphatic system is an accessory component of the circulatory system. It produces and stores *lymphocytes* and *lymph fluid* (which is derived from tissue fluid). Lymph vessels return lymph fluid to the circulation. Functions of the lymphatic system are as follows:

1. Returns excess tissue fluid that has leaked from the capillaries. If not removed, this fluid collects in spaces between the cells and results in *edema*.
2. Returns plasma proteins that have leaked out of the capillaries into the circulation. If not returned, these proteins would accumulate, increase the osmotic pressure in the tissue fluid, and upset capillary function.
3. Transports absorbed nutrients. Specialized lymph vessels transport nutrients, especially fats, from the digestive system to the blood.
4. Removes toxic substances and other cellular debris from circulation in tissues after infection or tissue damage.
5. Controls quality of tissue fluid by filtering it through lymph nodes before returning it to the circulation.

THE LYMPHATIC SYSTEM

Components of the System

Components of the lymphatic system include lymph fluid, lymph vessels, and lymph nodes. The functions of this system are as follows:

1. Transporting fluid from the tissues back to the bloodstream.
2. Assisting in controlling infection caused by microorganisms.
3. Transporting fats away from the digestive organs.

Parts and Functions of the System

Table 14–9

Term	Pronunciation	Definition
adenoids	add-eh-noyds	masses of lymph tissue near the opening into the pharynx
antibodies	an-tih-bod-eez	substances produced by the body in response to foreign organisms
Lymphatic	lim-fat-ic	
capillaries	cap-ih-lair-eez	smallest of the lymph vessels, they transport interstitial fluid back to the blood via large lymph vessels
ducts	ducts	the largest of the lymph vessels, point of entry to blood circulation

Term	Pronunciation	Definition
fluid		interstitial fluid in the lymph vessels
nodes		collections of lymphatic tissue
lymphocytes	lim-foh-sights	leukocytes originating from stem cells and developing in the bone marrow
macrophage	mack-roh-fayj	large cell involved in defending against infection; found in lymph nodes, liver, spleen, lungs, brain, and spinal cord
phagocytes	fag-oh-sights	cells that engulf and destroy bacteria
spleen		large organ located behind the stomach that filters blood to remove pathogens and serves as a blood reservoir
T cells		important part of the immune response; provide defense against disease by attacking foreign and abnormal cells
thymus gland	thigh-mus	endocrine gland that stimulates red bone marrow to produce T lymphocytes (T cells)
tonsils	ton-sills	three masses of lymphatic tissue that help protect against harmful substances from gaining entry through the mouth and nose

Pathological Conditions of the Lymph System

Table 14–10

Term	Pronunciation	Definition
carinii pneumonia	kah-rye'-nee-eye noo'-mon-ia	pneumonia caused by a common worldwide parasite to which most people have a natural immunity
hypersplenism	high'-per-splen-izm	enlargement of the spleen; splenomegaly
Kaposi's sarcoma	kap'-oh-seez'	malignant tumor of the blood vessels associated with AIDS
lymphadenopathy	lim-fad-en-noh-pa-thee	any disorder of the lymph nodes or lymph vessels
lymphoma	lim-foh'-mah	malignant tumor of the lymph nodes and lymph tissue
mononeucleosis	moh-oh-noo'-klee-oh-sis	benign self-limiting acute infection of B lymphocytes usually caused by Epstein-Barr virus
pneumonocystic pneumonia	noo-moh'-noh-sis-tik	a rare form of pneumonia in AIDS patients

Term	Pronunciation	Definition
sarcoidosis	sar-<u>koyd</u>-oh-sis	a systemic inflammatory disease characterized by small rounded lesions forming on the spleen, lymph nodes, and other organs
sarcoma	<u>sar</u>-kom'-ah	a malignant neoplasm of the connective and supportive tissues of the body

LESSON THREE   PROGRESS CHECK

■ DEFINITIONS

Define these cardiovascular diagnostic, surgical, or treatment terms:

1. angiography _X-ray examination of blood vessels_

2. angioplasty _A balloon-type catheter is used to exert pressure on the plaque in a vessel, opening up a blocked area_

3. anticoagulant _Medication to delay blood clotting_

4. cardiac catheterization _catheter passed into the ♡ through a vein in the arm & used to detect abnormal blood flow in arteries_

5. commissurotomy _cutting of a ♡ valve that is defective_

6. diuretic _medication that reduces intravascular blood volume, thus lowering BP_

7. Doppler _ultrasonic probe that checks blood flow_

8. electrocardiogram _picture of electrical impulse of the ♡_

9. endarterectomy _boring out the inner lining of an artery to increase the size of the lumen_

10. pacemaker _a battery powered device implanted to regulate ♡ beat_

11. sodium-restricted diet _adjunct treatment used to help reduce edema & BP_

12. vasodilator _a drug that causes a vessel to dilate_

13. vasopressor _a drug that causes a vessel to constrict_

14. venipuncture _puncture of a vein_

■ NAMING

Name the structure or fluid from the lymphatic system for the definitions given below:

1. large lymph vessel in the chest that drains lymph from the upper right part of the body _rt. lymphatic duct_

2. masses of lymph tissue in the nasopharynx _adnoids_

3. organ in the mediastinum that produces T cell lymphocytes and helps in the immune response _____
thymus gland

4. tiniest lymph vessels _lymph capillaries_

5. stationary lymph tissue along the path of lymph vessels all over the body _lymph Nodes_

6. large lymph vessel in the chest that drains lymph from the lower part and left side of the body above the diaphragm _thoracic duct_

7. fluid that lies between cells and becomes lymph as it enters lymph capillaries _Interstitial fluid_

8. organ near the stomach that produces, stores, and eliminates blood cells _spleen_

■ MATCHING

Match the following diagnostic procedures to their function:

_C_ **1.** echocardiogram

_G_ **2.** Holter monitor

_J_ **3.** treadmill test

_E_ **4.** angiography

_B_ **5.** arterial blood gases

_A_ **6.** CBC

_I_ **7.** cholesterol

_H_ **8.** ECG

_F_ **9.** prothrombin

_D_ **10.** angiocardiography

a. complete blood count: Hg, Hct, WBC, RBC, differential

b. measurement of O_2, CO_2, and pH

c. reflected sound waves from the heart

d. x-ray record of heart and blood vessels

e. x-ray record of an artery

f. blood coagulation test

g. recording device for ECG activity

h. electrical recording of heart activity

i. a fatlike substance found in vessel walls

j. evaluation of heart function by exercise

■ **MULTIPLE CHOICE**

Circle the letter of the correct answer:

1. The function(s) of the spleen is (are) to
   a. build up and destroy blood cells
   b. build bone marrow
   c. form antibodies
   d. manufacture lymph nodes

2. Which of these is *not* a function of circulation?
   a. carry oxygen and nutrients to the cell
   b. carry carbon dioxide and wastes from the cell
   c. carry blood to the heart
   d. carry electrical impulses

3. Erythrocytes are
   a. red blood cells
   b. blood fluids
   c. white blood cells
   d. blood clots

4. Leukocytes are
   a. red blood cells
   b. blood fluids
   c. white blood cells
   d. blood clots

5. Hemoglobin is
   a. an anticoagulant
   b. red blood cell pigment
   c. a protein that produces fibrin
   d. a protein that coagulates like egg white

6. Plasma is
   a. blood solids
   b. blood fluids
   c. blood clotting proteins
   d. blood cell pigments

7. Fibrinogen is
   a. a blood clotting protein
   b. an anticoagulant
   c. blood platelets
   d. an immature blood cell

8. Serum is
   a. blood solids
   b. blood fluid that does not clot
   c. a blood clotting protein
   d. an immature blood cell

9. Diastolic pressure is
    a. the top number in a blood pressure reading
    b. the measurement of blood viscosity
    c. an abnormal blood pressure reading
    d. the bottom number in a blood pressure reading

10. A sphygmomanometer is
    a. a test for cardiac function
    b. an instrument for performing venipuncture
    c. an instrument for measuring blood pressure
    d. a measuring device for counting white blood cells

■ ABBREVIATIONS

Define the following commonly used abbreviations:

1. ASD *atrial septal defect*
2. BP *blood pressure*
3. CBC *complete blood count*
4. CCU *coronary care unit*
5. CHF *congestive heart failure*
6. CO_2 *carbon dioxide*
7. CPR *cardiopulmonary resuscitation*
8. CVA *cerebrovascular accident (stroke)*
9. ECG, EKG *electrocardiogram*
10. MI *myocardial infarction (heart attack)*
11. O_2 *oxygen*
12. PVC *premature ventricular contraction*
13. RBC *red blood cell, red blood cell count*
14. TIA *transient ischemic attack*
15. WBC *white blood cell, white blood cell count*

■ WORD PUZZLE ON THE HEART

Find the 59 words related to the heart by reading forward, backward, up, down, and diagonally. When the 59 listed words have been circled, the remaining letters spell the word LIFE.

```
M  U  I  D  R  A  C  O  Y  M  U  I  D  R  A  C  I  R  E  P
E  I  M  P  U  L  S  E  S  A  R  D  O  S  L  E  H  N  B  U
D  S  T  S  D  N  U  O  S  V  O  E  P  A  D  Y  D  I  A  R
I  I  C  R  M  U  T  P  E  S  I  S  E  O  T  O  C  A  S  K
A  H  O  L  A  C  I  P  A  R  R  O  N  H  C  U  U  T  E  I
S  F  N  L  V  L  C  A  Y  E  E  L  M  A  S  R  S  R  A  N
T  O  T  A  E  T  A  C  R  B  F  C  R  P  I  R  I  I  E  I
I  E  R  W  N  R  I  E  A  I  N  D  I  C  E  E  N  O  N  E
N  L  A  R  A  I  D  M  N  F  I  D  L  Y  R  P  O  V  I  F
U  D  C  A  C  C  R  A  O  U  W  E  A  S  O  I  A  E  D  I
M  N  T  N  A  U  A  K  M  E  O  L  S  Y  I  C  T  N  N  B
C  U  I  U  V  S  C  E  L  L  L  E  E  S  R  A  R  T  E  E
I  B  F  L  A  P  S  R  U  C  F  L  V  T  E  R  I  R  T  R
L  T  O  I  T  I  I  C  P  I  C  C  L  O  P  D  A  I  E  S
O  R  R  M  F  D  N  I  R  R  U  Y  A  L  U  I  L  C  A  M
T  A  C  E  E  F  U  T  E  T  S  C  V  E  S  U  C  U  D  U
S  E  E  S  L  E  S  R  L  N  P  U  M  P  A  M  A  L  R  I
A  H  R  I  G  H  T  O  A  E  S  E  S  L  U  P  S  A  O  R
I  G  N  I  N  I  L  A  X  V  R  E  C  E  I  V  E  R  H  T
D  E  P  A  H  S  E  N  O  C  O  R  O  N  A  R  Y  X  C  A
```

WORDS TO LOOK FOR IN THE WORD PUZZLE

1. aortic
2. apex
3. apical
4. atrioventricular
5. atrium
6. auricle
7. AV
8. base
9. bicuspid
10. bundle of His
11. cardiac
12. chordae tendineae
13. closed
14. cone-shaped
15. contract
16. coronary
17. cusps
18. cycle
19. diastolic
20. endocardium
21. epicardium
22. fibers
23. flow
24. force
25. heart
26. inferior
27. impulses
28. layers
29. left
30. lining
31. mediastinum
32. mitral
33. myocardium
34. node
35. open
36. pacemaker
37. pericardium
38. pulmonary
39. pulses
40. pump
41. Purkinje fibers
42. receive
43. relax
44. rhythm
45. right
46. SA
47. sac
48. semilunar
49. septum
50. sinoatrial
51. sinus
52. sounds
53. superior
54. systole
55. tricuspid
56. valves
57. vena cava
58. ventricle
59. wall
LIFE

CHAPTER 15   Nervous System

OBJECTIVES

After completing this chapter and the exercises, the student should be able to:

1. Identify the organs of the nervous system (NS).
2. List the functions of the NS.
3. Identify and define clinical disorders affecting the NS.
4. List and explain laboratory tests and medical procedures used in diagnosing NS disorders.
5. Create new medical terms using combining forms and give their meanings.
6. Correctly spell and pronounce new medical terms .

OVERVIEW

The human NS provides functions not seen in other animal species, for instance, the formation of ideas. We are able to think and reason, i.e., judge right from wrong, separate logical from illogical, and plan for the future. Our NS is the center of all mental activity, including thought, learning, and memory (see Plate 11). It is no wonder, then, that any abnormal condition that affects the NS affects the entire body.

This chapter briefly describes the anatomy and physiology of the NS and its disorders. The study of the NS is called *neurology*. There are two physician specialties for the treatment of NS conditions: the *neurologist* diagnoses and treats diseases and disorders, while a *neurosurgeon* specializes in surgery involving the brain, spinal cord, or peripheral nerves. When studying materials in this chapter, refer to Figures 15–1 and 15–2.

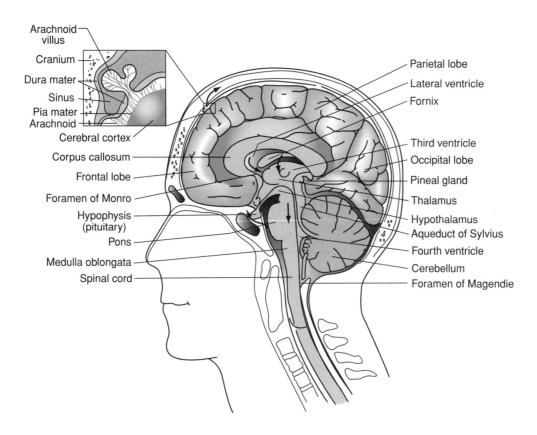

FIGURE 15–1 Midsagittal section of the human brain, showing circulation of cerebrospinal fluid in the brain and spinal cord. Inset: the cranial meninges.

ANATOMY AND PHYSIOLOGY

The nervous system consists of two main anatomical subdivisions, the central nervous system (CNS) and the peripheral nervous system (PNS). Its three main components are the brain, spinal cord, and nerves. There are 12 pairs of cranial nerves and 31 pairs of spinal nerves in the PNS. The brain and spinal cord constitute the CNS and are housed in the skull and vertebral canal, respectively. The brain and spinal cord receive, store, and process all sensory and motor data and control consciousness. The PNS transmits sensory and motor information back and forth between the CNS and the rest of the body.

The human brain comprises 2% of the body's total weight, consumes 25% of its oxygen, and receives 15% of its cardiac output (see Plate 11). The protective outer coverings of the brain are the bony skull and the *meninges,* the three connective tissue layers. The innermost covering, called the *pia mater,* is thin and delicate and closely adheres to the brain. The *arachnoid* is the middle layer and is separated from the pia mater by *subarachnoid* space. It contains

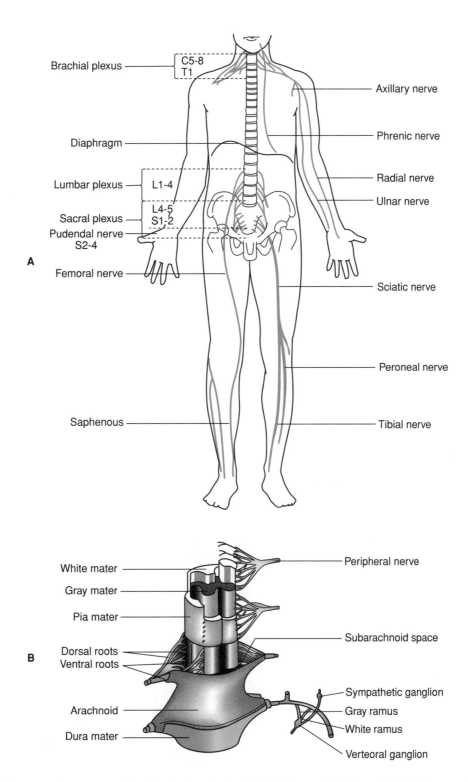

FIGURE 15–2 A, Sensory and motor tracts from the spinal cord to the brain. **B**, Diagram of spinal cord, showing three meningeal layers and association with sympathetic trunk.

cerebrospinal fluid, blood vessels, and weblike tissue that secure it to the pia mater. The *dura mater* is the thick outermost layer that adheres to the inner surface of the cranium.

Cerebrospinal fluid surrounds the *subarachnoid* spaces around the brain and spinal cord and fills the ventricles within the brain. White and gray matter are contained in the brain and spinal cord.

The *cerebrum* is the largest part of the brain. It has two hemispheres. The functional areas of the *cerebral cortex* include primary motor areas, primary sensory areas, and secondary areas that function at a higher level than the primary areas.

The *hypothalamus* lies inferior to the thalamus and forms the floor and lower part of the side walls of the third *ventricle*. It plays an important role in the regulation of appetite, heart rate, body temperature, water balance, digestion, and sexual activity.

The *cerebellum* lies inferior to the *pons* and is the second largest area of the brain. A cross-section of the cerebellum looks like a tree and is often referred to as *arbor vitae*, or tree of life.

Unconscious functions are housed in the cerebellum, hypothalamus, and brain stem. While consciousness resides in the cerebral cortex, many body functions, such as heartbeat and breathing, occur at the unconscious level.

This region of the brain controls unconscious actions. It sits below the cerebrum on the brain stem. The cerebellum controls muscle synergy and helps maintain posture. It receives impulses from the sense organs in the ear that detects body position and sends these impulses to the muscles to maintain or correct posture.

Inside the spinal cord is an inner section of gray matter associated with the PNS, and an outer section of white matter. The white matter is covered with a myelin sheath and conducts impulses to and from the brain. It carries all the nerves that affect the limbs and lower part of the body.

The cord of nervous tissue enclosed within the vertebral column is the spinal cord. It controls many of the reflex actions of the body and transmits impulses to and from the brain via ascending and descending tracts.

The PNS is all the nervous tissue found outside the brain and spinal cord. As outlined and defined in Lesson One, it includes the *optic, olfactory, trochlear, trigeminal, abducens, facial, vestibulo-ocular, glossopharyngeal, vagus, hypoglossal,* and *spinal accessory* nerves. Those nerves that control the special senses are discussed in the chapter pertaining to their functions and disorders. The PNS has two subsystems, the *somatic* nervous system and the *autonomic* nervous system. In general, the subdivisions of the autonomic nervous system (*sympathetic* and *parasympathetic*) exert opposing actions. Activation of the sympathetic portion causes the rate and intensity of reactions to increase, while the parasympathetic will slowly bring the body back to normal functions.

When studying this chapter, refer to Figures 15-1 and 15-2.

CENTRAL NERVOUS SYSTEM

The CNS is one of the two main divisions of the nervous system of the body, consisting of the brain and the spinal cord. The CNS processes information to and from the PNS and is the main network of coordination and control for the entire body.

Table 15–1

Term	Pronunciation	Definition
brain	brān	comprising the forebrain, midbrain, and hindbrain
cerebrum	ser-e-brum	main (largest) portion of the brain, occupying the upper part of the cranial cavity; its two hemispheres, united by the corpus callosum, form the largest part of the CNS in humans
cerebellum	ser'e-bel-um	situated on the back of the brain stem; consisting of a median lobe (vermis) and two lateral lobes (the hemispheres)
brain stem	brān stem	the stemlike portion of the brain connecting the cerebral hemispheres with the spinal cord and comprising the pons, medulla oblongata, and midbrain
encephalon	en-sef'-al-on	located between the cerebrum and midbrain, it contains the thalamus, hypothalamus, and pineal glands. Involved in controlling body temperature, sleep, appetite, blood pressure, and sexual activity
spinal cord	spi-nal kord	that part of the central nervous system lodged in the spinal column
meninges	men-in-jez	the three membranes covering the brain and spinal cord: dura mater, arachnoid, and pia mater
dura mater	du-rah ma-ter	the outermost, toughest of the three meninges (membranes) of the brain and spinal cord
arachnoid	ah-rak-noid	the delicate membrane interposed between the dura mater and the pia mater
pia mater	pi-ah ma-ter	the innermost of the three meninges covering the brain and spinal cord
cerebrospinal fluid	ser'a-bro-spi-nal floo-id	fluid within the ventricles of the brain, the subarachnoid space, and the central canal

AUTONOMIC NERVOUS SYSTEM (PERIPHERAL NERVOUS SYSTEM)

The PNS is composed of nerves and ganglia. Ganglia are groups of nerve cells outside of the CNS. It is divided into two subdivisions: the somatic and autonomic portions. The somatic portion (SNS) controls voluntary functions and certain reflex actions, such as knee jerk. The autonomic portion (ANS) controls the rest of the involuntary functions. The PNS contains both the SNS, which provides voluntary control over skeletal muscle, and the ANS, which controls smooth muscle, cardiac muscle, and gland secretions. The ANS is absolutely essential to survival.

Table 15–2

Term	Pronunciation	Definition
Cranial nerves	kra-ne-al nerves	the 12 pairs of nerves emerging from the cranial cavity through various openings in the skull, as follows:
olfactory	ol-fak-to-re	sense of smell
optic	op-tic	vision
oculomotor	ok'u-lo-mo-tor	movements of the eye
trochlear	trock-le-ar	muscles of the eyes
trigeminal	tri-jem-in-al	facial movements
abducens	ab-du-sens	muscles of the eye turning the eye outward
facial	fa-shal	muscles of the face, ears, and scalp
auditory	aw-di-to-re	pertaining to the ear or the sense of hearing
glossopharyngeal	glos'o-fah-rin-je-al	pertaining to the tongue and pharynx
pneumogastric vagus	nu'mo-gas-tric va-gus	voice and swallowing
spinal	spi-nal	neck muscles
hypoglossal	hi'po-glos-al	beneath the tongue
Spinal accessory nerves		the 31 pairs of nerves without special names that are connected to the spinal cord
Other components		
sympathetic	sim'pah-thet-ik	the part of the autonomic nervous system assisting the body in emergencies, defense, and survival

Term	Pronunciation	Definition
parasympathetic	par′ah-sim′pah-<u>thet</u>-ik	the part of the autonomic nervous system bringing body functions back to normal after a stressful situation has ended

CLINICAL DISORDERS

Table 15–3

Term	Pronunciation	Definition
abscess (brain)	<u>ab</u>-ses	secondary to infection in the body, e.g., ear, sinuses
Alzheimer's disease (presenile dementia)	<u>alts</u>-hi-merz di-<u>sez</u> pre-<u>se</u>-nīl de-<u>men</u>-she-ah	characterized by confusion, restlessness, agnosia, speech disturbances, inability to carry out purposeful movements, and hallucinations. The disease usually begins in later midlife with slight defects in memory and behavior and occurs with equal frequency in men and women. The cause is unknown
amyotrophic lateral sclerosis (ALS)	ah′mi-o-<u>trof</u>-ic <u>lat</u>-er-al skle-<u>ro</u>-sis	progressive degeneration of the upper and lower motor neurons; usually fatal
anencephaly	an′en-<u>sef</u>-ah-le	congenital absence of the brain; death occurs in 1–2 days
Bell's palsy	<u>pawl</u>-ze	unilateral facial paralysis of sudden onset caused by lesion of the facial nerve; facial distortion
carpal tunnel syndrome	car-pal tun-ell sin-drom	the disorder is largely due to repetitive overuse of the fingers, hands, or wrists, which causes inflammation of the median nerve in the tunnel. Symptoms are intermittent or continuous pain, especially at night. Treatment involves anti-inflammatory drugs, splints, physical therapy, and ceasing the overuse. If these measures fail, surgical measures to relieve the pressure may be necessary
cerebral palsy	<u>ser</u>-e-bral <u>pawl</u>-ze	paralysis from developmental defects or trauma; many symptoms; appearing before age 3, caused by nonprogressive damage to the brain

Term	Pronunciation	Definition
cerebrovascular accident (CVA)	ser'e-bro-<u>vas</u>-ku-lar	a decerease in blood flow supply to the brain, causing death to the specific portion of the brain tissue affected. The three types of CVA are hemorrhagic stroke, which occurs when a cerebral vessel ruptures, thrombotic stroke, which occurs when a blood clot in the arteries leading to the brain becomes occluded (blocked), and embolic stroke, which occurs when an embolus (fragment of blood clot, fat, bacteria, or tumor) lodges in a cerebral vessel and causes occlusion
concussion	kon-<u>kush</u>-un	a violent blow to the head; there may or may not be a loss of consciousness
convulsion (seizure)	kon-<u>vul</u>-shun (se-zhur)	an involuntary contraction or series of contractions of the voluntary muscles; sudden disturbances in mental functions and body movements, some with loss of consciousness
encephalitis	en'sef-ah-<u>li</u>-tis	inflammation of the brain
epilepsy	<u>ep</u>-i-lep'se	seizure disorder; cause usually unknown; symptoms can be managed with medication
fracture (skull)	<u>frak</u>-chur	a break in the bones of the skull; cause can be injury, gunshot wounds
grand mal seizure	grand mall seez'-yoor	also called tonic-clonic seizures; characterized by a sudden loss of consciousness, falling down, and involuntary muscle contractions. Often preceded by an aura, a peculiar sensation such as visual disturbance, numbness, or dizziness, which appears just before more definite symptoms
hematoma	he'mah-<u>to</u>-mah	blood "tumor" (clot); must be removed if large enough to cause pressure on brain
herpes zoster	<u>her</u>-peez <u>zos</u>-ter	"shingles"; an acute inflammatory disease of cerebral or spinal nerve due to viral infection; common in the elderly
hydrocephalus	hi'dro-<u>sef</u>-ah-lus	"water on the brain"; a congenital or acquired condition marked by dilation of the cerebral ventricles accompanied by an accumulation of cerebrospinal fluid within the skull. Typically, there is enlargement of the head, prominence of the forehead, mental deterioration, and convulsions

Term	Pronunciation	Definition
Huntington's chorea	ko-<u>re</u>-ah	ceaseless occurrence of rapid, jerky, involuntary movements; hereditary disease marked by chronic progressive chorea and mental deterioration
Korsakoff's syndrome	<u>kor</u>-suh-kufs <u>sin</u>-drom	an alcoholic psychosis with disorientation, progressing to complete amnesia
meningitis	men'in-<u>ji</u>-tis	inflammation of the meninges caused by bacterial, viral, or fungal infection
meningocele (myelomeningocele)	me-<u>ning</u>-go-sēl (mi'e-lo-me-<u>ning</u>-go-sēl)	hernial protrusion of the meninges through a bone defect in the cranium or vertebral column; may be repaired surgically
multiple sclerosis (MS)	<u>mul</u>-te-p'l skle-<u>ro</u>-sis	brain and cord contain areas of degenerated myelin. Symptoms of lesions include weakness, incoordination, speech disturbances, and visual complaints
myasthenia gravis (MG)	my-ass-thee'-nee-ah grav'-iss	a progressive neuromuscular disorder characterized by chronic fatigue and muscle weakness; considered to be an autoimmune disease. Antibodies block and destroy receptors at the myoneural junction because of a deficiency of acetylcholine. The onset of symptoms is gradual, with drooping eyelids, difficulty speaking and swallowing, and weakness of the facial muscles. The weakness may then extend to other muscles enervated by cranial nerves, especially the respiratory muscles. The disease occurs more often in women than men, with onset between ages 20-40, and in older men more often than in younger men. Onset is between ages 50 and 60
neuropathy	nu-<u>rop</u>-ah-the	disease of cranial and peripheral nervous system; motor, sensory, and reflex impairment
organic brain syndrome (chronic brain syndrome)	or-<u>gan</u>-ik	any mental disorder caused by impairment of brain tissue function; may be acute and reversible, caused by injury, infection, and nutritional deficiency, or chronic, resulting from relatively permanent organic impairment of brain tissue function
Parkinson's disease	<u>par</u>-kin-sunz di-<u>sez</u>	a slowly progressive, degenerative, neurologic disorder characterized by resting tremor

Term	Pronunciation	Definition
petit mal seizures	pet-ee-mall seez'-yoorz	also called absence seizure, the petit mal is a minor seizure lasting only a few seconds. The person has a momentary clouding of consciousness, may have a blank facial expression, and blink their eyes rapidly. The duration of the seizure is 5–10 s. The individual may not be aware of the episode. It is more frequent in children
poliomyelitis	po'le-o-mi'e-li-tis	an acute viral disease with fever, sore throat, headache, vomiting, and often stiffness of the neck and back; may be minor or major; can be prevented by vaccination
sciatica	si-at-i-kah	severe pain in the leg along the course of the sciatic nerve; also pain radiating into the buttock and lower limb, most commonly caused by herniation of a lumbar disk
shunt	shunt	to bypass, e.g., using a catheter to drain fluid from brain cavities to the spinal cord
spinal cord injuries	spi-nal kord in-ju-rez	a traumatic disruption of the spinal cord, with extensive musculoskeletal involvement. Spinal fractures and dislocations are common in car accidents and airplane crashes and can cause varying degrees of paraplegia and quadriplegia
subdural hematoma	sub-doo-ral hee-mah-toh-mah	the blood is usually a result of a closed head injury, acceleration-deceleration injury, use of anticoagulants, contusions, or chronic alcoholism. They are largely a result of venous bleeding. An acute subdural hematoma can occur within minutes or hours following an injury; a chronic subdural hemaoma takes weeks to months to evolve. Symptoms include drowsiness, headache, confusion, possible seizure, and signs of ICP and paralysis. Treatment involves surgical evacuation of the blood. In acute subdurals, it may be removed through bur holes in the skull, but chronic ones require a craniotomy because the blood has solidified and cannot be aspirated through bur holes

Term	Pronunciation	Definition
Tay-Sach's disease	tay'-sacks dih-zeez	an inherited inborn error of metabolism in which there is an enzyme deficiency causing altered lipid metabolism. Deficiency of this enzyme results in accumulation of a specific lipid in the brain, which leads to physical and mental retardation. It is a progressive disorder, marked by degeneration of brain tissue, dementia, convulsions, paralysis, blindness, and death. The symptoms begin around 6 months of age. Death occurs between 2 and 4 years of age. It is possible to test for this disease in the unborn fetus through amniocentesis. No therapy is available for the disease. Supportive and symptomatic care is indicated. Tay-Sach's primarily affects children of the Ashkenazic Jews
tumors (cord, brain)	too-morz	benign or malignant, primary or metastatic; may be classified by location, tissue type, or degree of malignancy, e.g., gliomas, neuromas
whiplash	hwip-lash	a popular term for an acute cervical sprain; acceleration extension injury of the cervical spine

TERMS USED IN DIAGNOSIS AND SURGERY

Table 15–4

Term	Pronunciation	Definition
angiogram (arteriogram), cerebral	an-je-o-gram (ar-te-re-o-gram') ser-e-bral	a radiopaque substance is injected into arteries in the neck, then x-ray films are taken
Babinski's sign	bah-bin-skez	reflex response; when sole of the foot is stroked, the big toe turns up instead of down (normal in newborn, but pathologic later on)
bur holes	ber	holes made with a drill creating openings in bone to permit access for biopsy, insertion of drains for relieving pressure, or for monitoring devices
computerized tomography (CT) brain scan. Also called CAT scan.		three-dimensional view of brain tissue obtained as x-ray beams pass through layers of the brain. Contrast medium may also be injected IV to better visualize abnormalities. CT scan will show areas of tumors, hemorrhage, blood clots, aneurysms, MS, and brain abscess

Term	Pronunciation	Definition
cordotomy	kor-<u>dot</u>-o-me	cutting of nerve fibers to relieve intractable pain
craniotomy	kra′ne-<u>ot</u>-o-me	any operation on the cranium, e.g., puncture of the skull and removal of its contents to decrease the size of the head of a dead fetus and aid in delivery
echoencephalogram (EEG)	ek′o-en-<u>sef</u>-ah-lo-gram′	use of ultrasound to show displacement of brain structures
electroencephalogram (EKG)	e-lek′tro-en-<u>sef</u>-ah-lo-gram′	record of electrical activity of the brain
laboratory procedures	<u>lab</u>-o-rah-tor′e pro-<u>se</u>-jurz	examination of cerebrospinal fluid (cell counts, culture, blood)
laminectomy	lam′i-<u>nek</u>-to-me	excision of the posterior arch of a vertebra to view the spinal cord or to relieve pressure
lumbar puncture (LP)	<u>lum</u>-bar <u>pungk</u>-chur	spinal tap
lumbar sympathectomy	<u>lum</u>-bar sim′pah-<u>thek</u>-to-me	a surgical interruption of part of the sympathetic nerve pathways, performed for the relief of chronic pain in vascular diseases, such as arteriosclerosis, claudication, and so on
magnetic resonance imaging (MRI) of the brain		noninvasive technique using magnetic waves to create an image of the brain. The MRI is far more precise and accurate than most diagnostic tools. It provides visualization of fluid, soft tissue, and bony structures. MRI and CT are used to complement each other in diagnosing brain and spinal cord lesions. Persons with any implanted metal devices such as a pacemaker, prosthesis, etc. cannot undergo MRI because the strong magnetic field will dislodge them
myelogram (myelography)	<u>mi</u>-e-lo-gram (mi′e-<u>log</u>-rah-fe)	the film produced by myelography, e.g., injection of a dye into the subarachnoid space to detect tumors or herniated disks
nerve block	nerv blok	injection of anesthetic into a nerve to produce the loss of sensation

Term	Pronunciation	Definition
nerve cells (neurons)	nerv selz (<u>new</u>-rons)	conducting cells of the nervous system, consisting of a cell body containing the nucleus and its surrounding cytoplasm, and the axon and dendrites; specialized cells for transmitting impulses
pneumoencephalogram (PEG)	nu'mo-en-<u>sef</u>-ah-lo-gram'	the radiograph obtained by visualization of the fluid-containing structures of the brain after cerebrospinal fluid is intermittently withdrawn by lumbar puncture and replaced by air, oxygen, or helium
positron emission tomography (PET) scan	pos'-ih-tron ee-miss'-shun toh-mog'-rah-fee	images of various structures show how the brain uses glucose and gives information about brain function. PET scans are used to assess Alzheimer's, stroke, epilepsy, and schizophrenia, as well as study and diagnose brain tumors
rhizotomy	ri-<u>zot</u>-o-me	cutting the roots of spinal nerves to relieve incurable pain
Romberg test	<u>rom</u>-berg	a test of the sense of balance, e.g., the patient may lose balance when standing erect, feet together, and eyes closed
trephination	tref'i-<u>na</u>-shun	drilling a hole in the skull to evacuate clots or inject air for a diagnostic procedure
vagotomy	va-<u>got</u>-o-me	surgical transection of the fibers of the vagus nerve
ventriculography	ven-trik'u-<u>log</u>-rah-fe	radiography of the cerebral ventricles after introduction of air or other contrast medium

PSYCHIATRIC TERMS

Table 15–5

Term	Pronunciation	Definition
affect	<u>af</u>-ekt	the feeling experienced in connection with an emotion
aggression	ah-<u>gresh</u>-un	hostile attitude; may be due to insecurity or inferiority feeling

Term	Pronunciation	Definition
ambivalence	am-<u>biv</u>-ah-lens	conflicting emotional attitudes toward a goal, e.g., hate and love
amnesia	am-<u>ne</u>-zhe-ah	loss of memory
autism	<u>aw</u>-tizm	complete withdrawal; inability to communicate
catatonia	kat'ah-<u>ton</u>-e-ah	excessive violent motor activity or lack of reaction and movement; observed in schizophrenia
delusion	de-<u>loo</u>-zhun	a false personal belief
delirium	de-<u>lir</u>-e-um	a mental disturbance of relatively short duration, e.g., illusions, hallucinations, and excitement
depression	de-<u>presh</u>-un	in psychiatry, a morbid sadness, dejection, or melancholy; a decrease of body functions
echolalia	ek'o-<u>la</u>-le-ah	automatic repetition by a patient of what is said to him or her
electroconvulsive therapy (ECT, EST)	e-lek'tro-con-<u>vul</u>-siv	introducing convulsions by means of electricity; used on patients with affective disorders
hallucination	hah-lu'si-<u>na</u>-shun	hearing or seeing things not really present
hypochondria	hi'po-<u>kon</u>-dre-ah	imaginary illnesses
hysteria	his-<u>te</u>-re-ah	extremely emotional state
involutional melancholia	in'vo-lu-shun-al mel'an-<u>ko</u>-le-ah	mental illness in late middle life, with agitation, worry, anxiety, and insomnia
malingering	mah-<u>ling</u>-ger-ing	make believe, e.g., pretending to be ill
manic-depressive	<u>man</u>'ik-de-<u>pres</u>-iv	major psychosis; fluctuation of behavior between mania and depression; also called bipolar disorder
megalomania	meg'ah-lo-<u>ma</u>-ne-ah	belief in one's own extreme greatness, goodness, or power
neurasthenia	nu'ras-<u>the</u>-ne-ah	a stage in the recovery from a schizophrenic experience during which the patient is listless and apparently unable to cope with routine activities and relationships
neurosis	nu-<u>ro</u>-sis	an emotional disorder caused by unresolved conflicts, anxiety being its chief characteristic; person is still in touch with reality
paranoid	<u>par</u>-ah-noid	a person who is overly suspicious (in trends or attitudes)

Term	Pronunciation	Definition
phobia	<u>fo</u>-be-ah	any persistent abnormal dread or fear
psychosis	si-<u>ko</u>-sis	a major mental disorder, with personality derangement and loss of contact with reality
rapid eye movements (REM)		occur during periods of dreaming
schizophrenia	skit'so-<u>fre</u>-ne-ah	any of a group of severe emotional disorders characterized by withdrawal from reality, delusions, hallucinations, ambivalence, inappropriate affect, and withdrawn, bizarre, and regressive behavior

SPECIAL TERMS

Table 15–6

Term	Pronunciation	Definition
aphasia	ah-<u>fa</u>-zhe-ah	loss of the ability to speak owing to injury or disease of the brain centers
ataxia	ah-<u>tak</u>-se-ah	failure of muscular coordination
biofeedback	bi'o-<u>fēd</u>-bak	the process of furnishing a person with information on the state of one or more physiologic variables, such as heart rate, blood pressure, or skin temperature, often enabling the person to gain some voluntary control over the body function
cauda equina	<u>kaw</u>-dah e-<u>kwi</u>-na	the collection of spinal roots descending from the lower spinal cord and supplying the rectal area
comatose	<u>ko</u>-mah-tōs	in a deep stupor; cannot be aroused
contrecoup	kon'truh-<u>koo</u>	denoting an injury to the brain, occurring at a site opposite to the point of impact
deep tendon reflex (DTR)	<u>ten</u>-don <u>re</u>-fleks	a reflex elicited by a sharp tap on the appropriate tendon or muscle to induce brief stretch of the muscle, followed by contraction
encephalon	en-<u>sef</u>-ah-lon	the brain
fissure	<u>fish</u>-er	many meanings; one refers to a deep furrow in the brain
flaccid	<u>flak</u>-sid	weak, lax, soft, flabby; poor muscle tone

Term	Pronunciation	Definition
foramen magnum	fo-<u>rah</u>-men <u>mag</u>-num	a large opening in the occipital bone through which the cord passes
ganglion	<u>gang</u>-gle-on	a knot. A group of nerve cell bodies, located outside the central nervous system
gyrus (pl., gyri)	<u>ji</u>-rus	convolutions of the cerebrum
hemisphere	<u>hem</u>-i-sfer	either half of the brain
ipsilateral	ip'si-<u>lat</u>-er-al	situated on or affecting the same side
limbic system	<u>lim</u>-bik <u>sis</u>-tem	the part of the brain associated with attitudes and emotional behavior
manometer	mah-<u>nom</u>-e-ter	an instrument for measuring the pressure, e.g., of spinal fluid
myelin	<u>mi</u>-e-lin	white, liquid, fatty substance surrounding some nerve fibers (white matter)
neurilemma (sheath of Schwann)	nu'ri-<u>lem</u>-ah (Shvan)	the membrane surrounding the peripheral nerves
paralysis	pah-<u>ral</u>-i-sis	inability to use muscles because of damage to the nervous system
paresis	<u>par</u>-e-sis	slight or incomplete paralysis
paresthesia	par'es-<u>the</u>-ze-ah	an abnormal sensation, such as burning or prickling
plexus	<u>plek</u>-sis	a network of nerves or blood vessels
reflex	<u>re</u>-fleks	an involuntary response to a stimulus
spastic	<u>spas</u>-ik	uncontrollable and forced contractions
stimulus	<u>stim</u>-u-lus	any agent, act, or influence that produces a reaction or response
sulcus (pl., sulci)	<u>sul</u>-kus (<u>sul</u>-ki)	a groove, trench, or furrow on the brain surface
syncope	<u>sin</u>-co-pe	a faint; temporary loss of consciousness
ventricle (brain)	<u>ven</u>-tri-k'l	a small cavity in the brain

LESSON TWO   PROGRESS CHECK

■ FILL-IN

Fill in the blanks to make a complete accurate sentence:

1. The ___Central___ nervous system consists of the brain and spinal cord.
2. The ___Central___ nervous system processes information, coordinates, and controls the body.
3. The ___autonomic___ nervous system regulates the activity of the cardiac muscle and glands.
4. The small cavities in the brain are called ___ventricles___.
5. The term used for the network of nerves or blood vessels is ___plexus___.
6. A groove or trench on the brain surface is a ___sulcus___.
7. The ___limbic___ system is the part of the brain associated with emotional behavior.
8. ___Ganglion___ refers to a group of nerve cell bodies.
9. Either half of the brain is called a ___hemisphere___.
10. ___Encephalon___ is the medical term for brain.
11. The foramen magnum is ___opening in occipital bone through which the spinal cord passes.___
12. The spinal roots that supply the rectal area are called ___cauda equina.___
13. The lobes located on the back of the brain are known as the ___cerebellum___.
14. The outermost membrane of the brain and spinal cord is called ___dura mater___.
15. ___Sympathetic___ is the term for the part of the nervous system that assists in defense and survival.

■ MATCHING: NERVES

Match the nerves on the left to their function on the right:

G **1.** olfactory   **a.** eye muscles
E **2.** optic   **b.** face movement
A **3.** trochlear   **c.** hearing
B **4.** trigeminal   **d.** beneath the tongue
C **5.** auditory   **e.** vision
F **6.** spinal   **f.** neck muscles
D **7.** hypoglossal **g.** smell

■ MATCHING: DISEASES

Match the disease state or condition at the left to its definition:

A **1.** Bell's palsy
F **2.** cerebral palsy
E **3.** concussion
G **4.** convulsion
H **5.** hematoma
D **6.** Huntington's chorea
C **7.** sciatica
B **8.** Parkinson's disease

a. unilateral facial paralysis
b. progressive neurologic disorder with tremors
c. severe leg pain
d. jerky involuntary movements with mental deterioration
e. violent blow to the head
f. paralysis from developmental defects
g. a seizure
h. a blood clot

■ TRUE/FALSE

T F **1.** Babinski's sign is normal in a newborn but pathologic in an adult.
T F **2.** A craniotomy is the cutting of nerve fibers.
T F **3.** A lumbar puncture is a spinal tap.
T F **4.** An EEG uses ultrasound to diagnose brain dysfunctions.
T F **5.** A myelogram uses dye injections to detect tumors.
T F **6.** A rhizotomy is surgery on the nose.
T F **7.** A vagotomy is surgical removal of the vagina.
T F **8.** Drilling a hole in the skull to remove a clot is called trephination.
T F **9.** The Romberg test determines a person's sense of balance.
T F **10.** A pneumoencephalogram (PEG) is a chest x-ray film to detect pneumonia.

■ DEFINITIONS

Briefly define the following psychiatric conditions:

1. ambivalence   _Conflicting emotional attitude_
2. autism   _Complete withdrawl_
3. delusion   _a false personal belief_
4. delirium   _Illusions, excitement, hallucinations (short duration)_
5. echolalia   _automatic repetition of what is said_
6. hypochondria   _~~Belief in~~ imaginary illness_

7. megalomania _belief in one's greatness, power_

8. paranoid _a person abnormally suspicious of others_

9. phobia _abnormal ~~dread~~ dread or fear_

10. schizophrenia _a group of severe emotional disorders characterized by delirium, delusions, hallucinations, + other bizarre behaviors_

■ SPELLING AND DEFINITION

Circle the letter of the correctly spelled term and then define the term:

1. **(a)** cerebrum **(b)** cerebrim **(c)** cherubim **(d)** cerabrem
   the largest portion of the brain; divided into L + rt. hemispheres
   Definition: _located in the upper part of the cranial cavity_

2. **(a)** meniges **(b)** meninjes **(c)** meninges **(d)** meneongis
   Definition: _the 3 membranes covering the brain + spinal cord_

3. **(a)** akraknoid **(b)** arachnoid **(c)** arachnid **(d)** arakenid
   Definition: _the ~~delicate~~ delicate membrane btwn the pia mater + dura mater_

4. **(a)** trochanter **(b)** trocklear **(c)** trichlear **(d)** trochlear
   Definition: _muscle ~~muscle~~ of the eyes_

5. **(a)** olfactory **(b)** audifactory **(c)** occulofactory **(d)** optifactory
   Definition: _sense of smell_

6. **(a)** hypogloseal **(b)** hypoglossal **(c)** hyperglossary **(d)** hydroglosal
   Definition: _beneath the tongue_

7. **(a)** anoncephaly **(b)** anoncephalon **(b)** anencephaly **(d)** acephalic
   Definition: _congenital absence of ~~the~~ a brain_

8. **(a)** hydrocephalus **(b)** hidrocephalon **(c)** hydroceptaly **(d)** hidrosephaly
   Definition: _accumulation of cerebrospinal fluid within the skull_

9. **(a)** menogenocele **(b)** myeongocele **(c)** menelomingocele **(d)** meningocele
   Definition: _hernial protrusion of the meninges through a defect in the skull or a vertebrae_

10. **(a)** poliomyelitis **(b)** poliomylitis **(c)** poliomilitis **(d)** poliomyleitis
    Definition: _an acute viral disease_

■ WORD PUZZLE ON THE NERVOUS SYSTEM (GENERAL TERMS)

The 53 words pertaining to the nervous system read forward, backward, up, down, and diagonally. When all of the 53 words have been circled, the remaining letters spell NERVES.

```
A  T  R  E  I  V  N  A  R  F  O  S  E  D  O  N  J  E  R  K
C  N  E  S  N  E  U  R  O  G  L  I  A  F  F  E  C  T  O  R
T  E  T  E  E  T  A  R  E  N  E  G  E  R  O  T  I  N  O  M
I  R  T  N  S  R  O  T  P  E  C  E  R  C  O  N  T  R  O  L
O  E  I  S  J  U  N  C  T  I  O  N  O  E  S  P  A  N  Y  S
N  F  M  O  C  N  S  N  P  A  M  M  E  L  O  R  U  E  N  E
P  F  S  R  C  H  A  R  G  E  M  U  I  L  U  M  I  T  S  G
O  E  N  Y  D  E  X  I  M  U  S  E  N  S  E  S  S  W  N  N
T  S  A  M  Y  E  L  I  N  S  H  E  A  T  H  C  I  N  O  A
E  N  R  O  T  O  M  I  I  T  L  U  S  P  R  T  S  E  I  H
N  O  T  R  E  A  C  T  R  A  T  E  A  A  H  S  P  U  T  C
T  R  O  N  E  A  E  A  N  O  H  T  X  D  K  N  A  R  C  T
I  U  R  R  T  V  N  I  N  C  H  E  R  E  N  O  C  O  U  C
A  E  U  E  R  S  M  O  N  W  L  A  C  N  O  X  E  N  D  E
L  N  E  E  M  R  M  A  A  F  W  V  L  D  B  A  S  S  N  T
S  R  N  I  E  I  R  Y  E  A  T  N  E  R  E  F  F  A  O  E
T  E  T  T  C  B  S  R  L  T  C  A  F  I  B  E  R  S  C  D
I  T  E  F  F  E  C  T  O  R  S  E  T  T  E  T  I  C  X  E
N  N  I  O  N  S  L  A  R  T  N  E  C  E  L  L  B  O  D  Y
U  I  I  N  F  O  R  M  A  T  I  O  N  N  A  W  H  C  S  S
```

WORDS TO LOOK FOR IN THE WORD PUZZLE

1. act
2. action potential
3. affector
4. afferent
5. autonomic
6. axons
7. branches
8. cell body
9. central
10. charge
11. cleft
12. CNS
13. communicate
14. conduction
15. control
16. dendrite
17. detect change
18. effectors
19. efferent
20. excite
21. fibers
22. information
23. interneurons
24. ions
25. jerk
26. junction
27. knob
28. mixed
29. monitor
30. motor
31. myelin sheath
32. nerve tissue
33. neuroglia
34. neurolemma
35. neurons
36. neurotransmitter
37. nodes of Ranvier
38. pathways
39. PNS
40. react
41. receptors
42. reflex arcs
43. regenerate
44. Schwann
45. senses
46. sensory
47. spaces
48. stimuli
49. synapse
50. terminal
51. transmit
52. units
53. withdrawal

NERVES

CHAPTER 16 — Genitourinary System

OBJECTIVES

After completing this chapter and the exercises, the student should be able to:

1. Identify the organs and describe the location and functions of the following sytems:

   a. urinary system (US)
   b. female reproductive system (FRS)
   c. male reproductive system (MRS)

2. Identify and define clinical disorders affecting:

   a. urinary system
   b. female reproductive system
   c. male reproductive system

3. Explain selected laboratory and medical procedures used in diagnosing diseases and disorders of the genitourinary (GU) system
4. Identify three secondary sex characteristics that occur in the male and female bodies at the onset of puberty
5. Identify six sexually transmitted diseases of the male and female reproductive systems

OVERVIEW

This chapter combines the urinary system and the reproductive system. To acquaint the student with the specifics of each system, this brief introduction will consider them separately (also see Plate 15).

URINARY SYSTEM

All living things produce waste and humans are no exception. Waste cannot accumulate in an organism without causing harm. There are several avenues by which waste excretion occurs. In humans, excretion of waste occurs in the lungs, skin, liver, intestines, and kidneys. Of all the organs that participate in removing waste, the kidneys are one of the most important, for they relieve the body of the greatest variety of dissolved wastes.

If the kidneys fail, there is no way for all the waste products to be eliminated from the body. Death will follow unless a kidney transplant replaces the failing kidney or the impurities are filtered out by dialysis (artificial kidney).

The urinary system consists of the organs that produce urine and eliminate it from the body. It is a major organ system in the maintenance of homeostasis.

The *urinary system* consists of two *kidneys,* which produce urine; two *ureters,* which carry urine to the urinary bladder for temporary storage; and the *urethra,* which carries urine to the outside of the body through an external *urethral orifice* (see Plate 15 for details). Lesson One defines and illustrates the system along with associated structures.

The kidney has many important functions. Among them are the following:

1. Elimination of organic wastes
2. Regulation of concentration of important ions
3. Regulation of acid-base balance
4. Regulation of RBC production
5. Regulation of blood pressure
6. Some control of blood glucose and blood amino acids
7. Elimination of toxic substances
8. Act as endocrine glands

The kidneys are bean-shaped, dark red organs approximately 5 in. long and 1 in. thick (about the size of a clenched fist). They are located high on the posterior abdominal wall adjacent to the last two pairs of ribs. They are *retroperitoneal.* Each is capped by an *adrenal* gland. Each kidney is surrounded by three layers of connective tissue. The *renal fascia* (outside covering) anchors the kidney to the surrounding structures and maintains its position. The *perirenal* fat is adipose tissue inside the renal fascia to cushion the kidney. The *renal capsule* is the smooth, transparent membrane that directly covers the kidney and can be easily stripped from it.

For a detailed explanation of the internal structure of the kidney, the structure of a nephron, and blood supply to the kidney, the student is referred to anatomy and physiology texts.

REPRODUCTIVE SYSTEM

The *reproductive* systems in males and females are concerned primarily with perpetuation of the species. In that respect, they differ from all other organ systems of the body, which are concerned with *homeostasis* and survival of the human body. Reproduction begins when the germ cells unite in a process called fertilization. In the female, the germ cell is the *ovum* (pl. *ova*); in the male, it is the *spermatozoon* (pl. *spermatozoa*).

Male Reproduction System

The male reproductive system function is to produce, nourish, and transport sperm from the penis into the female vagina during intercourse (*copulation*) and to produce the male hormone testosterone.

The primary male organs are the *gonads*, which are called *testes* (singular *testis* or *testicle*). They are responsible for production of *spermatozoa* and *testosterone*. The accessory organs of the MRS are a series of ducts, called *seminal vessels*, and the *prostate gland*. The *scrotum, penis*, and two *spermatic cords* support them.

The spermatozoon is a mature germ cell. It is microscopic in size and looks like a translucent tadpole. It has a flat epilliptical head section that contains the hereditary material, the chromosomes, and a long tail with which it propels itself in a rapid, lashing movement. The sex chromosome carried by the sperm determines the sex of the offspring. When mature, the sperm are carried in the semen.

From puberty on, the male reproductive organs produce and release billions of spermatozoa throughout the lifetime of the male. They also secrete testosterone, a male hormone, which is responsible for the secondary bodily changes that take place at puberty, such as pubic hair, beard, and deepening of the voice.

As you study this chapter, refer to Figures 16–1, 16–2, and 16–3, and be able to identify and label the structures. The male and female reproductive systems are detailed in Plate 15. The male and female organs are defined in Lesson One.

Female Reproductive System

Reproduction can only begin when the germ cells from the male (spermatozoa) unite with the germ cells from the female (ova). The reproductive role of the female is to produce eggs (ova) capable of being fertilized, and to provide a safe, nutrient-filled environment in which the fetus develops for 9 months if fertilization takes place. The ability to reproduce begins at puberty when mature ova can be released from the ovary and secondary sex characteristics appear, such as breast development, growth of pubic hair, widening of the pelvis ("developing hips," a sight not always welcome to young girls), and menstruation. Body build and stature difference between the male and female become pronounced. The hormones from the ovaries that play important roles in these processes are *estrogen* and *progesterone*. Other sex hormones are secreted by the pituitary gland and adrenal glands.

If fertilization occurs any time between puberty and cessation of the menses (menopause), the fertilized egg will grow and develop in the uterus. If fertilization does not occur, the uterine lining will shed through a bloody discharge, which is menstruation. The female has all of the eggs at birth she will produce in her lifetime, so this cycle will repeat itself monthly throughout the childbearing years. At the end of her reproduction cycle, menstruation will stop and she will no longer discharge eggs from the ovaries. This is known as menopause or climacteric. She will also have a decrease in hormone production. Medical terminology in relation to menopause is not given in the chapter. A brief explanation of this condition follows:

Menopause is cessation of menstrual cycles. It is considered complete after *amenorrhea* (absence of menstruation) for 1 year. The *climacteric* is the period during which the cycles are irregular before they stop.

The symptoms of menopause are related to decreased levels of estrogen and progesterone, which affect a number of organ systems and body chemistry:

1. Mammary glands, reproductive organs, and external genitalia decrease in size.
2. Vaginal lining thins and vaginal secretions become alkaline.
3. Vasodilation of blood vessels in the skin results in hot flashes and excessive perspiration in 75–80% of women during the climacteric.
4. Some women experience irritability, insomnia, headache, joint pains, and heart palpitations.
5. In approximately 25% of women, the accelerated loss of bone mass owing to diminished estrogen leads to osteoporosis. This is more likely to occur in small women with less bone mass. Diets low in calcium, especially during childbearing years, are another risk factor that promotes osteoporosis.

Female anatomy consists of external and internal genitalia. The external genitalia are the *mons pubis, labia majora, clitoris, labia minora, vestibule, urinary meatus, vaginal orifice, Bartholin's glands,* and *peritoneum.* Collectively, they are called the *vulva* or *pudendum.*

The internal genitalia consist of the *vagina, uterus, fallopian tubes,* and *ovaries.* The female also has mammary glands (breasts), and although they are not part of the reproductive process, they are part of the FRS because they are responsible for the production of milk (lactation).

The study of the FRS is called *gynecology. Obstetrics* is a specialty concerned with pregnancy and delivery.

URINARY SYSTEM

Organs and Structures

Table 16–1

Organ or Structure	Pronunciation	Definition
Bowman's capsule (renal capsule)	boh-muhnz cap-suhl	cup-shaped end of renal tubule containing the glomerulus
calyx	ka-liks	cup-shaped part of the renal pelvis through which urine passes from the renal tubules
cortex	kawr-teks	the outer layer of the kidney
glomerulus	gloh-mer-yah-luhs	collection of coiled intertwined capillaries located in the kidney cortex
kidneys	kid-nez	two organs on the posterior abdominal wall that filter the blood, excreting the end products of body metabolism in the form of urine, and regulating body mineral levels
medulla	me-dul-ah	the inner layer of the kidney
nephron	nef-ron	the structural and functional unit of the kidney, the parenchyma, numbering about a million and capable of forming urine
renal artery	ree-nal ar-teh-ree	one of two large arteries branching from the abdominal aorta that supplies blood to kidneys, adrenals, and ureters
renal pelvis	ree-nal pel-vis	the funnel-shaped expansion of the upper end of the ureter
renal tubule	ree-nal toob-yool	long, twisted tube leading from glomerulus to collecting tubules
renal vein	ree-nal vain	one of two large veins that carries blood from the kidneys to the inferior vena cava
ureter	u-re-ter	the tubular structure through which urine passes from the kidney to the bladder
urethra	yoo-ree-thruh	the passage through which urine is discharged from the bladder to the body exterior
urinary bladder	yoor-uh-ner-ee blad-er	musculomembranous sac that stores urine, receiving it through the ureters and discharging it through the urethra

Organ or Structure	Pronunciation	Definition
urinary meatus	<u>yoor</u>-uh-ner-ee me-<u>a</u>-tus	opening of the urethra to the exterior

Clincal Conditions and Procedures

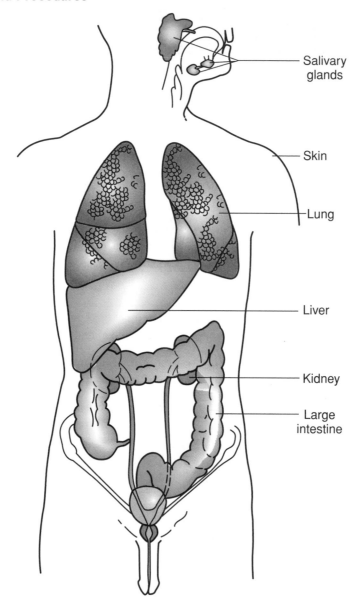

FIGURE 16–1A Organs of the excretory system.

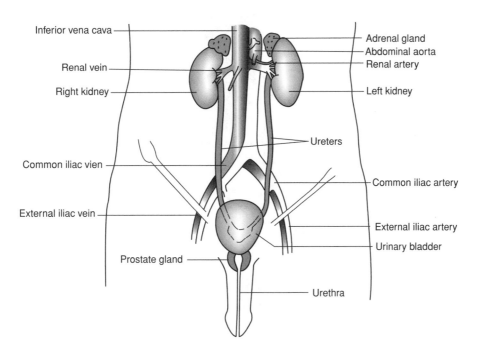

FIGURE 16–1B Urinary system with blood vessels.

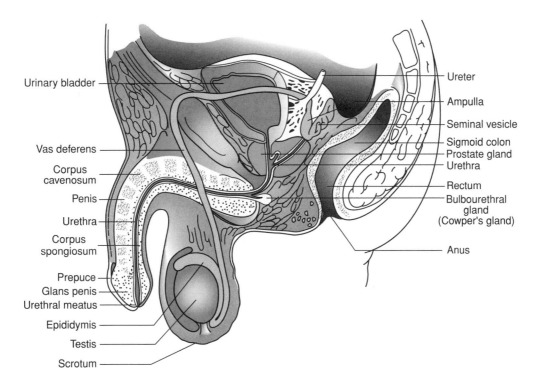

FIGURE 16–2 Midsagittal section of the male reproductive system.

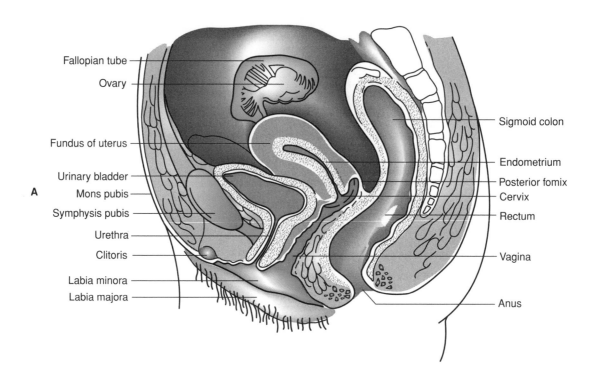

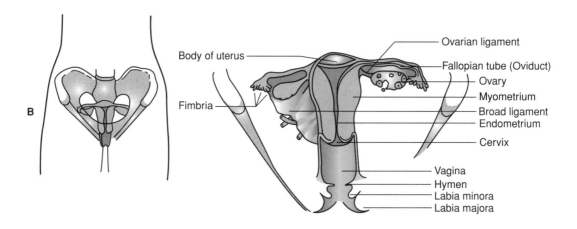

FIGURE 16–3 Female reproductive system. **A,** Midsagittal section of the reproductive organs of the human female. **B,** Anterior aspect of the female reproductive organs, with the left tube, ovary, and the entire ureters cut away to show their internal anatomy. At the left is the position of the female reproductive organs in the pelvis.

Clincal Conditions and Procedures

Table 16–2

Clinical Condition	Pronunciation	Definition
azoturia	az′o-tu-<u>re</u>-ah	excess urea (or other nitrogen compounds) in urine
calculus (renal) (pl., calculi)	<u>kal</u>-ku-lus (<u>re</u>-nal)	kidney stone(s)
cystitis	sis-<u>ti</u>-tis	inflammation of the urinary bladder
dialysis	di-<u>al</u>-i-sis	the process of using an artificial kidney to filter waste materials from the body
"floating kidney"	<u>flōt</u>-ing <u>kid</u>-ne	a kidney not securely fixed in the usual location because of birth defect or injury
glomerulonephritis	glo-mer′u-lo-ne-<u>fri</u>-tis	nephritis with inflammation of the capillary loops in the renal glomeruli
hydronephrosis	hi-dro-ne-<u>fro</u>-sis	distention of the renal pelvis with urine, caused by obstruction of the ureter
nephrolithiasis	nef′ro-li-<u>thi</u>-ah-sis	a condition marked by the presence of renal calculi (stones)
nephroptosis	nef′rop-<u>to</u>-sis	downward displacement of a kidney
nephrorrhaphy	nef-<u>ror</u>-ah-fe	suture of the kidney
pyelitis	pi′e-<u>li</u>-tis	inflammation of the renal pelvis
renal failure	<u>re</u>-nal <u>fāl</u>-yer	kidney fails to function normally, e.g., in excretion of body waste
renal transplant	<u>re</u>-nal <u>trans</u>-plant	transferring a kidney surgically from one person to another to replace a diseased structure
uremia	u-<u>re</u>-me-ah	the retention of toxic body waste in blood
ureterostomy	u-re′ter-<u>os</u>-to-me	creation of a new outlet for a ureter through the abdominal wall to the outside
urethritis	u′re-<u>thri</u>-tis	inflammation of the urethra
urinary tract infection (UTI)	<u>yoor</u>-uh-ner-ee trakt in-<u>fek</u>-shun	an infection of the urinary tract
Wilms' tumor	vilmz <u>too</u>-mor	a malignant tumor of the kidney, usually affecting children under age 5

Diagnostic Medical Terms

Table 16–3

Term	Pronunciation	Definition
albuminuria	al-bu'mi-<u>nu</u>-re-ah	abnormal presence of serum albumin (protein) in the urine
anuria	ah-<u>nu</u>-re-ah	no urine produced
bladder distention	<u>blad</u>-der dis-<u>ten</u>-shun	full urinary bladder
blood chemistries	blud <u>kem</u>-is-treez	blood tests for kidney function, especially blood urea nitrogen (BUN) and creatinine
blood urea nitrogen (BUN)	blud u-<u>re</u>-ah <u>ni</u>-tro-jin	the urea (in terms of nitrogen) concentration of serum or plasma; an important indicator of renal function
catheterization	kath'e-ter-i-<u>za</u>-shun	passage of a catheter (tube) into the bladder to relieve bladder distention or for other purposes
Clinitest	<u>klin</u>-i-test	popular test for urine glucose or other substances
continent	<u>kon</u>-ti-nent	able to control urination (and/or defecation)
cystoscopy	sis-<u>tos</u>-ko-pe	visual examination of the urinary tract with a cystoscope
diuresis	di'u-<u>re</u>-sis	increased excretion of urine
dysuria	dis-<u>u</u>-re-ah	painful or difficult urination
enuresis	en'u-<u>re</u>-sis	uncontrolled urination while sleeping (bed-wetting)
frequency (urgency)	<u>fre</u>-kwen-se (<u>ur</u>-jen-se)	desire to urinate at short intervals, but discharging small amounts because of reduced bladder capacity
hematuria	hem'ah-<u>tu</u>-re-ah	the presence of blood in the urine
incontinent	in-<u>kon</u>-ti-nent	inability to control urination (and/or defecation)
intravenous pyelogram (IVP)	in'trah-<u>ve</u>-nus <u>pi</u>-e-lo-gram	a technique in radiology for examining the structures and evaluating the function of the urinary system
I & O		intake and output. The amount of fluids (usually) ingested and excreted in a given period of time, measured and charted
KUB		abbreviation for kidney, ureter, and bladder
micturate	mik-<u>tu</u>-rāt	urinate
nocturia, nycturia	nok-<u>tu</u>-re-ah, nik-<u>tu</u>-re-ah	excessive urination at night

Term	Pronunciation	Definition
oliguria	ol'i-gu-re-ah	excreting a small amount of urine
pyuria	pi-u-re-ah	pus in the urine
retrograde pyelogram	re-tro-grād pi-e-lo-gram'	a technique in radiology for examining the structures of the collecting system of the kidneys that is especially useful in locating an obstruction in the urinary tract
scan (renal)	skan (re-nal)	an image produced after the patient is injected with a radioactive substance. It determines kidney shape and function
Testape	tes-tap	special paper that changes color when dipped in urine
ultrasonography	ul'trah-son-og-rah-fe	imaging body structures by recording the echoes of high-frequency sound waves reflected by body tissues on a paper or other device
urinalysis (UA)	u'ri-nal-i-sis	analysis of the urine, e.g., acidity, sugar level
urinary retention	yoor-uh-ner-ee re-ten-shun	inability to urinate for various reasons. Body retains urine waste
vesico-	ves-i-ko	a combining form meaning "pertaining to the bladder"
void	void	to empty the bladder, urinate

REPRODUCTIVE SYSTEM

Male Organs

Table 16–4

Organ	Pronunciation	Definition
Cowper's glands	ku'pers glandz	pea-sized glands that secrete lubricating fluid during intercourse. Also called bulbourethral glands
glans penis	glanz pee-nis	tip of the penis
penis	pee-nis	the organ of copulation
perineum	per-uh-nee-uhm	area between the scrotum and anus
prepuce	pree-pyoos	fold of skin covering the glans penis at birth; foreskin
prostate gland	pross-tayt gland	gland surrounding the neck of the bladder and urethra; contributes secretions that enhance sperm motility and neutralizes acid vaginal secretions

Organ	Pronunciation	Definition
scrotum	scrow-tum	two-compartment sac outside the body that houses the testes
testis (pl., testes)	<u>tes</u>-tis (<u>tes</u>-tez)	one of the pair of male gonads that produce semen
Ducts	duks	narrow tubular structures for excretion of semen and spermatozoa
epididymis	ep'i-<u>did</u>-i-mis	a duct bordering the testes for storage, transit, and maturation of spermatozoa
vas deferens	vas <u>def</u>-er-enz	extension of the epididymis that joins the seminal vesicle to form the ejaculatory duct
seminal duct	<u>sem</u>-in-al duk	the passages for conveyance of spermatozoa and semen
ejaculatory duct vesicle	e-<u>jak</u>-u-<u>la</u>-tor'e duk <u>ves</u>-i-cul	the duct formed by union of the vas deferens and the duct of the seminal vesicle
urethra	yoo-<u>ree</u>-thruh	opening for sperm and urine passage to the outside of the body
accessory glands	ak-<u>ses</u>-o-re glandz	their secretions mix with sperm to form seminal fluid
external genitalia	eks-<u>ter</u>-nal jen'i-<u>ta</u>-le-ah	scrotum and penis

Female Organs

Table 16–5

Organ	Pronunciation	Definition
Bartholin's glands	bar'-teh-linz' glandz	small mucus-secreting glands located near the vagina
clitoris	klit'-or-is	erectile tissue at junction of labia majora and labia minora; equivalent to male penis
hymen	high'-men'	thin elastic connective tissue covering the vaginal opening
Internal genitalia		
cervix	ser'-viks	necklike section at lower end of uterus
fallopian tubes (oviducts)	fah-loh-pee-an toobs (oh-vih-duks)	ducts in which fertilization occurs and passageway for ova to the uterus

Organ	Pronunciation	Definition
ovary	oh'-vay'-ree	the female gonad: either of the paired female sex glands in which ova are formed and released, and which produce the female hormones
uterus	yoo'-ter'-us	cavity opening into the vagina below and into a fallopian tube on either side; organ for nourishing the fetus
vagina	vaj-in-nah	birth canal and receptacle for copulation
labia majora	lay'-bee-ah mah'-jor-ah	two outer folds of skin on either side of the vaginal orifice
labia minora	lay'-bee-ah mih'-nor-ah	two thin folds of skin within the folds of the labia majora
mammary glands	mam'-oh-ree glandz	female breasts; considered accessory glands to the FRS, they are necessary for breast-feeding of the infant (lactation)
mons pubis	monz' pew-biss	mound of fatty tissue over the pubis
perineum	par-ih-nee-um	area between vaginal orifice and anus

Male Clinical Conditions

Table 16–6

Clinical Condition	Pronunciation	Definition
benign prostatic hypertrophy (BPH)	bi-<u>nin</u> pros-<u>tat</u>-ic hi-<u>per</u>-tro-fe	enlargement of the prostate gland, common among men by the age of 50
circumcision	ser'kum-<u>sizh</u>-un	removing foreskin, or prepuce
cryptorchidism	krip'<u>tor</u>-ki-dizm	undescended testicle(s)
epididymitis	ep'i-did'i-<u>mi</u>-tis	inflammation of the epididymis; from venereal disease
hydrocele	<u>hi</u>-dro-sel'	fluid collected in the testes
orchiectomy	or'ke-<u>ek</u>-to'-me	castration
orchiopexy	<u>or</u>-ke-o-pek'se	fixation of an undescended testis in the scrotum
orchitis	or-<u>ki</u>-tis	inflammation of a testis

Clinical Condition	Pronunciation	Definition
prostatectomy	pros'tah-<u>tek</u>-to'-me	excision of all or part of the prostate
varicocele	<u>var</u>-i-ko-sel'	varicose veins near the testes
vasectomy	vah-<u>sek</u>-to-me	male sterilization by cutting or tying the vas deferens

Female Clinical Conditions

Table 16–7

Clinical Condition	Pronunciation	Definition
abortion (AB)	ah'-<u>bor</u>-shun	expulsion from the uterus of the products of conception before the fetus is viable
Bartholin's cyst or abscess	<u>bar</u>-tel-inz' sist or ab'ses	chronic or acute inflammation of Bartholin's gland
colporrhaphy	kol-<u>por</u>-ah-fe	suture of the vagina; to correct cystocele and rectocele
colposcopy	kol-<u>pos</u>-ko-pe	examination of the cervix by means of a colposcope
cystocele	<u>sis</u>-to-sel	hernia of the bladder into the vagina
dilatation and curettage (D&C)	dil'ah-<u>ta</u>-shun ku're-<u>tahzh</u>	dilating the uterine cervix and using a curette to scrape the endometrium of the uterus; to diagnose disease, to correct vaginal bleeding, or to produce abortion
endometriosis	en'do-me'tre-<u>o</u>-sis	cells of the lining of the uterus spreading into the pelvis (peritoneal cavity)
fibroids	<u>fi</u>-broidz	colloquial term for benign tumor (leiomyoma) of the uterus
fistula	<u>fis</u>-tu-lah	an abnormal passage between two internal organs, e.g., vesicovaginal (between bladder and vagina) fistula
hydrosalpinx	hi'dro-<u>sal</u>-pinks	fluid collecting in the uterine tube, causing distention
hysterectomy	his'te-<u>rek</u>-to-me	excision of the uterus
hysterosalpingogram	his'ter-o-sal-<u>ping</u>-go-gram	an x-ray film of the uterus and the fallopian tubes to allow visualization of the cavity of the uterus and the passageway of the tubes
laparoscopy	lap'-ah-<u>ro</u>-sko'-pe	laparoscopic visualization of the peritoneal cavity

Clinical Condition	Pronunciation	Definition
leukorrhea	loo-ko-<u>re</u>-ah	a whitish, viscid discharge from the vagina
miscarriage	mis'-<u>kar</u>-ij	spontaneous abortion
monilia (moniliasis)	mo'-<u>nil</u>-e-ah (mon'i-<u>li</u>-ah-sis)	yeastlike fungus infection of the vagina and other body parts
oophorectomy	o'of-o-<u>rek</u>-to-me	excision of one or both ovaries; female castration
pelvic examination	<u>pel</u>-vic eg'-zam'i-<u>na</u>-tion	a diagnostic procedure in which the external and internal genitalia are physically examined using inspection, palpation, etc.
pelvic inflammatory disease (PID)	<u>pel</u>-vic in-<u>flam</u>-a-to-ry di-sez'	any inflammatory condition of the female pelvic organs, especially one caused by bacterial infection
prolapse of uterus	<u>pro</u>-laps of <u>u</u>-ter-us	downward displacement of the uterus into the vagina
salpingectomy	sal'pin-<u>jek</u>-to-me	excision of one or both fallopian tubes
salpingitis	sal'pin-<u>ji</u>-tis	inflammation of one or both fallopian tubes
trichomonas infection	trik'o-<u>mo</u>-nas in-<u>fek</u>-shun	inflammation of the vagina by a parasite, with itching and foul discharge
tubal ligation	<u>tu</u>-bal li-<u>ga</u>-shun	sterilization by "tying" both fallopian tubes
vaginal speculum	<u>vaj</u>-i-nal <u>spek</u>-u-lum	an instrument used to dilate the vagina during a pelvic examination

Male and Female Conditions

Sexually transmitted diseases (STDs)

The following conditions occur in both men and women and are the most communicable diseases in the world. They are spread through sexual contact with body fluids such as blood, semen, and vaginal secretions. STDs may be contracted during vaginal, oral, or anal intercourse, or by direct contact with infected skin. AIDS can also be transmitted through sharing of needles by drug users, placenta of the infected mother to the baby during birth, and through breast milk of an infected mother when nursing the baby. The incidence of STDs in the United States is extremely high and may reach epidemic proportions, as the latest figures indicate that AIDS is again on the rise after a period of decline.

Table 16–8

Term	Pronunciation	Definition
acquired immunodeficiency syndrome (AIDS)		a fatal disease caused by the human immunodeficiency virus (HIV), which destroys the body's immune system by invading the helper T-cells (T-lymphocytes). HIV replicates itself in the T-cell, destroying the cell, and then invades other T-cells
chlamydia	klah'-mid-ee-ah	a widespread sexually transmitted bacterial infection that invades the urethra of men and the vagina and cervix of women The disease is asymptomatic in the early stages, which makes possible the spread of chlamydia as the partners are unaware that they have it
gonorrhea	gon-oh'-ree-ah	inflammation of the mucous membranes of the genital tract, affecting both male and female, caused by gonococci (berry-shaped) bacteria. Gonorrhea is spread by intercourse with an infected partner, or passed from an infected mother to her infant during birth
genital herpes	jen-ih'-tal her-peez	a highly contagious venereal disease caused by the type 2 herpes simplex virus (HSV-2), although it may be caused by HSV-1, the virus associated with oral infections (cold sores). Genital herpes is transmitted by direct contact with infected body secretions. Remissions and relapses occur and no drug is known to be effective as a cure
genital warts	jen-ih'-tal warts	Small, fleshy growths on the external genitalia.Genital warts are transmitted from person to person through sexual intercourse. They are caused by the human papilloma virus (HPV) and appear from 1 to 6 months after the initial contact
syphilis	sif-ih'-lis	a chronic, infectious disease caused by spirochete bacteria, and transmitted by sexual intercourse with an infected partner. This is a highly infectious disease that can affect any body organ. A chancre (hard ulcer) appears on the external genitalia a few weeks after exposure. It usually develops on the penis of the male and on the labia of the female

Pregnancy and Birth

Table 16–9

Term	Pronunciation	Definition
amniocentesis	am'ne-o-sen-<u>te</u>-sis	taking a sample of amniotic fluid during pregnancy for various reasons
amnion (BOW)	<u>am</u>-ne-on	amniotic sac; bag of waters
anesthesia (OB)	an'es-<u>the</u>-ze-ah	loss of feeling or sensation, especially the loss of pain sensation induced to permit the performance of surgery or other painful procedures
antepartum	an-te-<u>par</u>-tum	period from conception to onset of labor
Apgar	<u>ap</u>-gar	the evaluation of an infant's physical condition, usually performed 1 and 5 min after birth, based on a rating of five factors that reflect the infant's ability to adjust to extrauterine life
bloody show	<u>blud</u>-e sho	appearance of blood forerunning labor
caesarean (C-section)	si-<u>zar</u>-i-en	a surgical procedure in which the abdomen and uterus are incised and a baby is delivered
cephalopelvic disproportion (CPD)	sef'ah-lo-<u>pel</u>-vik dis-pruh-<u>pawr</u>-shuhn	a condition in which the fetal head is too large for the mother's pelvis
Coombs' test	Kumz test	a blood test to diagnose hemolytic anemias in a newborn
dystocia	dis-<u>to</u>-se-ah	abnormal labor or childbirth
ectopic pregnancy (extrauterine)	ek-<u>top</u>-ik (eks'trah-<u>u</u>-ter-in)	pregnancy outside the uterus, usually in the fallopian tube
EDC		expected date of confinement (due date)
episiotomy	e-piz'e-<u>ot</u>-o-me	surgical incision into the perineum and/or vagina for obstetric purposes
fetal heart tones (FHT, fht)	<u>fe</u>-tal hart tonz	the fetal heart sounds heard through the mother's abdomen in pregnancy
forceps delivery	<u>for</u>-seps de-<u>liv</u>-er-e	applying forceps to fetal head; *low* or *midforceps* delivery according to the degree of engagement of the fetal head and *high* when engagement has not occurred
gestation	jes-<u>ta</u>-shun	period from conception to birth
gravida	<u>grav</u>-i-dah	a pregnant woman; gravid means "pregnant"
ICN		intensive care nursery

Term	Pronunciation	Definition
induction	in-<u>duk</u>-shun	labor is initiated artificially, e.g., by a drug
insemination	in-sem'i-<u>na</u>-shun	the depositing of seminal fluid within the vagina or cervix
intrapartum	in-tra-<u>par</u>-tum	period from onset of labor through first hour after delivery
LMP		last menstrual period (due date)
lochia	<u>lo</u>-ke-ah	a vaginal discharge during the first week or two after childbirth
meconium	me-<u>ko</u>-ne-um	dark green mucilaginous material in the intestine of the full-term fetus, expelled as first stool
multigravida	mul-ti-<u>grav</u>-i-dah	a woman who has had more than one pregnancy
multipara	mul-<u>tip</u>-ah-rah	a woman who has borne more than one viable infant
neonatal period	ne'o-<u>na</u>-tal	the first 4 weeks after birth
obstetrical index (OB index)	ob-<u>stet</u>-ri-cal <u>in</u>-deks	the number of pregnancies, term deliveries, abortions, and stillbirths a woman has experienced
pelvimeter (pelvimetry)	pel-<u>vim</u>-e-ter (pel-<u>vim</u>-e-tre)	an instrument used to measure the capacity and diameter of the pelvis for delivery
placenta	plah-<u>sen</u>-tah	organ for exchange of nutrients and wastes between mother and fetus; called the afterbirth
postpartum	post-<u>par</u>-tum	6-week period following childbirth
prenatal	pre-<u>na</u>-tal	before birth
presentation	prez'en-<u>ta</u>-shun	the position of a baby in utero with reference to the part of the baby that is directed toward or into the birth canal
primipara	pri-<u>mip</u>-ah-rah	a woman bearing her first viable child
stillborn (sb)	<u>stil</u>-born	born dead
test-tube baby		the fertilization of an ovum outside of the uterus
toxemia	tok-<u>se</u>-me-ah	a group of pathologic conditions, essentially metabolic disturbances, occurring in pregnant women, manifested by hypertension, edema, etc. May be preeclampsia or eclampsia
trimester	tri-<u>mes</u>-ter	a period of 12 weeks
vernix caseosa	<u>ver</u>-niks ca-see-<u>o</u>-suh	a "cheesy" white substance on the skin of the newborn

LESSON TWO   PROGRESS CHECK

■ LISTS

1. List the organs of the urinary system:

   a. two _____

   b. two _____

   c. one _____

   d. one _____

2. List three important functions of the urinary system:

   a. _____

   b. _____

   c. _____

3. List the important function of the reproductive system: _____

4. List the sex organs of female reproduction:

   a. two _____

   b. two _____

   c. two _____

   d. one _____

   e. one _____

   f. one _____

5. List the sex organs of male reproduction:

   a. two _____

   b. three _____

   c. four _____

   d. one _____

   e. one _____

   f. one _____

■ **MULTIPLE CHOICE**

Circle the letter of the correct answer:

1. Which of the following statements describes the cortex?
   a. membranous sac containing urine
   b. outer layer of the kidney
   c. upper end of the ureter
   d. the renal pelvis

2. The medulla is:
   a. the inner part of the kidney
   b. the outer layer of the kidney
   c. the renal pelvis
   d. the urinary meatus

3. The functional unit of the kidney that produces urine is called a
   a. ureter
   b. bladder
   c. nephron
   d. urethra

4. The urinary bladder receives urine through the _____ and discharges it through the
   _____ .
   a. ureter, nephron
   b. bladder, urethra
   c. medulla, meatus
   d. ureter, urethra

■ **COMPARE AND CONTRAST**

Explain the *differences* in the following conditions of the urinary tract:

EXAMPLE: calculi/cystitis
Calculi are kidney stones, but cystitis is inflammation of the urinary bladder.

1. albuminuria/anuria _____

2. enuresis/diuresis _____

3. incontinence/urinary retention _____

4. hydronephrosis/nephrolithiasis _____

5. nycturia/oliguria/dysuria _____

6. pyelitis/glomerulonephritis _____

■ MATCHING: CLINICAL PROCEDURES

Match the procedure with its definition:

1.	catheterization	**a.**	imaging with sound waves
2.	Clinitest	**b.**	radiologic examination of the kidneys' collecting system
3.	cystoscopy	**c.**	determination of acidity and sugar levels of urine
4.	IVP	**d.**	measure of the amount of glucose in the urine
5.	I & O	**e.**	tube in the bladder for urine drainage
6.	UA	**f.**	visual examination of the bladder
7.	ultrasonography	**g.**	measuring and charting all ingested and excreted fluids
8.	retrograde pyelogram	**h.**	radiologic technique for examining kidney function

■ COMPLETION

Write in the medical term for each of the following meanings:

1. _____ a male gonad that supplies sperm to the semen

2. _____ the scrotum, penis, vulva, clitoris, and urethra

3. _____ extension of the epididymis and part of the ejaculatory duct

4. _____ gland surrounding the neck of the bladder in males

5. _____ the gland that is used for storage and maturation of spermatozoa

6. _____ passage for spermatozoa and semen

7. _____ a female gonad that produces eggs

8. _____ duct where fertilization occurs

9. _____ female organ that nourishes the fetus

10. _____ birth canal and receptacle for coitus

■ MATCHING: MALE CLINICAL CONDITIONS

Match these clinical conditions that occur in the *male* to their best definition:

1.	circumcision	**a.**	sterilization
2.	cryptorchidism	**b.**	excision of the prostate gland
3.	orchiectomy	**c.**	removal of the prepuce
4.	prostatectomy	**d.**	undescended testicle(s)
5.	vasectomy	**e.**	castration

■ MATCHING: FEMALE CLINICAL CONDITIONS

Match these clinical conditions that occur in the *female* to their best definition:

1. cystocele   **a.** castration

2. endometriosis   **b.** sterilization

3. hysterectomy   **c.** hernia of the bladder into the vagina

4. oophorectomy   **d.** excision of the uterus

5. tubal ligation   **e.** endometrial tissue spread into the peritoneal cavity

■ DEFINITIONS

These medical terms are specific to pregnancy and childbirth. Name the term that means:

1. Taking a sample of amniotic fluid _____

2. Evaluation of an infant's condition at birth _____

3. The fetal head is too large for the mother's pelvis _____

4. Abnormal labor or childbirth _____

5. A pregnancy outside the uterus _____

6. Period from conception to birth _____

7. A pregnant woman _____

8. First 4 weeks after birth (infant) _____

9. Six-week period after birth (mother) _____

10. The afterbirth _____

■ WORD PUZZLE ON THE GENITOURINARY SYSTEM

Find the 50 words related to the genitourinary system by reading forward, backward, up, down, and diagonally. When the 50 listed words have been circled, the remaining letters spell the words URINARY SYSTEM.

```
R E D D A L B Y R A N I R U C O R T E X
S E T Y L O R T C E L E D I C A C I R U
U G T R A M S P O R T C I T O M S O E R
T L F R A L U B U T I R E P L U D R A I
A O I B O W M A N S C A P S U L E P B N
E M L A C P A F F E R E N T M O S O S A
M E T R R U E Y E N D I K E N O C O O T
N R R T E R U R E T E R T T N P E L R I
O U A E A E E N I R U S S E O O N G P O
I L T R T A D H T Y V E R R F D N T N
T U E I I H I N T S O C C C H H I I I O
A S N O N R A N Y L A N R X P E N D O I
R R I L I A E R U L E S E E N G N N T
T E N E N R A M Y R R I T A N L L E R I
N N E S E L E X Y S U V E Y L E O C E R
E A R F L T U B U L E L C E L L O S T U
C L F I S D I U L F S E T S A W P A L T
N E P P R O X I M A L P D I S T A L I C
O A S T D I M A R Y P M E D U L L A F I
C O N V O L U T E D E M E N O G I R T M
```

WORDS TO LOOK FOR IN THE WORD PUZZLE

1. ADH
2. afferent
3. arterioles
4. ascending loop
5. Bowman's capsule
6. calyx
7. capillary system
8. cell
9. column
10. concentration
11. convoluted
12. cortex
13. creatinine
14. descending loop
15. distal
16. efferent
17. electrolytes
18. excrete
19. filter
20. filtrate
21. fluids
22. glomerulus
23. kidney
24. Loop of Henle
25. meatus
26. medulla
27. micturition
28. nephron
29. osmotic
30. pelvis
31. peritubular
32. proximal
33. pyramid
34. reabsorption
35. renal
36. renin
37. retroperitoneal
38. secrete
39. transport
40. trigone
41. tubule
42. urea
43. ureter
44. urethra
45. uric acid
46. urinary bladder
47. urination
48. urine
49. volume
50. wastes

URINARY SYSTEM

CHAPTER 17 Musculoskeletal System

OBJECTIVES

After completing this chapter and the exercises, the student should be able to:

1. Locate and name the major bones of the body by labeling the diagram provided.
2. Locate and name the major muscles of the body by labeling the diagram provided.
3. Classify the joints found in the musculoskeletal system (MSS).
4. Identify the types of bone fractures.
5. Identify and describe the types of muscles.
6. Define and explain various pathological conditions of the musculoskeletal system.
7. Identify important laboratory tests and procedures relating to the musculoskeletal system.

OVERVIEW

The musculoskeletal system includes the bones, muscles, and joints. All have important functions in the body. The human skeleton consists of 206 bones. Bones provide internal structural support, giving shape to our bodies and enabling us to stand upright. Some bones protect internal organs. The rib cage, for example, protects the lungs and heart, and the skull protects the brain. The skeleton plays an important role in purposeful movement as the site of attachment for tendons of many skeletal muscles. The skeletal muscles' action on bones results in movement or stabilizes the skeleton. Bones are home to cells that give rise to red blood cells, white blood cells, and platelets (hematopoiesis). They are a storage depot for fat, which is necessary for cellular energy production, and they are a reservoir for minerals, especially calcium and phosphorus. Bones release and absorb calcium as needed to help maintain normal blood levels. Calcium is essential to muscle contraction, and disturbances in calcium levels can impair their function.

The adult human skeleton contains about 206 bones that make up the solid framework of the body. The skeleton is completed in certain areas by cartilage. The skeleton is organized into the *axial* skeleton, the *appendicular* skeleton, and the joints between bones (see Plates 1 and 2). *Axis* and *appendicular* are defined in the first chart in Lesson One.

The axial skeleton is composed of 80 bones that make the long axis of the body and protect the organs of the heart, neck, and torso.

1. The *vertebral column* has 26 vertebrae separated by intervertebral disks.
2. The *skull* is balanced on the vertebral column.

    a. *Cranial* bones enclose and protect the brain.
    b. *Facial* bones give shape to the face or contain teeth.
    c. Six *auditory* (ear) *ossicles* transmit sound.
    d. The *hyoid* supports the tongue and larynx.

3. The *thoracic* cage includes the ribs and sternum.

The appendicular skeleton is composed of 126 bones that make up arms, legs, and the pectoral and pelvic girdles that anchor them to the axial skeleton.

Joints are *articulations* between two or more bones. They connect the bones of the skeleton and are classified by the degree of movement they permit. Immovable joints permit no movement. Skull bones, for example, are held together by immovable joints, as is the pubic symphysis that is formed by the two pubic bones. Freely movable joints allow movement, such as the vertebrae. The joints between vertebrae allow some movement so that we can bend or curl up in our beds. The most freely moving joint is the *synovial* joint. This is the ball and socket hip joint or the joints in the femur. Synovial joints differ in structure but share many features. It is a complex joint.

The functions of the skeletal system are:

1. to support and shape the body.
2. to provide movement. Bones and joints act as levers. As the muscles that are anchored to bones contract, the force applied to the levers results in movement.
3. for protection. The skeletal system protects soft delicate organs of the body.
4. for blood cell formation (*hematopoiesis*). The red bone marrow is the site of production of red blood cells (*erythrocytes*), white blood cells (*leukocytes*), and *platelets* of the blood.
5. for storage of minerals, primarily calcium phosphate and calcium carbonate. The bones contain 99% of the body's calcium. Calcium and phosphorus in the bone are withdrawn as needed for other body functions. They must be replenished through nutrition.

Muscles, whether attached to bones or to internal organs and blood vessels, are responsible for movement. Most muscles cross one or more joints, and when they contract they cause movement. Internal movement is the contraction and relaxation of visceral muscles. Some muscles steady the joints, helping to maintain upright posture against the pull of gravity. Other muscles anchored to the bones of the skull and face allow us to frown, smile, open and close our eyes, and move our lips. Muscles also produce enormous amounts of heat as a by-product of metabolism. A physician who specializes in bone and joint diseases is called an *orthopedist*.

Muscle tissue constitutes 40–50% of body weight. It consists predominantly of contractile cells called muscle fibers. Through contraction, muscles produce movement and do work (see Plates 4 and 5).

Muscles have these properties: *contractility, excitability* (response when stimulated by nerve impulses), *extensibility* (will stretch beyond their relaxed length), and elasticity (will return to their original length). Mammals are the only animals with facial muscles, and the human body contains the same number of muscles from birth to death.

There is special classification and terminology related to muscles. These are explained and defined in Lesson One.

The functions of the muscular system are:

1. movement
2. body support and maintenance of posture
3. heat production

The energy sources for muscle contraction are an interesting part of muscle physiology involving the citric acid cycle. Additional energy sources are formed by the metabolism of glucose and fatty acids through anaerobic (glycolytic pathway) and aerobic reactions. The value of exercise in weight control can be verified with these facts.

Many injuries, diseases, and disorders affect the musculoskeletal system. These are defined in Lesson One.

Lessons to be learned are separated into sections for better identification and clarity:

1. head and body bones, joints, and accessories
2. body muscles
3. pathological conditions of MSS and the procedures and tests used to diagnose and treat them (medical management)

LESSON ONE　　　MATERIALS TO BE LEARNED

The musculoskeletal system serves the following functions in the body:

1. *Support and protection.* The forms and shapes of the body are maintained and vital organs are protected from injury.
2. *Movement.* Body movement is made possible by a coordination of different components of the musculoskeletal system.
3. *Red blood cell turnover.* Marrow from the large bones serves as the site for turnover (destruction and rebuilding) of red blood cells.
4. *Storage.* Bones store minerals and muscles store nutrients for energy production.

Refer to Figures 17–1 to 17–4 when studying the following charts.

THE SKELETAL SYSTEM

Division

Table 17–1

Main Division	Pronunciation	Definition
appendicular	ap'en-<u>dik</u>-u-lar	an appendage; limbs
axis (n.) (axial [adj.])	<u>ak</u>-sis (<u>ak</u>-si-el)	a line that passes through the center of the body traversing skull, thorax, and vertebral column
ethmoid	<u>eth</u>-moid	the light and spongy bone at the base of the cranium; the upper nasal bone between the eyes
frontal	<u>frun</u>-tal	forehead
mandible	<u>man</u>-di-b'l	large bone constituting the lower jaw
maxilla	mak-<u>sil</u>-ah	one of a pair of large bones forming the upper jaw
occipital	ok-<u>sip</u>-i-tal	the cuplike bone at the back of the skull
parietal	pah-<u>ri</u>-e-tal	bone of the skull (top of the head)
sphenoid	<u>sfe</u>-noid	bone at the base of the skull, anterior to the temporal bones
temporal	<u>tem</u>-po-ral	large bones forming part of the temples
turbinate	<u>ter</u>-bi-nat	cone-shaped nasal bone

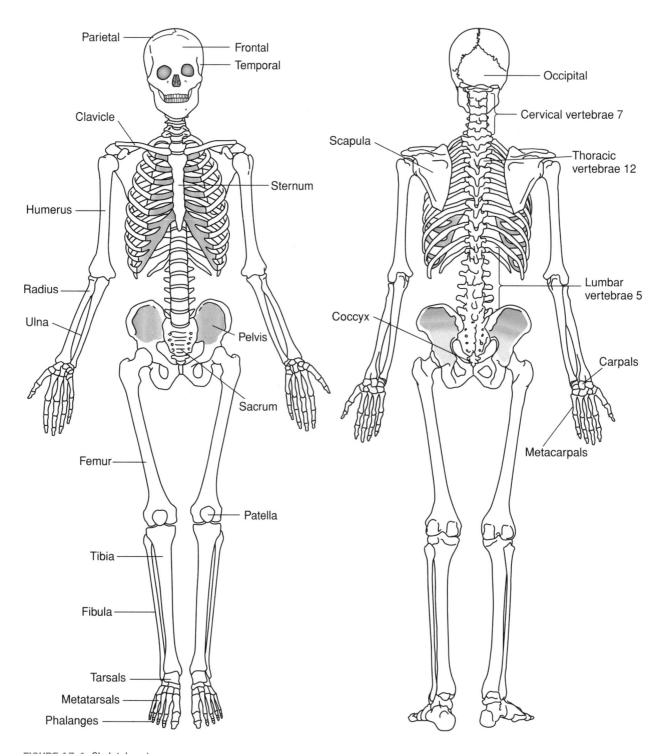

FIGURE 17–1 Skeletal system.

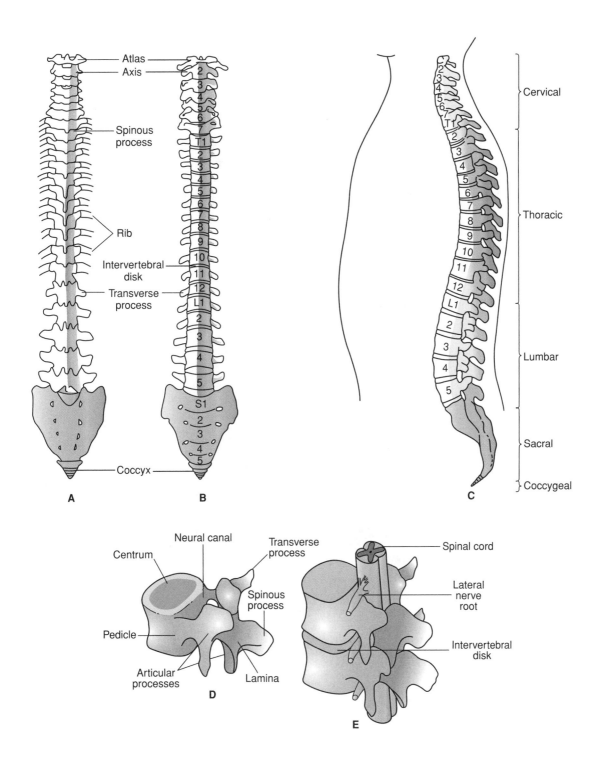

FIGURE 17–2 A, Vertebral column, posterior aspect. **B**, Vertebral column, anterior aspect. **C**, Vertebral column, lateral aspect. **D**, Vertebral column, diagonal view from top. **E**, Vertebral column, two vertebrae held in position by an intervertebral disk. Shows position of spinal cord and its peripheral nerves.

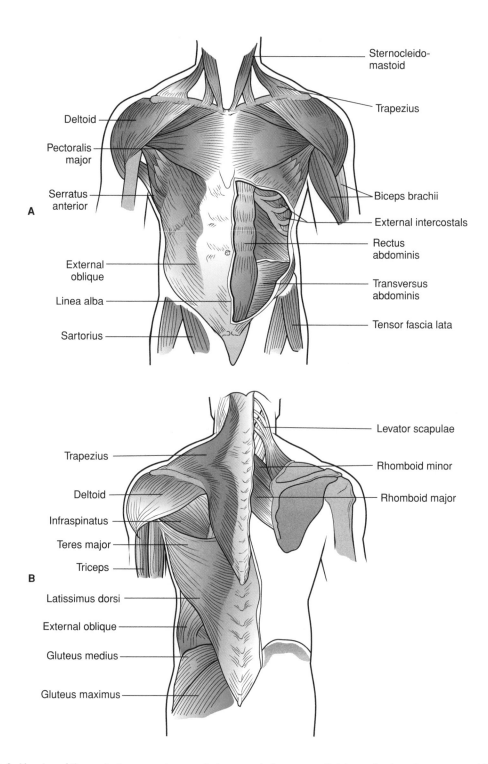

FIGURE 17–3 A, Muscles of the neck, thorax, and arm, anterior aspect. Some superficial muscles have been removed from the left side to permit exposure of the deep muscles. **B**, Muscles of the neck, thorax, and arm, posterior aspect. The superficial muscles have been removed on the right side to permit exposure of the deep muscles connecting the scapula to the spinal vertebrae.

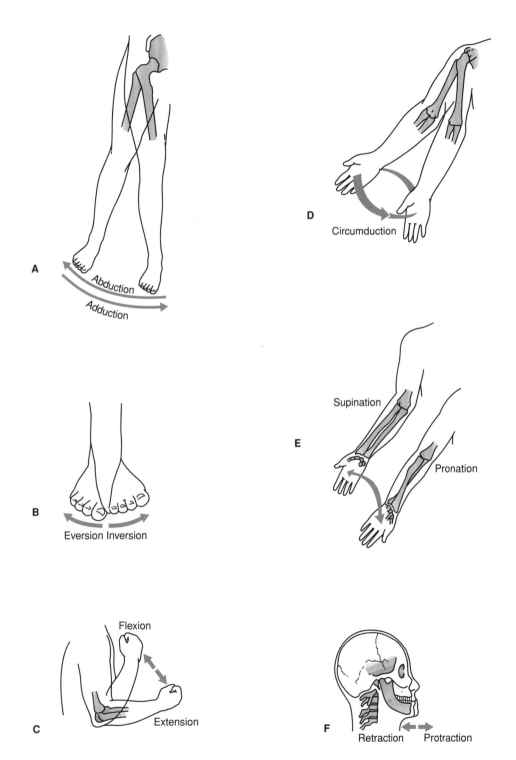

FIGURE 17–4 Movements of diarthrodial joints. **A**, Abduction-adduction. **B**, Eversion-inversion. **C**, Flexion-extension. **D**, Circumduction. **E**, Supinationpronation. **F**, Protraction-retraction.

Body Bones

Table 17–2

Part	Pronunciation	Definition
clavicle	klav-i-k'l	a long, curved, horizontal bone just above the first rib (collar bone)
femur	fe-mur	the thigh bone, extending from the pelvis to the knee
fibula and tibia	fib-u-lah and tib-e-ah	the fibula is the smallest of the bones of the leg; the tibia is the second longest bone of the skeleton, located at the medial side of the leg
humerus	hu-mer-us	upper-arm bone, consisting of a body, a head, and the condyle
radius and ulna	ra-de-us and ul-nah	the radius is the larger of the two bones of the forearm; the ulna is the bone on the medial or little-finger side of the forearm, lying parallel with the radius
scapula	skap-u-lah	shoulder blade
sternum	ster-num	the elongated, flattened bone forming the middle portion of the thorax (breastbone)
vertebral column	ver-te-bral kol-em	the flexible structure that forms the longitudinal axis (backbone) of the skeleton; it consists of 26 separate vertebrae arranged in a straight line from the base of the skull to the coccyx (tailbone)

Head Bones

Table 17–3

Part	Pronunciation	Definition
ethmoid	eth-moid	a very light and spongy bone at the base of the cranium; the upper nasal bone between the eyes
frontal	frun-tal	forehead
hyoid	hahy-oid	point of attachment for muscles of head and throat
lachrymal	lak-ruh-muhl	two bones that house the tear ducts
mandible	man-dih-bel	large bone constituting the lower jaw
maxilla	mak-sil-ah	one of a pair of large bones forming the upper jaw
nasal	ney-zuhl	two bones that shape the nose
occipital	ock-sip-it-al	the cuplike bone at the back of the skull
palatine	pal-uh-tahyn	forms the hard palate (roof of the mouth)

Part	Pronunciation	Definition
parietal	pah-<u>ri</u>-et-al	parietal bone of the skull (top of the head)
sphenoid	<u>sfne</u>-noid	bone at the base of the skull, anterior to the temporal bones
temporal	<u>tem</u>-poor-al	large bones forming part of the temples
turbinate	<u>ter</u>-beh-nate	cone-shaped nasal bone
vomer	voh-mer	lower part of the nasal septum
zygomatic	zahy-guh-<u>mat</u>-ik	two bones, one on each side of the face, which form the high part of the cheek bones and outer eye socket

Joints and Accessory Parts

Table 17–4

Part	Pronunciation	Definition
ball and socket	bawl and <u>sok</u>-et	a joint in which the globular head of an articulating bone is received into a cuplike cavity, e.g., the hip and shoulder
hinge	hinj	hinge joint, e.g., elbow, knees, and fingers
sutures	<u>su</u>-cherz	lines of junction between the bones of the skull
intervertebral	in-ter-<u>ver</u>-te-bral	the fibrous substance between the disks of the spinal vertebrae
aponeurosis	ap'o-nu-<u>ro</u>-sis	a flattened tendon, connecting a muscle with the parts it moves
bursa (pl., bursae)	<u>ber</u>-sah (<u>ber</u>-see)	a fluid-filled sac located in tissues to reduce friction
fascia (pl., fasciae)	<u>fash</u>-e-ah (<u>fash</u>-shee-ee)	a sheet of fibrous tissue holding muscle fibers together
interphalangeal	in'ter-fah-<u>lan</u>-je-al	between two contiguous joints and phalanges, e.g., between the fingers and toes
lamina (pl., laminae)	<u>lam</u>-i-nah <u>lam</u>-i-nee	the flattened part of the vertebral arch (thinnest part of a vertebra)
ligament	<u>lig</u>-ah-ment	a band of fibrous tissue connecting bones or cartilages
meniscus (pl., menisci)	me-<u>nis</u>-kus (me-<u>nis</u>-ki)	a crescent-shaped fibrocartilage in the knee joint

Part	Pronunciation	Definition
synovial fluid	si-<u>no</u>-ve-al	the transparent, viscid fluid found in joint cavities, bursae, and tendon sheaths
tendon	<u>ten</u>-don	a fibrous cord of connective tissue attaching the muscle to bone or cartilage
theca	<u>the</u>-kah	a case or sheath of a tendon

Bone Processes, Depressions, and Holes

Bone processes are enlarged tissues that extend out from the bones to serve as attachments for muscles and tendons. The bone head is the rounded end of a bone separated from the body of the bone by a neck. Many bones have a small rounded process called a tubercle for attachment of tendons or muscles. Below the neck of the femur is a large bony process called a trochanter, and at the end of the bone is a rounded knuckle-like projection that fits into the fossa (bone depression) of another bone to form a joint.

Bone depressions are the openings or cavities in a bone that help to join one bone to another and are the passageway for the blood vessels and nerves. As noted above, the fossa is a shallow cavity in or on a bone. The foramen is an opening for blood vessels and nerves. A fissure, or suture, is a deep, narrow, slitlike opening. A sinus is a hollow space in a bone, for example, the paranasal sinuses.

Table 17–5

Structure	Pronunciation	Definition
acetabulum	as'e-<u>tab</u>-u-lum	the cup-shaped cavity (socket) receiving the head of the femur
foramen (pl., foramina)	fo-<u>ra</u>-men (fo-<u>ram</u>-i-nah)	holes in a bone for large vessels and nerves to pass through
fossa (pl., fossae)	<u>fos</u>-ah (<u>fos</u>-ee)	a hollow or depressed area
groove	groov	a narrow, linear hollow or depression in bone
malleolus	mah-<u>le</u>-o-lus	a rounded process, such as the protuberance on either side of the ankle joint, at the lower end of the fibula or the tibia
olecranon	o-<u>lek</u>-rah-non	bony projection of the ulna at the elbow
prominence	<u>prom</u>-i-nens	protrusion or projection
sinus	<u>si</u>-nus	one definition is a recess, cavity, or channel, such as one in bone
tuberosity	too'be-<u>ros</u>-i-te	an elevation or protuberance, especially of a bone

THE MUSCULAR SYSTEM

Basically there are three categories of muscles in the body:

1. Heart or cardiac muscle.
2. Striated or striped muscles, e.g., skeletal muscles. These muscles are voluntary muscles that a person has control over.
3. Nonstriated or nonstriped muscles, e.g., smooth muscles. These muscles are involuntary and there is no way to have control over them, e.g., movement of the stomach and intestine.

Body muscles are identified in the following manner:

1. Function—a muscle name has two parts: The first part is a word root, ending in a suffix (-or or -ens); the second part is the name of the affected body structure. An example is extensor carpi, or extension of the wrist.
2. Points of origin and attachment—the muscle name joins the names of points of origin and attachment with a word terminal (-eus or -is). An example is sternoclavicularis, for sternum and clavicle.
3. Form or position—the muscle name contains a descriptive word and the name of the muscle location. An example is pectoralis minor, for small chest muscle.
4. Resemblance to an object for which the muscle is used—an example is buccinator. This refers to the cheek muscle, which is used in blowing a trumpet.

When studying the following information refer to Figures 17–3, 17–4, and 17–5.

Muscles of the Body

Table 17–6

Medical Term	Pronunciation	Definition
biceps brachii	bye'-seps bray-kee-eye	muscle extending from scapula to radius. Used to flex lower arm and turn palm of hand upward
buccinator	buck-sin-ay-tor	fleshy part of the cheek. Used to smile, blow outward, and whistle
cardiac muscle	kar'-de-ac' muhs-uhl	specialized muscle found in the walls of the heart. Involuntary muscles, controlled by the ANS
deltoid	dell-toyd	muscle covering the shoulder joint. Extends from clavicle and scapula to humerus. Extends the arm
gastrocnemius	gas-trok'-nee-mus	main calf muscle. Attaches to heel bone
gluteus maximus	gloo'-tee-us max'-ih-mus	fleshy part of the buttocks. Extends from ilium to femur. Adducts and rotates thigh laterally

Medical Term	Pronunciation	Definition
hamstring	ham-string	muscle in posterior thigh used for flexing, as in kneeling, and for extension
latissimus dorsi	lah'-<u>tis</u>-ih-<u>mus</u> dor'-see	muscle extending from lower vertebrae to humerus. Used for swinging the arms
masseter	<u>mass</u>-see'-ter	muscle at angle of jaw. Used for biting and chewing
orbicularis occuli	or-<u>bick</u>-yoo'-<u>lar</u>-iss <u>ock</u>-yool-eye	body of the eyelid, opens and closes the eye, wrinkles forehead
orbicularis oris	or-<u>bick</u>-yoo'-<u>lar</u>-iss or-iss	muscle surrounding the mouth. Closes and purses the lips
pectoralis major	<u>peck</u>-tor'-<u>ray</u>-lis	large, fan-shaped muscle across front of the chest. Adducts, flexes, and rotates the arms inward
quadriceps femoris	<u>kwod</u>-rih-<u>seps</u>' <u>fem-or</u>-is	anterior thigh muscle. Part of a five-muscle group that extends the thigh
skeletal muscles	<u>skel</u>-i-tl <u>muhs</u>-uhl	also called striated (striped) or voluntary muscles. Muscles attached to skeletal bones except for face, eyes, tongue, and throat. Under concious control
smooth muscles	smooth <u>muhs</u>-uhl	muscles found in the wall of the stomach, intestine, blood vessels, and respiratory tract. Also called involuntary or visceral muscle (not under concious control)
sternomastoid	stir'-no-<u>mass</u>-toyd	muscle extending from sternum to side of the neck. Used for turning the head
temporal	<u>tem</u>-por'-al	muscle above the ear. Used for opening and closing the jaw
trapezius	trap-<u>pee</u>-zee'-us	triangular muscle extending from back of shoulder to clavical. Used to raise shoulders
triceps brachii	<u>tri</u>-seps <u>bray</u>-kee'-eye	muscle extending from scapula to ulna. Responsible for adducting the elbow

Motion

Table 17–7

Movement	Pronunciation	Definition
flexion	<u>flek</u>-shun	bending
extension	ek-<u>sten</u>-shun	the movement by which the two ends of any jointed part are drawn away from each other; straightening

Movement	Pronunciation	Definition
adduction	ad-<u>duk</u>-shun	to draw toward the axial (median) line of a limb
abduction	ab-<u>duk</u>-shun	to draw away from the axial (median) line of a limb
pronation	pro-<u>na</u>-shun	the prone position (palm down, face down)
supination	su'pi-<u>na</u>-shun	palm or face upward
proximal	<u>prok</u>-si-mal	nearest to a point of reference or origin
distal	<u>dis</u>-tal	farthest from any point of reference or origin

Physiological Status of Muscles

Table 17–8

Condition	Pronunciation	Definition
contracture	kon-<u>trak</u>-chur	permanent contraction of a muscle
muscle atrophy	<u>muhs</u>-uhl <u>at</u>-ro-fe	wasting away of muscle from disuse
muscle hypertrophy	<u>muhs</u>-uhl hi-<u>per</u>-tro-fe	muscle enlargement from overuse
muscle tone	<u>muhs</u>-uhl tōn	normal degree of vigor and tension in a muscle; muscles partially contracted
paralysis	pah-<u>ral</u>-i-sis	loss of muscular contraction because of nerve damage
paresis	pah-<u>re</u>-sis	slight or incomplete paralysis

Injuries

Table 17–9

Type	Pronunciation	Definition
fracture	<u>frak</u>-chur	the breaking of a bone; there are many types
skull fracture	skul <u>frak</u>-chur	a fracture of the bony structure of the head
torn ligament, tendon, or cartilage	<u>lig</u>-ah-ment <u>ten</u>-don <u>kar</u>-ti-lij	a complete or partial tear of a ligament, tendon, or cartilage; common sports injuries
subluxation	sub'luk-<u>sa</u>-shun	partial dislocation
spondylolisthesis	spon'di-lo-lis-<u>the</u>-sis	forward displacement of a vertebra over a lower segment; a type of dislocation

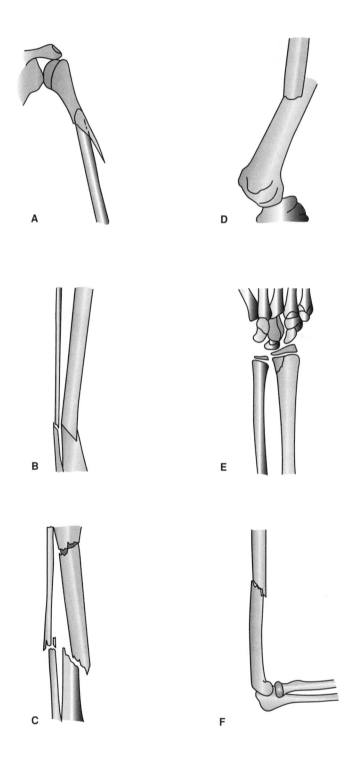

FIGURE 17-5 Types of fractures. **A**, Longitudinal, through upper shaft of right humerus. **B**, Spiral, of tibia and fibula. **C**, Comminuted, of tibia and fibula. **D**, Transverse, through lower shaft of femur. **E**, Impacted. **F**, Pathologin, through area of destruction secondary to metastatic carcinoma.

Clinical Disorders

Table 17–10

Disorder	Pronunciation	Definition
arthritis	ar-<u>thri</u>-tis	inflammation of a joint; there are 4 common types
bursitis	ber-<u>si</u>-tis	inflammation of a bursa
carpal tunnel syndrome	<u>kar</u>-pal <u>tun</u>-el <u>sin</u>-drom	a common painful disorder of the wrist and hand, caused by pressure on the median nerve in the wrist
collagen disease	<u>kol</u>-ah-jen di-<u>zez</u>	a group of diseases with widespread pathologic changes in connective tissue, e.g., lupus erythematosus, dermatomyositis
gout	gowt	a hereditary form of arthritis caused by accumulation of uric acid crystals, especially in the great toe
herniated nucleus pulposus	<u>her</u>-ne-at'ed <u>nu</u>-kle-us pul-<u>po</u>-sus	a rupture of the fibrocartilage surrounding an intervertebral disk, releasing the nucleus pulposus that cushions the vertebrae above and below
kyphosis	ki-<u>fo</u>-sis	humpback or hunchback; a spinal deformity
Legg-Calvé-Perthes disease	leg-kal-<u>vay</u>-<u>per</u>-tes di-<u>zez</u>	osteochondrosis of the head of the femur in children
lordosis	lor-<u>do</u>-sis	forward curvature of the lumbar spine; swayback
lupus erythematosus (LE)	<u>loo</u>-pus er-i'the-ma-<u>to</u>-sus	see systemic lupus erythematosus
muscular dystrophy	<u>mus</u>-ku-lar <u>dis</u>-tro-fe	genetic diseases with progressive atrophy of skeletal muscles
myasthenia gravis	mi-as-<u>the</u>-ne-ah <u>gra</u>-vis	lack of muscle strength
myositis	mi'o-<u>si</u>-tis	inflammation of a voluntary muscle
Osgood-Schlatter disease	<u>oz</u>-good-<u>shlat</u>-er di-<u>zez</u>	inflammation of the tibial tubercle caused by chronic irritation and seen primarily in muscular, athletic adolescents; characterized by swelling and tenderness over the tibial tubercle that increases with exercise
osteochondritis	os'te-o-kon-<u>dri</u>-tis	inflammation of the bone and cartilage
osteochondrosis	os'te-o-kon-<u>dro</u>-sis	disease of the bone and cartilage

Disorder	Pronunciation	Definition
osteomalacia	os′te-o-mah-<u>la</u>-she-ah	softening of the bones resulting from vitamin D deficiency
osteomyelitis	os′te-o-mi′e-<u>li</u>-tis	inflammation of bone and marrow caused by bacterial invasion
osteoporosis	os′te-o-po-<u>ro</u>-sis	porous condition of bones; occurs primarily in postmenopausal women
rheumatism	<u>roo</u>-ma-tizm	disorders marked by inflammation, degeneration, or metabolic derangement of the connective tissue structures, especially the joints and related structures, and attended by pain, stiffness, or limitation of motion
rickets	<u>rik</u>-ets	vitamin D deficiency, especially in infancy and childhood, marked by bending and distortion of the bones
sarcoma (osteogenic)	sar′<u>ko</u>-mah (os′te-o-<u>jen</u>-ik)	a malignant tumor of bone
scoliosis	sko′le-<u>o</u>-sis	lateral curvature of the spine
spina bifida	<u>spi</u>-nah <u>bi</u>-fid-a	a congenital defect in the spine
spondylitis (ankylosing)	spon′di-<u>li</u>-tis (ang′ki-<u>lo</u>-sing)	inflammation of the vertebrae, commonly progressing to eventual fusion of the involved joints
systemic lupus erythematosus (SLE)	sis-<u>tem</u>-ik <u>loo</u>-pus er-i′the-ma-<u>to</u>-sus	a chronic inflammatory disease affecting many systems of the body
tendinitis	ten′di-<u>ni</u>-tis	inflammation of a tendon

Medical Management

Table 17–11

Procedure	Pronunciation	Definition
amputation	am′pu-ta′shun	removal of a limb or other appendage of the body
arthrocentesis	ar′thro-sen-te′sis	puncture of a joint cavity to remove fluid
arthroscopy	ahr-thros-kuh-pee	examination of the interior of a joint with an endoscope
arthrotomy	ar-throt′o-me	surgical creation of an opening into a joint, such as for drainage

Procedure	Pronunciation	Definition
electrical stimulation	e-<u>lek</u>-tri-k'l stim'u-<u>la</u>-shun	a process used to heal fractures more quickly
electromyogram (electromyography)	e-lek'tro-<u>mi</u>-o-gram (e-lek'tro-mi-<u>og</u>-rah-fe)	the film record made and the study of muscular contraction
external fixation	eks-<u>ter</u>-nal fik-<u>sa</u>-shun	the process of making a bone immovable
fracture reduction	<u>frak</u>-chur re-<u>duk</u>-shun	the correction of a fracture, luxation, or hernia
laminectomy with diskectomy	lam'i-<u>nek</u>-to-me dis-<u>kek</u>-to-me	excision of the posterior arch of a vertebra; excision of an intervertebral disk
meniscectomy	men'i-<u>sek</u>-to-me	excision of a meniscus, e.g., of the knee joint
myelogram	<u>mi</u>-e-lo-gram	the film produced by radiography of the spinal cord after injection of a dye into the spinal cavity
myogram	<u>mi</u>-o-gram	a record produced by myography; same as electromyogram
replantation	re'plan-<u>ta</u>-shun	the insertion of an organ or tissue in a new site in the body
spondylosyndesis	spon'di-lo-<u>sin</u>-de-sis	surgical creation of ankylosis between contiguous vertebrae; spinal fusion
total hip replacement		replacement of the hip joint with an artificial ball and socket joint, performed to relieve a chronically painful and stiff hip caused by certain clinical disorders
traction	<u>trak</u>-shun	the act of drawing or pulling

Abbreviations (Musculoskeletal System)

Table 17–12

Abbreviation	Definition
ANA	antinuclear antibodies; a laboratory serum test; ANA is associated with many diseases
ASO	antistreptolysin O
CRP	C-reactive protein
DJD	degenerative joint disease

Abbreviation	Definition
ORIF	open reduction internal fixation; reduction of a fracture after incision into the fracture site
RA	rheumatoid arthritis
RA factor	rheumatoid arthritis factor
SLE (LE)	systemic lupus erythematosus; lupus erythematosus
SR (ESR)	sedimentation rate; erythrocyte sedimentation rate

LESSON TWO   PROGRESS CHECK

■ LIST THE FUNCTION

List the four major functions of the musculoskeletal system and one example of each:

Function	*Example*
1. Support + protection	vital organs protected
2. Movement	all body muruts
3. red blood cell turnover	bone marrow in the site
4. storage	minerals + nutrients

■ MATCHING: LOCATIONS

Match the main divisions of the musculoskeletal system listed on the left to their locations listed at the right:

F **1.** axis   **a.** lower jaw

G **2.** frontal   **b.** upper jaw

I **3.** temporal   **c.** bone at base of the skull

H **4.** parietal   **d.** nasal bone

J **5.** occipital   **e.** spongy bone at base of the cranium

A **6.** mandible   **f.** skull, thorax, vertebrae

B **7.** maxilla   **g.** forehead

C **8.** sphenoid   **h.** top of the head

D **9.** turbinate   **i.** bones at the temples

E **10.** ethmoid   **j.** cuplike bone at the back of the skull

■ MULTIPLE CHOICE

Circle the letter of the correct answer:

1. The clavicle is
   a. the rib bone
   (b) the collar bone
   c. the breastbone
   d. the thigh bone

2. The sternum is
   a. the collar bone
   (b) the breastbone
   c. the thigh bone
   d. the nasal bone

3. The femur is
   (a) the thigh bone
   b. the nasal bone
   c. the breastbone
   d. a bone in the forearm

4. The radius and ulna are
   a. leg bones
   b. shoulder blades
   (c) bones in the forearm
   d. thigh bones

5. The fibula and tibia are
   a. bones in the forearm
   b. breastbones
   c. thigh bones
   (d) leg bones

6. There are _____ separate vertebrae in the vertebral column.
   a. 18
   b. 22
   (c) 26
   d. 30

7. The longitudinal axis is commonly called
   a. the tailbone
   (b) the backbone
   c. the lower leg
   d. the upper arm

8. The bone that goes from pelvis to knee is the
   a. coccyx
   b. humerus
   (c) femur
   d. tibia

9. The radius is to the ulna as the
   a. maxilla is to the mandible
   b. clavicle is to the sternum
   c. occipital is to the parietal
   (d.) tibia is to the fibula

■ NAME THE STRUCTURE

Name the following joints and accessory parts from the word pool given below the descriptions:

1. A fluid-filled sac located in tissues *bursa*
2. A sheet of fibrous tissue holding muscles together *fascia*
3. Flattened part of the vertebral arch *lamina*
4. Band of fibrous tissue *ligament*
5. A flattened connecting tendon *aponeurosis*
6. Elbows, knees, and fingers *hinges*
7. Lines of junction between the bones of the skull *sutures*
8. Hip and shoulder joints *ball & socket*
9. Fibrous cord of connective tissue *tendon*
10. Crescent-shaped fibrous cartilage in the knee *Meniscus*

WORD POOL

aponeurosis, ball and socket, bursa, fascia, hinge joint, lamina, ligament, meniscus, sutures, tendons

■ MATCHING

Match the muscle conditions at the left to their definitions on the right:

C 1. atrophy   a. permanent drawing together – *contracture (A)*
D 2. hypertrophy   b. loss of contraction caused by nerve damage – *paralysis (B)*
E 3. tone   c. wasting away from disuse – *atrophy (C)*
B 4. paralysis   d. enlargement from overuse – *hypertrophy (D)*
A 5. contracture   e. normal vigor and tension – *tone (E)*

Match the musculoskeletal injury to its clinical name:

D 6. common sports injury   a. subluxation – *partial dislocation*
A 7. partial dislocation   b. spondylolisthesis – *displacement of a vertebra*
B 8. displacement of a vertebra   c. skull fracture – *broken bone in head*
E 9. broken bone anywhere   d. torn ligament – *common sports injury*
C 10. broken bone in the head e. fracture – *broken bone anywhere*

The musculoskeletal system is prone to many types of inflammation. Match the condition listed at the left to its *location* in the right column:

G **11.** arthritis   **a.** in a tendon – *tendonitis*

F **12.** bursitis   **b.** in the bone and marrow – *osteomyelitis*

D **13.** myositis   **c.** in a vertebra – *spondylitis*

E **14.** osteochondritis   **d.** in a voluntary muscle – *myositis*

B **15.** osteomyelitis   **e.** in the bone and cartilage – *osteochondritis*

C **16.** spondylitis   **f.** in a bursa – *bursitis*

A **17.** tendonitis   **g.** in a joint – *arthritis*

■ COMPARE AND CONTRAST

Explain the differences in the following clinical disorders:

EXAMPLE: Osgood-Schlatter disease/Legg-Calvé-Perthes disease. Osgood-Schlatter disease is inflammation of the tibia caused by chronic irritation; Legg-Calvé-Perthes disease is inflammation of the head of the femur in children.

1. kyphosis/lordosis *Kyphosis – humpback (or hunchback) lordosis – curvature of the lumbar spine (swayback)*

2. gout/rickets *gout – a form of arthritis rickets: a deficiency of Vit. D*

3. carpal tunnel syndrome/collagen disease *CTS: a painful disorder of the wrist & hand CD: a disease of connective tissue*

4. muscular dystrophy/myasthenia gravis *MD: progressive atrophy of the skeleton MG: lack of muscle strength*

5. osteomalacia/osteoporosis *Osteomalacia: softening of the bones osteoporosis: brittle porous bones*

6. sarcoma/scoliosis *sarcoma: a malignant bone tumor scoliosis: lateral curvature of the spine*

7. spina bifida/spondylitis *SB: a congenital defect in the spine S: inflammation of the vertebra*

■ WORD PUZZLE ON THE MUSCULOSKELETAL SYSTEM

There are 63 words on the musculoskeletal system in this puzzle. They read forward, backward, up, down, and diagonally. When the 63 words have been circled, the remaining letters spell SKELETAL SYSTEM.

```
S  I  S  E  L  C  I  V  A  L  C  I  T  A  M  O  G  Y  Z  N
E  S  P  E  C  T  O  R  A  L  G  I  R  D  L  E  B  S  O  M
G  C  E  S  S  H  Y  O  I  D  E  N  I  P  S  O  U  T  A  U
N  H  L  C  K  L  A  T  I  P  I  C  C  O  N  L  E  N  N  L
A  I  V  A  O  M  A  X  I  L  L  A  E  E  A  L  U  O  A  O
L  U  I  P  M  R  F  R  O  N  T  A  L  T  E  B  I  R  S  C
A  M  S  U  A  I  P  X  Y  C  C  O  C  K  R  M  O  U  V  L
H  U  I  L  N  D  R  D  D  E  N  S  S  I  O  P  R  O  C  A
P  I  B  A  D  I  I  C  I  L  E  R  U  R  M  E  M  L  I  R
A  L  U  P  I  O  B  T  A  O  A  M  C  E  M  E  X  A  C  D
T  I  P  A  B  M  T  S  E  L  L  A  T  U  R  C  I  C  A  E
E  L  D  L  L  H  I  A  U  U  L  Y  H  N  S  A  P  I  R  T
L  A  I  A  E  T  B  C  M  U  A  S  T  A  U  R  H  V  O  R
L  T  O  T  C  E  I  B  A  L  L  U  K  S  I  P  O  R  N  E
A  E  N  I  O  D  A  M  L  N  U  Y  S  A  D  A  I  E  T  V
S  I  E  N  N  R  X  U  L  A  B  T  E  L  A  L  D  C  A  I
A  R  H  E  C  S  I  R  E  L  I  V  N  A  R  S  I  A  R  N
L  A  P  G  H  B  A  C  U  M  F  R  U  M  E  F  S  X  S  C
T  P  S  A  A  R  L  A  S  M  U  N  R  E  T  S  X  I  A  U
A  X  O  C  S  O  S  S  I  C  L  E  S  E  P  A  T  S  L  S
```

WORDS TO LOOK FOR IN THE WORD PUZZLE

1. acromion	14. dens	27. malleus	40. pelvis	53. styloid process
2. appendicular skeleton	15. disk	28. mandible	41. phalanges	54. talus
3. anvil	16. ethmoid	29. manubrium	42. pubis	55. tarsal
4. atlas	17. femur	30. maxilla	43. radius	56. temporal
5. axial	18. fibula	31. nasal	44. rib	57. thoracic
6. axis	19. frontal	32. occipitals	45. sacrum	58. tibia
7. bone	20. humerus	33. orbs	46. scapula	59. vertebral column
8. cage	21. hyoid	34. os coxa	47. sella turcica	60. vomer
9. carpals	22. ilium	35. ossicles	48. skull	61. ulna
10. cervical	23. incus	36. palatine	49. sphenoid	62. xiphoid
11. clavicles	24. ischium	37. parietal	50. spine	63. zygomatic
12. coccyx	25. lacrimal	38. patella	51. stapes	**SKELETAL SYSTEM**
13. concha	26. lumbar	39. pectoral girdle	52. sternum	

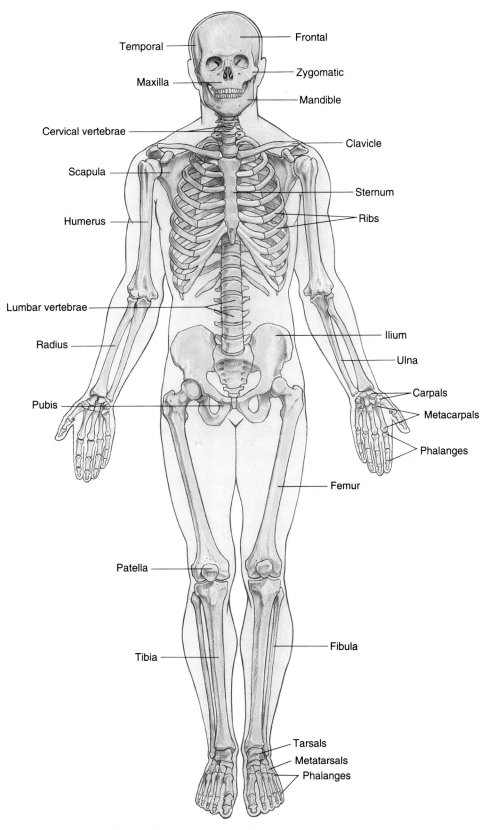

PLATE 1

THE
SKELETAL
SYSTEM
(front view)

Temporal

Frontal

Maxilla

Zygomatic

Mandible

Cervical vertebrae

Clavicle

Scapula

Sternum

Humerus

Ribs

Lumbar vertebrae

Ilium

Radius

Ulna

Carpals

Pubis

Metacarpals

Phalanges

Femur

Patella

Fibula

Tibia

Tarsals

Metatarsals

Phalanges

PLATE 2

THE SKELETAL SYSTEM
(side and back views)

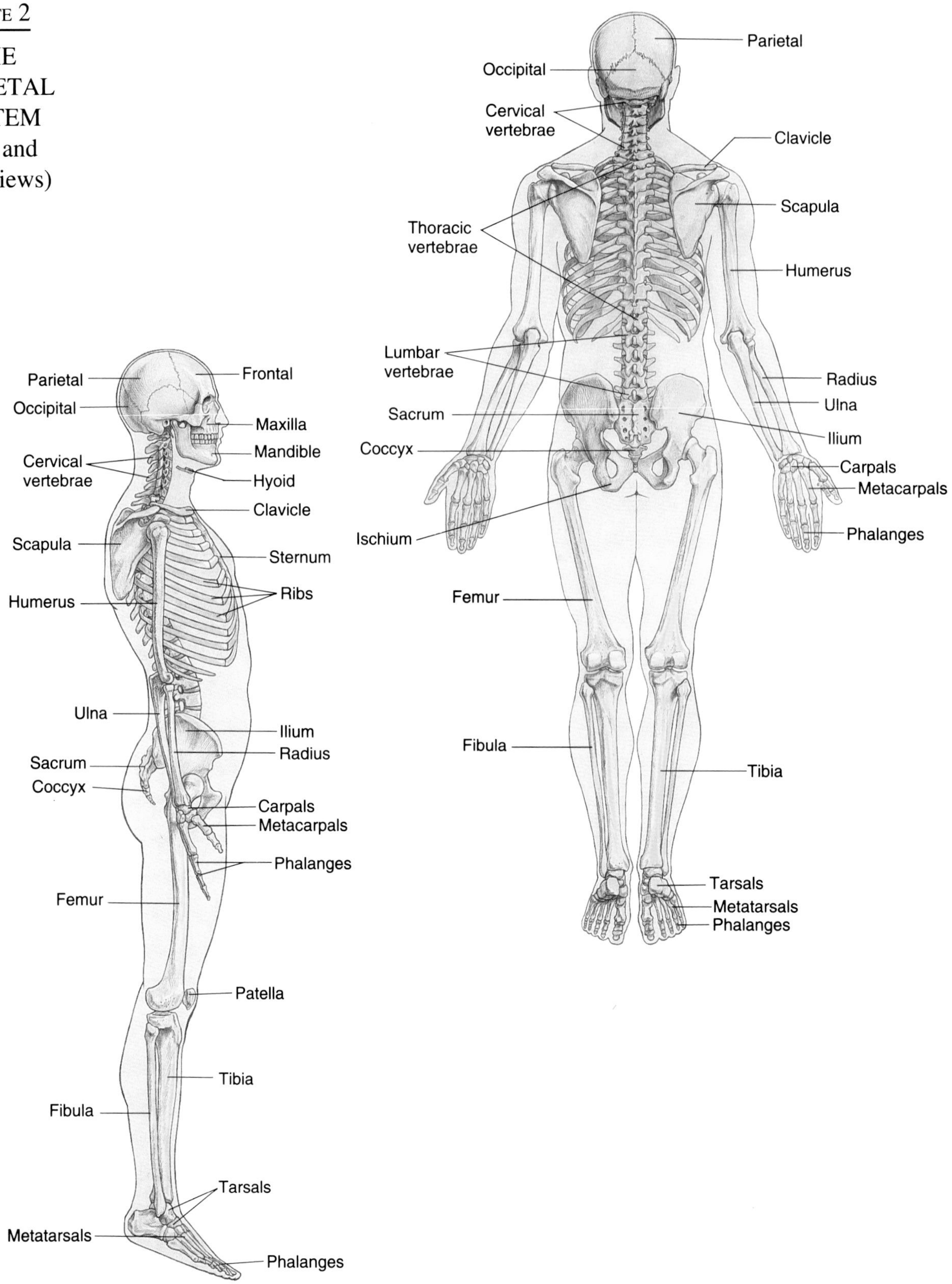

Back view labels (right figure):
- Parietal
- Occipital
- Cervical vertebrae
- Clavicle
- Scapula
- Thoracic vertebrae
- Humerus
- Lumbar vertebrae
- Sacrum
- Radius
- Ulna
- Coccyx
- Ilium
- Ischium
- Carpals
- Metacarpals
- Phalanges
- Femur
- Fibula
- Tibia
- Tarsals
- Metatarsals
- Phalanges

Side view labels (left figure):
- Parietal
- Frontal
- Occipital
- Maxilla
- Mandible
- Cervical vertebrae
- Hyoid
- Clavicle
- Scapula
- Sternum
- Humerus
- Ribs
- Ulna
- Ilium
- Radius
- Sacrum
- Coccyx
- Carpals
- Metacarpals
- Phalanges
- Femur
- Patella
- Tibia
- Fibula
- Tarsals
- Metatarsals
- Phalanges

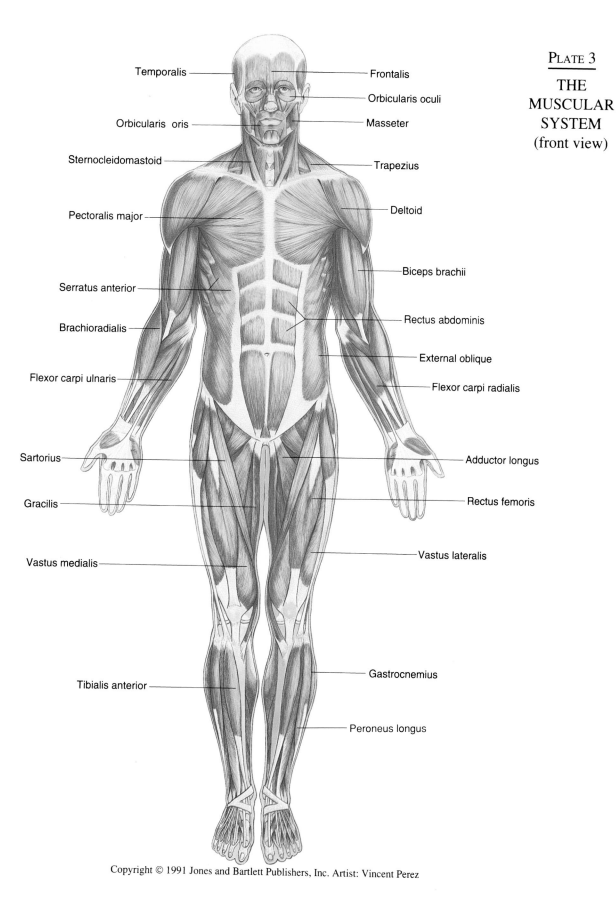

Temporalis

Frontalis

Orbicularis oculi

Orbicularis oris

Masseter

Sternocleidomastoid

Trapezius

Pectoralis major

Deltoid

Biceps brachii

Serratus anterior

Rectus abdominis

Brachioradialis

External oblique

Flexor carpi ulnaris

Flexor carpi radialis

Sartorius

Adductor longus

Gracilis

Rectus femoris

Vastus medialis

Vastus lateralis

Tibialis anterior

Gastrocnemius

Peroneus longus

PLATE 3

THE
MUSCULAR
SYSTEM
(front view)

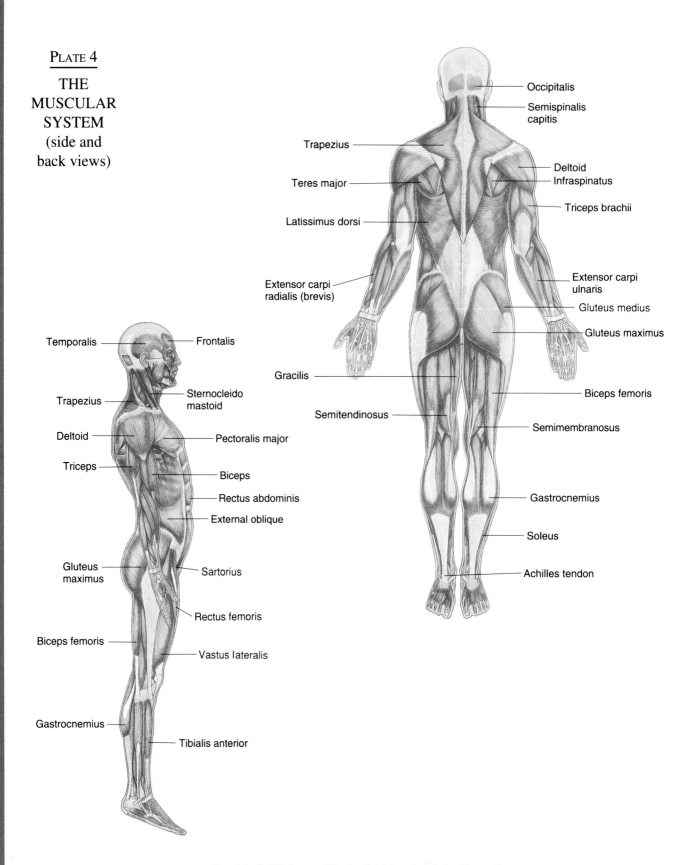

PLATE 4

THE
MUSCULAR
SYSTEM
(side and
back views)

Occipitalis

Semispinalis
capitis

Trapezius

Deltoid

Infraspinatus

Teres major

Triceps brachii

Latissimus dorsi

Extensor carpi
ulnaris

Gluteus medius

Gluteus maximus

Extensor carpi
radialis (brevis)

Gracilis

Biceps femoris

Semitendinosus

Semimembranosus

Temporalis

Frontalis

Gastrocnemius

Trapezius

Sternocleido
mastoid

Soleus

Deltoid

Achilles tendon

Pectoralis major

Triceps

Biceps

Rectus abdominis

External oblique

Gluteus
maximus

Sartorius

Rectus femoris

Biceps femoris

Vastus lateralis

Gastrocnemius

Tibialis anterior

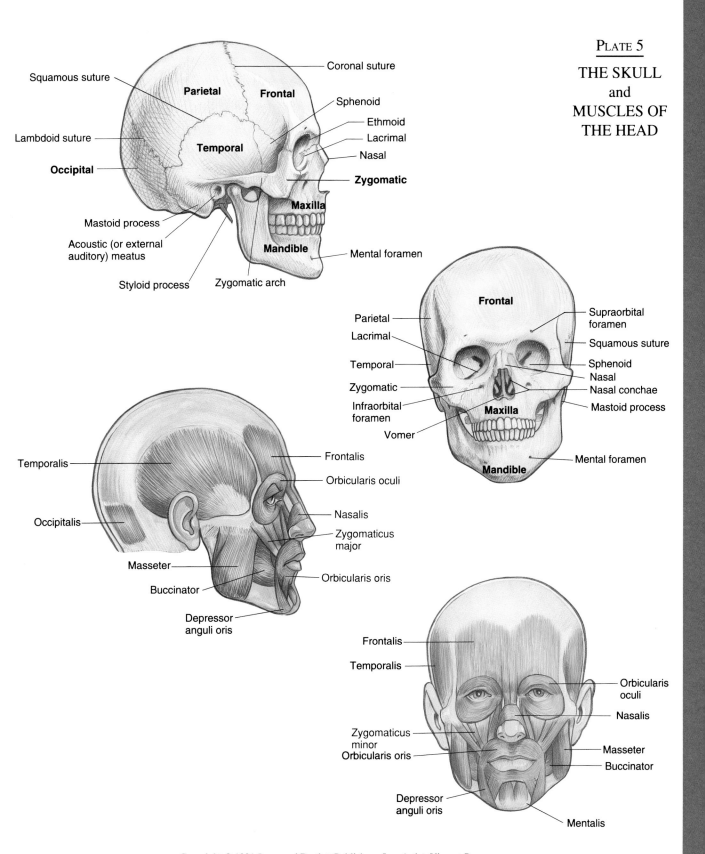

PLATE 5

THE SKULL
and
MUSCLES OF
THE HEAD

Coronal suture

Squamous suture

Parietal **Frontal**

Sphenoid

Ethmoid

Lacrimal

Lambdoid suture

Nasal

Temporal

Zygomatic

Occipital

Maxilla

Mastoid process

Mandible

Mental foramen

Acoustic (or external auditory) meatus

Styloid process Zygomatic arch

Frontal

Parietal

Supraorbital foramen

Lacrimal

Squamous suture

Temporal

Sphenoid

Zygomatic

Nasal

Nasal conchae

Infraorbital foramen

Maxilla

Mastoid process

Vomer

Mental foramen

Mandible

Temporalis

Frontalis

Orbicularis oculi

Nasalis

Occipitalis

Zygomaticus major

Masseter

Orbicularis oris

Buccinator

Depressor anguli oris

Frontalis

Temporalis

Orbicularis oculi

Nasalis

Zygomaticus minor

Orbicularis oris

Masseter

Buccinator

Depressor anguli oris

Mentalis

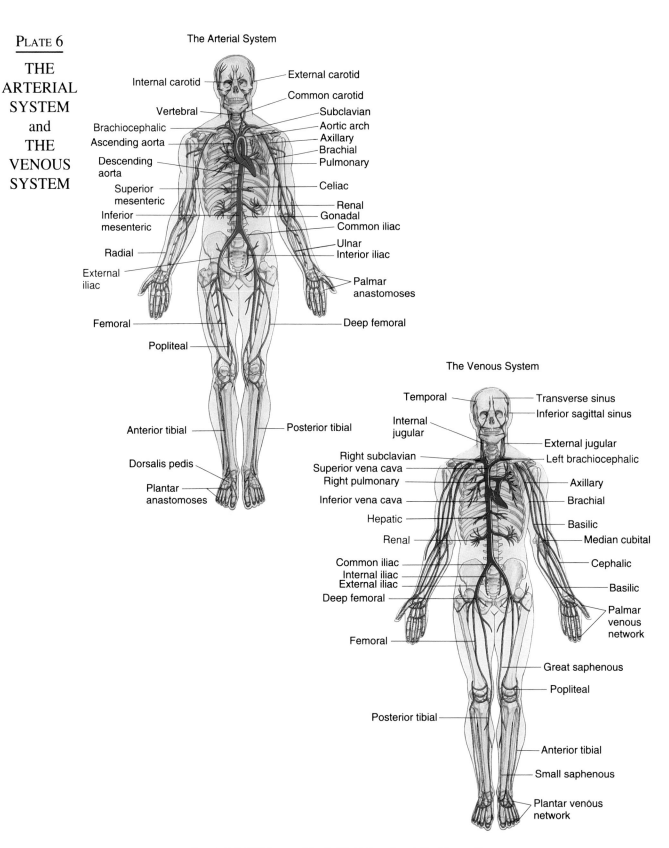

PLATE 6

THE
ARTERIAL
SYSTEM
and
THE
VENOUS
SYSTEM

The Arterial System

Internal carotid
External carotid
Common carotid
Vertebral
Subclavian
Brachiocephalic
Aortic arch
Ascending aorta
Axillary
Descending aorta
Brachial
Pulmonary
Superior mesenteric
Celiac
Inferior mesenteric
Renal
Gonadal
Common iliac
Radial
Ulnar
Interior iliac
External iliac
Palmar anastomoses
Femoral
Deep femoral
Popliteal
Anterior tibial
Posterior tibial
Dorsalis pedis
Plantar anastomoses

The Venous System

Temporal
Transverse sinus
Inferior sagittal sinus
Internal jugular
External jugular
Right subclavian
Left brachiocephalic
Superior vena cava
Axillary
Right pulmonary
Brachial
Inferior vena cava
Basilic
Hepatic
Median cubital
Renal
Common iliac
Cephalic
Internal iliac
External iliac
Basilic
Deep femoral
Palmar venous network
Femoral
Great saphenous
Popliteal
Posterior tibial
Anterior tibial
Small saphenous
Plantar venous network

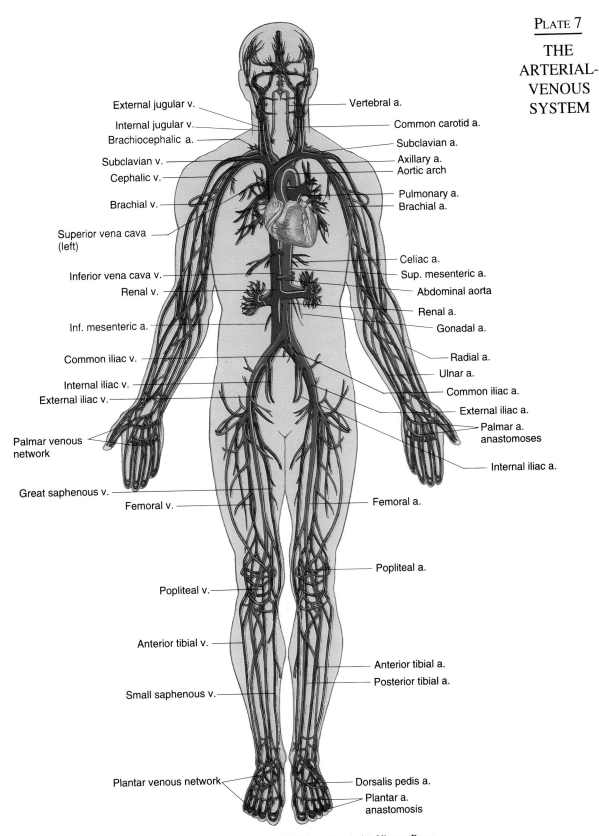

PLATE 7

THE
ARTERIAL-
VENOUS
SYSTEM

External jugular v.

Internal jugular v.

Brachiocephalic a.

Subclavian v.

Cephalic v.

Brachial v.

Superior vena cava
(left)

Inferior vena cava v.

Renal v.

Inf. mesenteric a.

Common iliac v.

Internal iliac v.

External iliac v.

Palmar venous
network

Great saphenous v.

Femoral v.

Popliteal v.

Anterior tibial v.

Small saphenous v.

Plantar venous network

Vertebral a.

Common carotid a.

Subclavian a.

Axillary a.

Aortic arch

Pulmonary a.

Brachial a.

Celiac a.

Sup. mesenteric a.

Abdominal aorta

Renal a.

Gonadal a.

Radial a.

Ulnar a.

Common iliac a.

External iliac a.

Palmar a.
anastomoses

Internal iliac a.

Femoral a.

Popliteal a.

Anterior tibial a.

Posterior tibial a.

Dorsalis pedis a.

Plantar a.
anastomosis

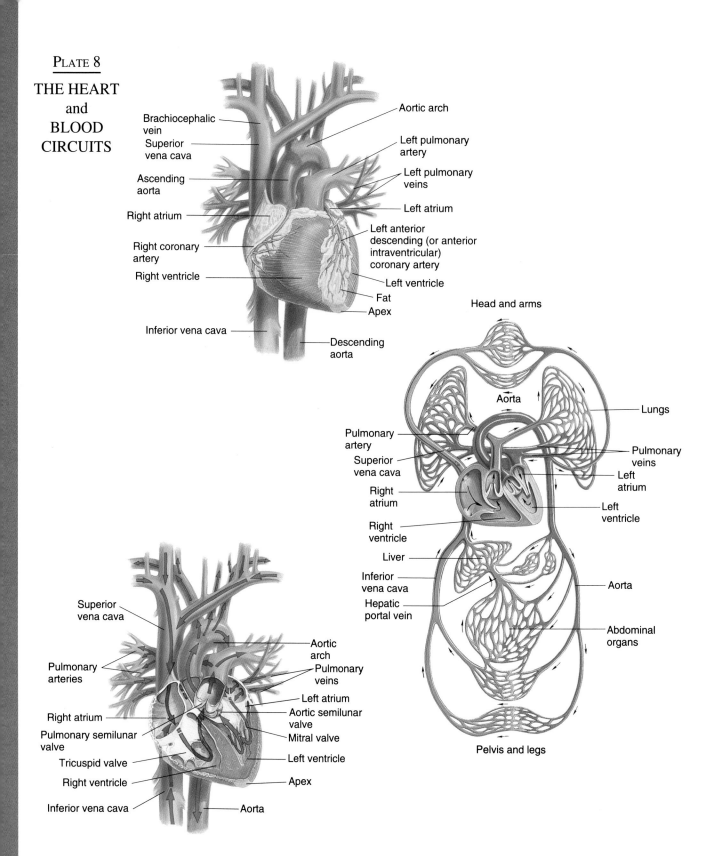

PLATE 8

THE HEART
and
BLOOD
CIRCUITS

Brachiocephalic vein
Superior vena cava
Ascending aorta
Right atrium
Right coronary artery
Right ventricle
Inferior vena cava

Aortic arch
Left pulmonary artery
Left pulmonary veins
Left atrium
Left anterior descending (or anterior intraventricular) coronary artery
Left ventricle
Fat
Apex
Descending aorta

Head and arms
Aorta
Lungs
Pulmonary artery
Pulmonary veins
Superior vena cava
Left atrium
Right atrium
Left ventricle
Right ventricle
Liver
Inferior vena cava
Aorta
Hepatic portal vein
Abdominal organs
Pelvis and legs

Superior vena cava
Pulmonary arteries
Right atrium
Pulmonary semilunar valve
Tricuspid valve
Right ventricle
Inferior vena cava

Aortic arch
Pulmonary veins
Left atrium
Aortic semilunar valve
Mitral valve
Left ventricle
Apex
Aorta

PLATE 9

THE
ENDOCRINE
SYSTEM

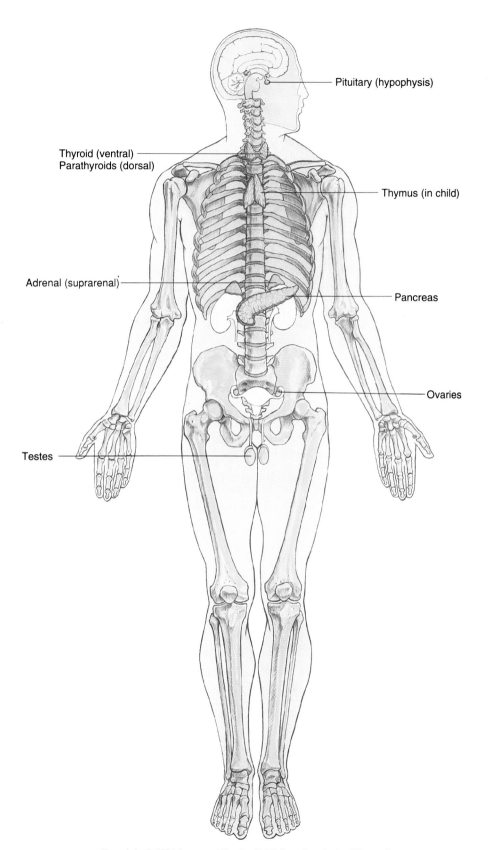

Pituitary (hypophysis)

Thyroid (ventral)
Parathyroids (dorsal)

Thymus (in child)

Adrenal (suprarenal)

Pancreas

Ovaries

Testes

PLATE 10

THE
LYMPHATIC
SYSTEM

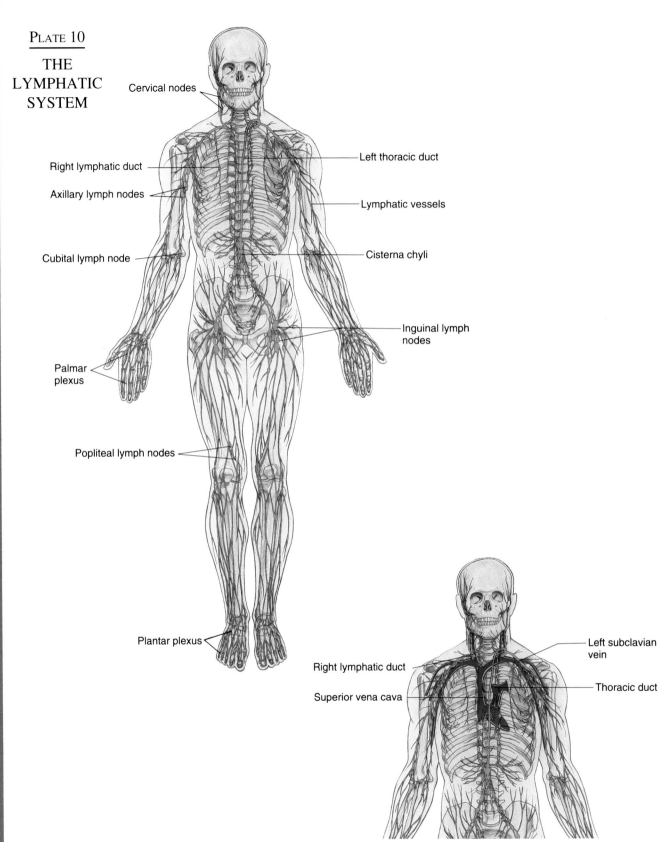

Cervical nodes

Right lymphatic duct

Axillary lymph nodes

Cubital lymph node

Palmar
plexus

Popliteal lymph nodes

Plantar plexus

Left thoracic duct

Lymphatic vessels

Cisterna chyli

Inguinal lymph
nodes

Right lymphatic duct

Superior vena cava

Left subclavian
vein

Thoracic duct

Copyright © 1991 Jones and Bartlett Publishers, Inc. Artist: Vincent Perez

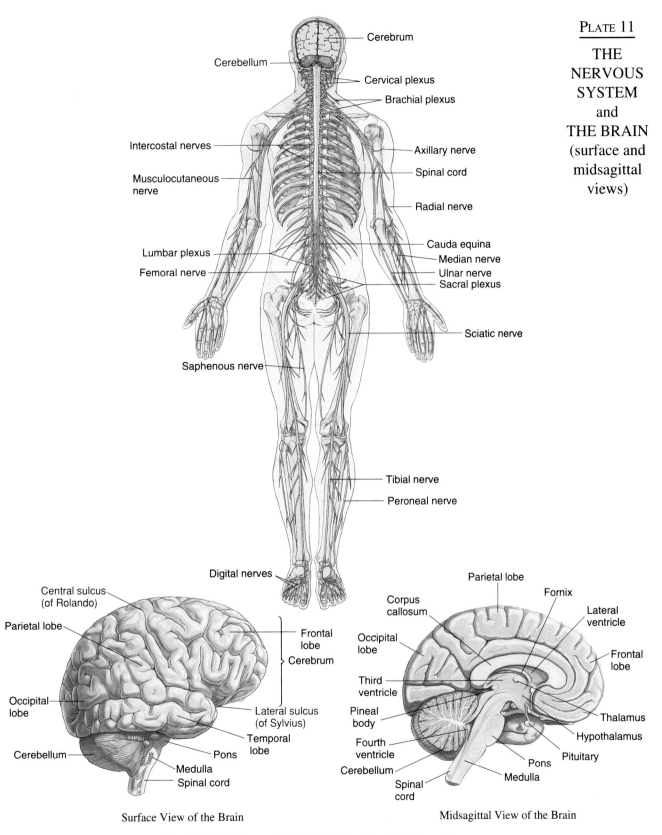

Cerebrum

Cerebellum

Cervical plexus

Brachial plexus

Intercostal nerves

Axillary nerve

Musculocutaneous nerve

Spinal cord

Radial nerve

Cauda equina

Median nerve

Lumbar plexus

Ulnar nerve

Femoral nerve

Sacral plexus

Sciatic nerve

Saphenous nerve

Tibial nerve

Peroneal nerve

Digital nerves

Central sulcus (of Rolando)

Parietal lobe

Occipital lobe

Cerebellum

Frontal lobe

Cerebrum

Lateral sulcus (of Sylvius)

Temporal lobe

Pons

Medulla

Spinal cord

Surface View of the Brain

Parietal lobe

Corpus callosum

Fornix

Lateral ventricle

Occipital lobe

Frontal lobe

Third ventricle

Thalamus

Pineal body

Hypothalamus

Fourth ventricle

Pituitary

Cerebellum

Pons

Spinal cord

Medulla

Midsagittal View of the Brain

Copyright © 1991 Jones and Bartlett Publishers, Inc. Artist: Vincent Perez

PLATE 12

THE
VISCERA

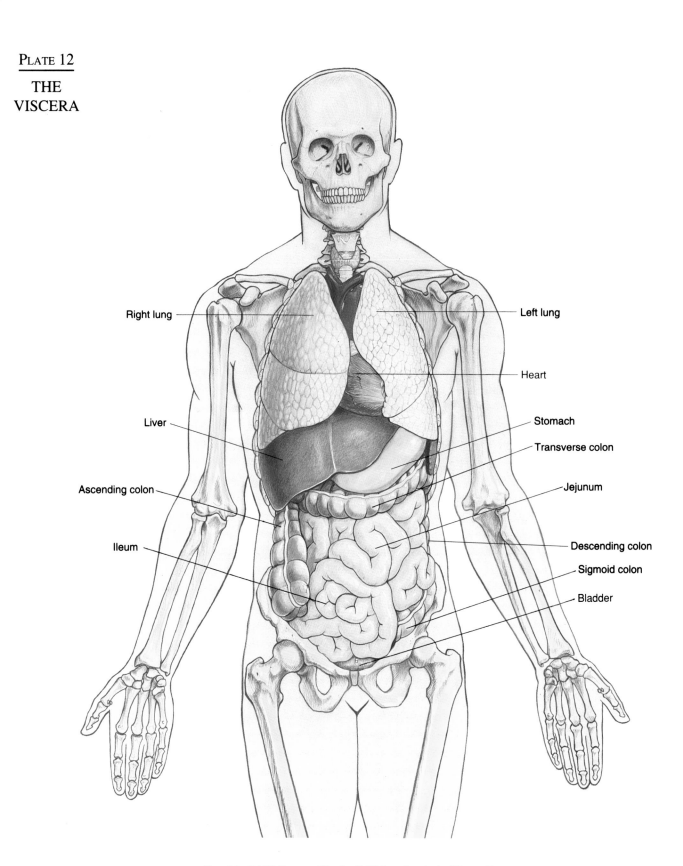

Right lung

Left lung

Heart

Liver

Stomach

Transverse colon

Ascending colon

Jejunum

Ileum

Descending colon

Sigmoid colon

Bladder

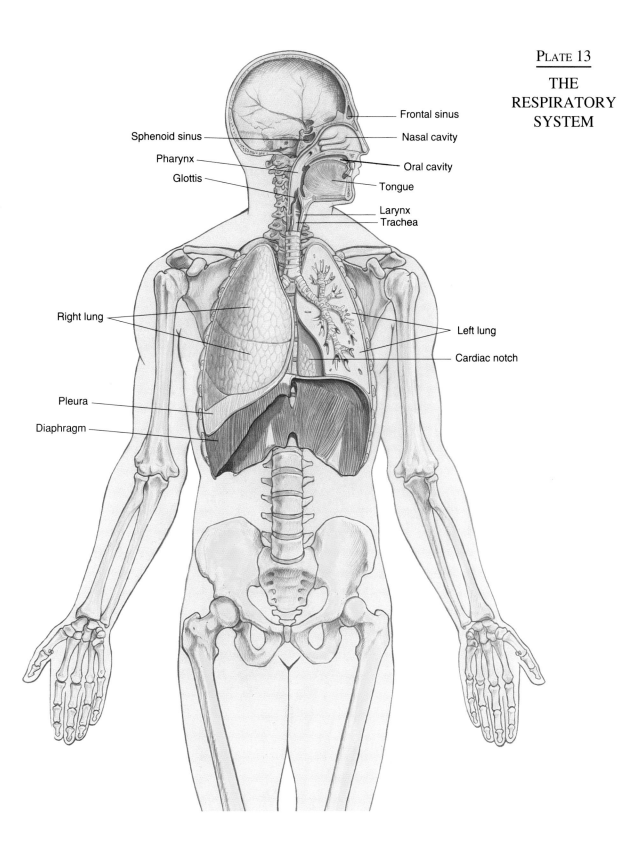

PLATE 13

THE
RESPIRATORY
SYSTEM

Frontal sinus

Sphenoid sinus

Nasal cavity

Pharynx

Oral cavity

Glottis

Tongue

Larynx
Trachea

Right lung

Left lung

Cardiac notch

Pleura

Diaphragm

PLATE 14

THE DIGESTIVE SYSTEM

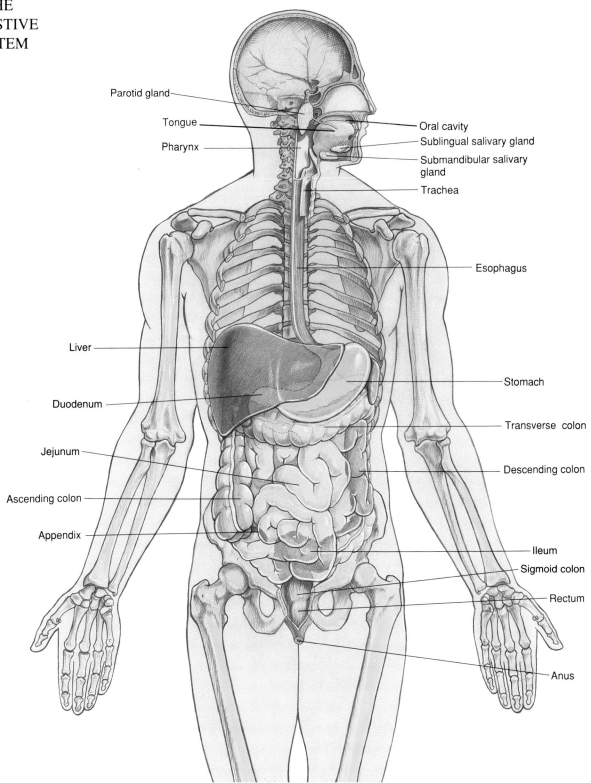

Parotid gland

Tongue

Pharynx

Oral cavity

Sublingual salivary gland

Submandibular salivary gland

Trachea

Esophagus

Liver

Stomach

Duodenum

Transverse colon

Jejunum

Descending colon

Ascending colon

Appendix

Ileum

Sigmoid colon

Rectum

Anus

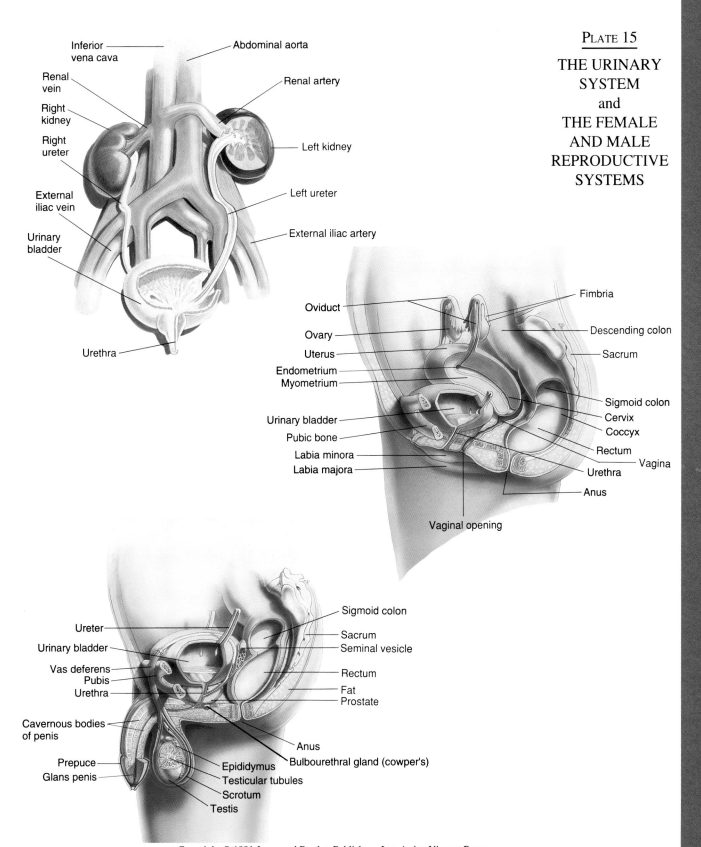

PLATE 15

THE URINARY
SYSTEM
and
THE FEMALE
AND MALE
REPRODUCTIVE
SYSTEMS

Inferior vena cava

Abdominal aorta

Renal vein

Renal artery

Right kidney

Left kidney

Right ureter

External iliac vein

Left ureter

Urinary bladder

External iliac artery

Urethra

Oviduct

Fimbria

Ovary

Descending colon

Uterus

Sacrum

Endometrium

Myometrium

Urinary bladder

Sigmoid colon

Pubic bone

Cervix

Coccyx

Labia minora

Rectum

Labia majora

Vagina

Urethra

Anus

Vaginal opening

Ureter

Sigmoid colon

Urinary bladder

Sacrum

Vas deferens

Seminal vesicle

Pubis

Urethra

Rectum

Cavernous bodies of penis

Fat

Prostate

Anus

Prepuce

Bulbourethral gland (cowper's)

Glans penis

Epididymus

Testicular tubules

Scrotum

Testis

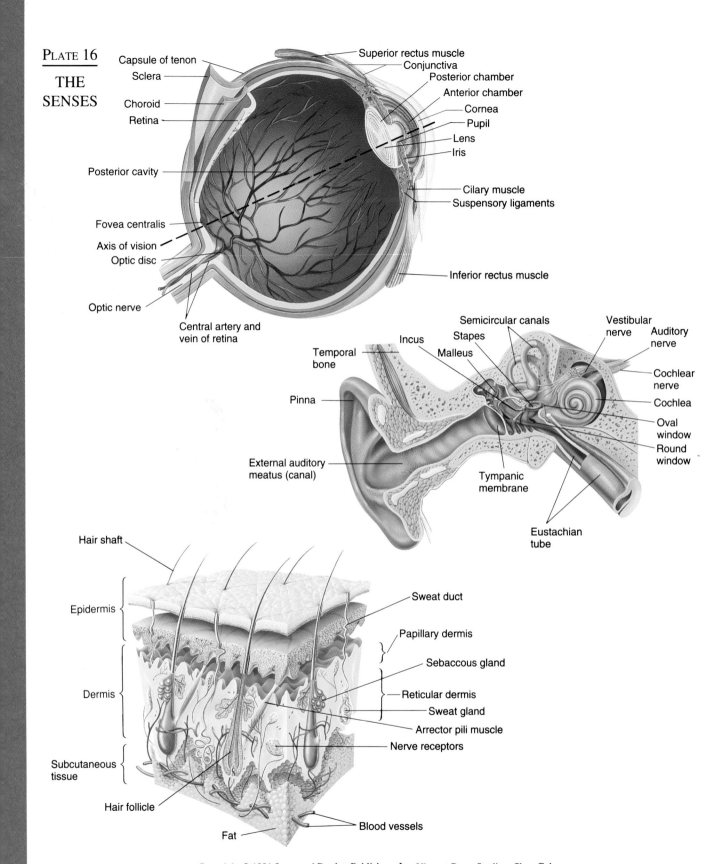

PLATE 16

THE
SENSES

Eye diagram labels:
Capsule of tenon
Sclera
Choroid
Retina
Posterior cavity
Fovea centralis
Axis of vision
Optic disc
Optic nerve
Central artery and vein of retina
Superior rectus muscle
Conjunctiva
Posterior chamber
Anterior chamber
Cornea
Pupil
Lens
Iris
Cilary muscle
Suspensory ligaments
Inferior rectus muscle

Ear diagram labels:
Temporal bone
Pinna
External auditory meatus (canal)
Incus
Malleus
Stapes
Semicircular canals
Tympanic membrane
Vestibular nerve
Auditory nerve
Cochlear nerve
Cochlea
Oval window
Round window
Eustachian tube

Skin diagram labels:
Hair shaft
Epidermis
Dermis
Subcutaneous tissue
Hair follicle
Fat
Sweat duct
Papillary dermis
Sebaccous gland
Reticular dermis
Sweat gland
Arrector pili muscle
Nerve receptors
Blood vessels

CHAPTER 18 Eyes and Ears

OBJECTIVES

After completing this chapter and the exercises, the student should be able to:

1. Identify and label the structures of the eyes and ears.
2. Describe the functions of the eyes and ears.
3. Define and explain various pathological conditions affecting the eyes and ears.
4. Identify important laboratory tests and procedures related to the diagnosis and treatment for conditions of these special sense organs.
5. Use correctly spelled terminology to build medical words related to structure, function, and pathological conditions of these special sense organs.
6. Define commonly used abbreviations.

OVERVIEW

The eyes and ears are part of special senses that stem from the peripheral nervous system (PNS). When studying this chapter, refer to Figures 18–1 and 18–2.

The eye is an optical system that focuses light rays on photoreceptors, which change light energy to nerve impulses. Human eyes are spherical organs located in bony orbits, or eye sockets, cavities formed by the bones of the skull. The eye is embedded in orbital fat for insulation and protection. It is attached to the orbit by six muscles, the extrinsic eye muscles, which control eye movement. Small tendons connect these muscles to the outermost layer of the eye. Structures of the eye include the following:

1. The *sclera* is the tough, white outer layer of the eyeball that protects the interior of the eye. At the front of the eye, the sclera forms a domed transparent orb called the *cornea.* The cornea has a curved surface that focuses light coming into the eye.

2. The *uvea* is the vascular layer below the sclera. It supplies blood to muscles and nerves within the eye and gives the eye its color. It contains three structures: the choroid, the ciliary body, and the iris.

3. The *choroid,* a darkly pigmented layer of tissue, houses many tiny blood vessels and acts to absorb light within the eye. This prevents blurring of visual images. The *ciliary body,* an extension of the choroid, enables the eye to focus on objects of varying distances. Another extension of the choroid is the *iris.* The pigmentation of the iris is what determines eye color. At the center of the iris is an opening called the *pupil.* The pupil of the eye expands and contracts, regulating the amount of light entering the eye.

4. On the inner surface of the choroid is the *retina,* light-sensitive receptor cells. The retina contains rods and cones that detect color stimuli (photopigments), which it sends to the brain for interpretation.

5. The *optic nerve* carries impulses from the retina to areas of the brain that are responsible for processing visual information.

6. Although not involved in vision directly, the eyelids and eyelashes protect the eyeball from physical trauma. A thin membrane known as *conjunctiva* lines the inside of each eyelid.

7. The *lacrimal* glands of the eye produce tears, which keep the eye lubricated (see Plate 16 for further details).

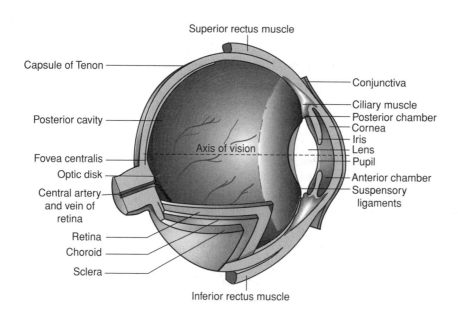

FIGURE 18–1 Structure of the eye, transverse section.

The ear has three distinct and anatomically separate sections—the outer, middle, and inner ears. Please refer to the appropriate figure(s) to visualize each as we discuss their structure and functions. See Plate 16 and Figure 18–2.

The middle ear lies within the temporal bones of the skull. It contains three tiny bones, the auditory ossicles. They are named for their shapes. Starting from the outside they are the *malleus* (hammer), *incus* (anvil), and *stapes* (stirrup). The malleus is connected to the *tympanic membrane.*

The middle ear cavity opens to the pharynx via the *eustachian tube,* also called the auditory tube. The eustachian tube serves as a pressure valve. Yawning and swallowing open the tube to equalize pressure within the middle ear.

The inner ear is a mazelike structure that occupies a large cavity in the temporal bone. It consists of bony and membranous structures surrounded by fluid. It contains two sensory organs—the *cochlea,* a snail-shell-shaped bony structure that houses the organs of hearing, and the *vestibular apparatus.*

The *cochlea* is a a hollow, bony spiral containing three fluid-filled canals—the *upper vestibular canal,* the *middle cochlear canal,* and the *lower tympanic canal.*

The *organ of Corti* contains the receptor cells, tiny hair cells that are stimulated by sound vibrations. The sound vibrations are then converted to nerve impulses that are transmitted to the brain for interpretation.

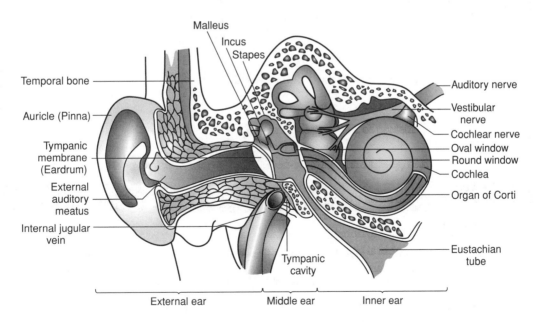

FIGURE 18–2 Frontal diagram of the outer ear, middle ear, and internal ear. A section of the cochlear duct has been cut away to show the position of the organ of Corti.

To summarize briefly how we hear, let us create a pathway of sound waves through the ear by structure and function:

1. The outer ear auricle (*pinna*) funnels sound waves into the external auditory canal, which directs it to the tympanic membrane (eardrum), causing it to vibrate.
2. The middle ear, which contains the eardrum ossicles, the malleus, incus, and stapes, vibrate when struck by the sound waves and transmit the sound to the cochlea in the inner ear by causing the oval window to vibrate the fluids within the canals.
3. The cochlea converts the fluid waves to nerve impulses. The semicircular canals, the *sacculi* and *utricle*, detect head movement and linear acceleration.
4. The auditory nerve fibers that lie close to the hair cells of the organ of Corti pick up the sound wave impulses and transmit them to the cerebral cortex of the brain, where they are interpreted and we are able to hear.

All the structures and functions pertaining to the eyes and ears are defined and illustrated throughout the chapter. Major disorders and diseases are also defined and discussed.

| LESSON ONE | MATERIALS TO BE LEARNED |

Figures 18–1 and 18–2 describe the anatomic parts of the eyes and ears.

EYES

Structure of the Eye

Table 18–1

Structure	Pronunciation	Definition
sclera	<u>skle</u>-rah	tough white outer coat of the eyeball
conjunctiva	kon'junk-<u>ti</u>-vah	membrane lining the eyelids and covering the eyeball
cornea	<u>kor</u>-ne-ah	transparent anterior part of the eye
choroid	<u>ko</u>-roid	the middle, vascular coat of the eye, between the sclera and the retina
iris	<u>i</u>-ris	pigmented membrane behind the cornea, perforated by the pupil
pupil	<u>pu</u>-pil	opening in the center through which light enters the eye
lens	lenz	transparent body separating the posterior chamber and constituting the refracting mechanism of the eye

Structure	Pronunciation	Definition
ciliary muscle	<u>sil</u>-e-er'e <u>mus</u>-el	eye muscle capable of changing lens shape during contraction and relaxation
aqueous humor	<u>a</u>-kwe-us <u>hu</u>-mor	watery liquid in chamber in the front of the lens; it circulates through the anterior chamber of the eye
vitreous humor	<u>vit</u>-re-us <u>hu</u>-mor	jellylike transparent substance in the posterior chamber
retina	<u>ret</u>-i-nah	innermost layer of the eyeball, containing elements for reception and transmission of visual stimuli

Eye Disorders

Table 18–2

Disorder	Pronunciation	Definition
amblyopia	am'ble-<u>o</u>-pe-ah	dimness of vision without a detectable organic lesion of the eye; related to absence, weakness, or paralysis of an eye muscle
astigmatism	ah-<u>stig</u>-mah-tism	condition characterized by irregular cornea and lens of the eye; corrected with lenses
blepharitis	blef'ah-<u>ri</u>-tis	inflammation of the eyelids
blepharoptosis	blef'ar-op-<u>to</u>-sis	drooping of upper eyelid
cataract	<u>kat</u>-ah-rakt	opaque (not clear) lens of the eye
chalazion	kah-<u>la</u>-ze-on	a small eyelid mass resulting from chronic inflammation of a meibomian gland
color blindness	<u>kul</u>-er <u>blind</u>-nes	popular term for any deviation from normal perception of color
conjunctivitis	kon-junk'ti-<u>vi</u>-tis	inflammation of the conjunctiva
corneal ulcer	<u>kor</u>-ne-al <u>ul</u>-ser	a local inflammation of the cornea caused by injury or inflammation
dacryoadenitis	dak're-o-ad'e-<u>ni</u>-tis	inflammation of a lacrimal gland
dacryocystitis	dak-re-o-sis-<u>ti</u>-tis	inflammation of the lacrimal sac
dacryolith	<u>dak</u>-re-o-lith'	a lacrimal calculus (stone)

Disorder	Pronunciation	Definition
detached retina	de-<u>tacht</u> <u>ret</u>-i-nah	separation of the inner layers of the retina from the pigment epithelium
diabetic retinopathy	<u>dye</u>-ah'-bet-ic' <u>reh</u>-tin-op'-ah-thee'	scarring of the capillaries of the retina as a consequence of DM of long duration. Retinal effects of DM include abnormal dilation of the retinal veins, hemorrhage, microaneurysms, and neovascularization (new blood vessels forming near the optic disk causing leakage of blood). These effects cause a permanent decline in vision and will lead to blindness. Diabetic retinopathy is a leading cause of blindness in the U.S.
floaters (in vitreous)	<u>flo</u>-ters	"spots before the eyes"; these deposits in the vitreous of the eye usually move about and are probably a benign degenerative change. Also seen in hypertension
foreign body in the eye	<u>for</u>-in <u>bod</u>-e	any object not belonging to the eye; hazards depending on circumstances
glaucoma	glaw-<u>ko</u>-mah	eye disease characterized by an increase in intraocular pressure related to alterations in circulation of vitreous humor, causing pathologic changes and visual defects
hemorrhage (subconjunctival)	<u>hem</u>-o-rij (sub'-kon-junk-<u>ti</u>-val)	blood escaping from the vessels, and bleeding from beneath the conjunctiva
herpes zoster (ophthalmic)	<u>her</u>-pez <u>zos</u>-ter (of-<u>thal</u>-mic)	involving the fifth cranial nerve (forehead, eyelid, and cornea), this infection by a herpes virus can be serious
hyperopia	hi'per-<u>o</u>-pe-ah	farsightedness, e.g., the person cannot read a book
injury	<u>in</u>-ju-re	eye injuries include foreign bodies, contusions, lacerations, burns, etc.
iritis	i-<u>ri</u>-tis	inflammation of the iris
keratoconus	ker'ah-to-<u>ko</u>-nus	conical protrusion of the central part of the cornea
macular degeneration	mah'-<u>cull</u>-lar de-<u>jen</u>-er-aye-<u>shun</u>	deterioration of the macula of the eye, resulting in a severe loss of central vision in the affected eye
meibomian cyst	mi-<u>bo</u>-me-an	a small localized swelling of the eyelid resulting from obstruction and retained secretions of the meibomian glands. A nonmalignant condition; often requires surgery for correction
nystagmus	nis-<u>tag</u>-mus	involuntary rapid movement (horizontal, vertical, rotary, or mixed, i.e., of two types) of the eyeball
papilledema	pap'il-e-<u>de</u>-mah	edema of the optic disk

Disorder	Pronunciation	Definition
presbyopia	pres-be-<u>o</u>-pe-ah	diminution of accommodation of the lens of the eye caused by loss of elasticity, normally occurring with aging; farsightedness
ptosis	<u>to</u>-sis	drooping of upper eyelid
retinitis	ret′i-<u>ni</u>-tis	inflammation of the retina
retinoblastoma	ret′i-no-blas-<u>to</u>-mah	a tumor arising from the retinal cells
retinopathy	ret′i-<u>nop</u>-ah-the	any disease of the retina
strabismus	strah-<u>biz</u>-mus	squint; deviation of the eye from normal; crossed eyes; usually correctable
stye (or hordeolum)	sti (hor-<u>de</u>-o-lum)	inflammation of the sebaceous glands of the eyelid
trachoma	trah-<u>ko</u>-mah	a contagious disease of the conjunctiva and cornea, producing photophobia, pain, and lacrimation; uncommon
uveitis	u′ve-<u>i</u>-tis	inflammation of the uvea (iris and blood vessels)

Eye Diagnosis and Surgery

Table 18–3

Diagnosis or Surgery	Pronunciation	Definition
cataract extraction	<u>kat</u>-ah-rakt eks-<u>trak</u>-shun	a surgical excision of the lens of the eye. Special lenses or glasses are prescribed
cryoextraction	kri′o-eks-<u>trak</u>-shun	application of extremely low temperature for the removal of a cataractous lens
cryoretinopexy	kri′o-<u>ret</u>-i-no-pex-ee	fixation of a detached retina using extremely low temperature instead of the laser beam
dacryocystotomy	dak′re-o-sis-<u>tot</u>-o-me	incision of the lacrimal sac and duct
enucleation	e-nu′kle-<u>a</u>-shun	surgical removal of the eye
fundoscopy	fun-<u>dus</u>-ko-pe	examination and study of the fundus of the eye by means of an ophthalmoscope
gonioscopy	go′ne-<u>os</u>-ko-pe	instrument for demonstrating ocular motility and rotation
iridectomy	ir′i-<u>dek</u>-to-me	excision of part of the iris
iridencleisis	ir′i-den-<u>kli</u>-sis	excision of part of the iris in glaucoma

Diagnosis or Surgery	Pronunciation	Definition
keratoplasty	ker-ah-to-plas'te	plastic surgery of the cornea; corneal grafting
laser photocoagulation	la-zer fo'to-ko-ag'u-la-shun	using the laser beam to treat retinal detachment
pterygium surgery	te-rig-e-um ser-jer-e	growth of the conjunctiva: neovascularization that invades the cornea; it can be removed surgically
slit lamp		an instrument used in ophthalmology for examining the conjunctiva, lens, vitreous humor, iris, and cornea. A high-intensity beam of light is projected through a narrow slit and a cross-section of the illuminated part of the eye is examined through a magnifying lens
tonometer	to-nom-e-ter	instrument for measuring tension or pressure, especially intraocular pressure
tonometry	to-nom-e-tre	measurement of tension or pressure, e.g., intraocular pressure
trabeculectomy	trah-bek'u-lec-to-me	excision of fibrous bands or connective tissue
vitrectomy	vi-trek-to-me	aspiration of vitreous fluid and replacement with saline solution

Common Medical Eye Terms

Table 18–4

Term	Pronunciation	Definition
accommodation	ah-kom'o-da-tion	adjustment of the eye for seeing objects at various distances
anisocoria	an'i-so-ko-re-ah	inequality in size of the pupils of the eyes
Braille	brāl	a system of printing for the blind consisting of raised dots and prints that can be read by touch
canal of Schlemm	kah-nal of Shlem	opening through which aqueous humor must flow out or pressure in the eye increases resulting in glaucoma
canthus (pl., canthi)	kan-thus	the angle at either end of the fissure between the eyelids
CC		with correction (glasses or lenses)
cryoprobe	kri-o-prob	an instrument for applying extreme cold to tissue
cystitome	sis-ti-tome	an instrument for opening the lens capsule

Term	Pronunciation	Definition
diopter	di-<u>op</u>-ter	unit of measure for lenses
electronystagmography	e-lek'tro-nis'tag-<u>mog</u>-rah-fe	recordings of eye movements to provide objective documentation of induced and spontaneous nystagmus
emmetropia	em'e-<u>tro</u>-pe-ah	normal vision
eye bank		storage for donor organs
fundus	<u>fun</u>-dus	the back portion of the interior of the eyeball, visible through the pupil by use of the ophthalmoscope
funduscope (or ophthalmoscope)	<u>fun</u>-dus-skōp (of-<u>thal</u>-mo-skōp)	an instrument containing a perforated mirror and lenses used to examine the interior of the eye; also spelled "fundoscope"
guide dogs		trained dogs for the blind; also called seeing-eye dogs
lacrimation	lak'ri-<u>ma</u>-shun	secretion and discharge of tears
laser	<u>la</u>-zer	a device that transfers light of various frequencies into an extremely intense, small beam of radiation. It is used as a tool in surgery, in diagnosis, and in physiologic studies
lensometer	lenz-<u>om</u>-e-ter	device for obtaining eyeglass prescriptions
miotic (or myotic)	mi-<u>ot</u>-ik	a drug that causes contraction of the pupil
mydriatic	mid're-<u>at</u>-ik	a drug that dilates the pupil
OD		abbreviation for oculus dexter (right eye)
ophthalmoscope	of'<u>thal</u>-mo-skop	instrument containing a perforated mirror and lenses, used to examine the interior of the eye; also called funduscope
OS		abbreviation for oculus sinister (left eye)
OU		abbreviation for oculus uterque (each eye) or oculus unitas (both eyes)
peripheral vision	pe-<u>rif</u>-er-al <u>vizh</u>-un	vision at the outer edges when the eyes are looking straight ahead
PERRLA (or PERLA)		acronym for Pupils Equal, Round, React to Light, Accommodation
refractive error	re-<u>frak</u>-tiv	the determination of the refractive errors of the eye and their correction with glasses or lenses

Term	Pronunciation	Definition
SC		without correction (glasses or lenses)
Snellen eye chart		one of several charts used in testing visual acuity. Letters, numbers, or symbols are arranged on the chart in decreasing size from top to bottom
visual acuity (VA)	vizh'<u>u</u>-al ah-<u>ku</u>-i-te	clarity or clearness of vision
20/20 vision		a person who can read what the average person can read at 20 feet has 20/20 vision

EARS

Structure of the Ear

Table 18–5

Structure	Pronunciation	Definition
external ear		auricle (or pinna) or ear canal
middle ear		separated from the external ear by the tympanic membrane; consists of three bones: malleus, incus, and stapes
inner ear		the complex inner structure of the ear: vestibule, semicircular canals, and cochlea, composing the membranous labyrinth
tympanic membrane	tim-<u>pan</u>-ik <u>mem</u>-brane	the thin partition between the external acoustic meatus and the middle ear
tympanum	<u>tim</u>-pan-um	eardrum (middle ear)
cerumen	se-<u>roo</u>-men	earwax
eustachian tube	u-<u>stay</u>-shen	a tube, lined with mucous membrane, that joins the nasopharynx and the tympanic cavity; accomplishes equalization of air pressure

Ear Disorders

Table 18–6

Disorder	Pronunciation	Definition
acoustic neuroma	ah'-<u>koos</u>-tic new-rom-ah	A benign tumor arising from the acoustic nerve in the brain. This tumor causes tinnitus, vertigo, and decreased hearing. Small tumors may be surgically resected or removed by radiation therapy

Disorder	Pronunciation	Definition
cholesteatoma	koh-les-tee′-ah-toh-mah	a collection of skin cells and cholesterol in a sac within the middle ear. These cystlike masses are most often the result of chronic otitis media, but may also be a congenital defect. Cholesteatoma can lead to conductive hearing loss, occlusion of the middle ear, destruction of ossicles, and inner ear erosion. Symptoms include weakness of facial muscles, drainage from the affected ear, vertigo, and earache
conduction deafness	kon-duk-<u>shun</u>	hearing loss that occurs when the conduction of sound waves through the external and middle ear to the inner ear is impaired
deafness	<u>def</u>-nes	lacking the sense of hearing; hearing impairment
eustachian salpingitis	u-<u>stay</u>-shen sal′pin-<u>ji</u>-tis	inflammation of the eustachian tubes
furunculosis	fu-rung′ku-<u>lo</u>-sis	a skin infection affecting the ear canal
impacted cerumen	im-<u>pak</u>-ted se-<u>roo</u>-men	cerumen (earwax) impacted firmly into the ear
labyrinthitis	lab′i-rin-<u>thi</u>-tis	inflammation of the labyrinth (inner ear); otitis interna
mastoiditis	mas′toi-<u>di</u>-tis	inflammation of the mastoid antrum and cells (of the temporal bone)
Meniere's disease	Men′e-<u>ārz</u> di-<u>zez</u>	deafness, tinnitus, and dizziness; causes unknown
myringitis	mir′in-<u>ji</u>-tis	inflammation of the tympanic membrane (eardrum)
otitis externa	o-ti-tis ex-<u>ter</u>-na	inflammation of the external ear
otitis media	o-ti-tis <u>me</u>-di-a	inflammation of the middle ear
otosclerosis	o′to-skle-<u>ro</u>-sis	ankylosis of the stapes, resulting in conductive hearing loss
presbycusis	pres′bĭ-<u>ku</u>-sis	progressive hearing loss in some elderly persons
sensorineural deafness	<u>sen</u>-soh′-ree-<u>noo</u>-ral	also called nerve deafness, this type of hearing loss results from physical damage to the hair cells, the vestibulocochlear nerve, or the auditory cortex. This condition may occur because of aging. Explosions, extremely loud noises, such as from machinery or loud music, and some antibiotics can damage the hair cells in the organ of Corti, creating partial to complete deafness. Other causes include brain tumors, strokes, infections, trauma, vascular disorders, and degenerative diseases

Ear Surgery

Table 18–7

Surgery	Pronunciation	Definition
fenestration	fen′es-<u>tra</u>-shun	the surgical creation of a new opening in the labyrinth of the ear for restoration of hearing in otosclerosis
mastoidectomy	mas′toi-<u>dek</u>-to-me	excision of the mastoid cells or the mastoid process
myringotomy	mir′ing-<u>got</u>-o-me	incision of the tympanic membrane; tympanotomy with placement of tubes to maintain drainage
otoplasty	<u>o</u>-to-plas′te	plastic surgery of the ear (pinna)
stapedectomy	sta′pe-<u>dek</u>-to-me	excision of the stapes
tympanoplasty	tim′pah-no-<u>plas</u>-te	plastic surgery on the eardrum
tympanotomy	tim′pah-<u>not</u>-o-me	myringotomy; incision of the tympanic membrane

Common Medical Ear Terms

Table 18–8

Term	Pronunciation	Definition
acoustic meatus	ah-<u>koos</u>-tik me-<u>a</u>-tus	opening or passage in the ear
AD		auris dextra, right ear
AS		auris sinistra, left ear
AU		aures unitas (both ears) or auris uterque (each ear)
audiometer	aw′de-<u>om</u>-e-ter	a device for testing the hearing
audiometrist	aw′de-<u>om</u>-e-trist	person who performs hearing tests
auditory (or acoustic)	<u>aw</u>-di-to′re (ah-<u>koos</u>-tik)	pertaining to the ear; sense of hearing
decibel	<u>des</u>-i-bel	a unit of measure of the intensity of sound
hearing aid	<u>hēr</u>-ing	a device used to increase the intensity of sound
hearing-ear dogs		dogs trained to respond to sounds and alert the hearing-impaired person
otoscope	<u>o</u>-to-skōp	an instrument used for inspecting the ear

Term	Pronunciation	Definition
otoscopy	o-<u>tos</u>-ko-pe	examination of the ear by means of the otoscope
sign language	sine <u>lan</u>-gwij	communication by means of manual signs and gestures
tinnitus	ti-<u>ni</u>-tus	a noise (ringing) in the ears
tuning fork	<u>too</u>-ning	a small metal instrument consisting of a stem and two prongs used to test hearing
vertigo	<u>ver</u>-ti-go	a sensation of rotation or dizziness

LESSON TWO — PROGRESS CHECK

■ MATCHING: EYE STRUCTURES

For the list of terms on the left, select the correct definition on the right:

1.	sclera	**a.**	watery liquid in front of the lens
2.	conjunctiva	**b.**	jellylike substance behind the lens
3.	cornea	**c.**	innermost layer of the eyeball
4.	iris	**d.**	refracting mechanism of the eye
5.	pupil	**e.**	white outer coating of the eye
6.	lens	**f.**	membrane lining the eyelids
7.	aqueous humor	**g.**	transparent anterior part of the eye
8.	vitreous humor	**h.**	pigmented membrane behind the cornea
9.	retina	**i.**	opening through which light enters

■ MULTIPLE CHOICE: EYE

Circle the letter of the correct answer:

1. Impairment of vision with aging, caused by loss of elasticity, is a condition known as
- **a.** strabismus
- **b.** nystagmus
- **c.** presbyopia
- **d.** trachoma

2. Which of the following conditions describes the drooping of the lower eyelid?
    a. chalazion
    b. blepharoptosis
    c. dacrycystoptosis
    d. hyperopia

3. Deviation from normal color perception is a condition of
    a. herpes zoster
    b. floaters
    c. cataracts
    d. color blindness

4. Foreign bodies, contusions, lacerations, and burns to the eye are conditions of
    a. detached retinas
    b. blepharoptosis
    c. injuries
    d. retinopathies

5. A small hard mass on the eyelid formed by sebaceous gland enlargement is a
    a. chalazion
    b. sty
    c. corneal ulcer
    d. foreign body in the eye

6. Astigmatism is a condition in which
    a. the eyeball is too long
    b. there is an increase in intraocular pressure
    c. there is a defective curvature in the eye cornea
    d. there is dilation of the retinal veins

7. The transparent anterior part of the eye is the
    a. cornea
    b. iris
    c. lens
    d. pupil

8. An enucleation is a (an)
    a. cataract removal
    b. excision of the iris
    c. removal of the eye
    d. examination of the conjunctiva

9. A tonometer measures
    a. intraocular pressure
    b. amount of light entering the eye
    c. adjustments for various distances
    d. inequality of size of the pupils

■ EAR STRUCTURES

Identify the location of the following structures of the ears:

Structure   *Location*

1. external ear   _____

2. middle ear   _____

3. inner ear   _____

4. tympanic membrane   _____

5. eustachian tube   _____

6. cerumen   _____

■ MULTIPLE CHOICE: EAR

Circle the letter of the correct answer:

1. Which of the following terms denotes the creation of a new opening in the labyrinth of the ear?
   a. fenestration
   b. acoustic meatus
   c. otoplasty
   d. myringotomy

2. Plastic surgery on an eardrum is called
   a. tympanotomy
   b. tympanoplasty
   c. otoplasty
   d. stapedectomy

3. The unit of measure of the intensity of sound is called a (an):
   a. electronystagnometry
   b. audiometry
   c. decibel
   d. tuning fork

4. Which of the following terms describes tinnitus?
   a. dizziness
   b. nausea
   c. intense sound
   d. ringing of the ears

5. Vertigo is the term used for
   a. a sensation of rotation
   b. ringing of the ears
   c. intense sound
   d. sign communication

■ WORD PUZZLE ON THE SENSORY SYSTEM

Find the 69 words related to the senses by reading forward, backward, up, down, and diagonally. When the 69 words have been circled, the remaining letters will spell SENSES.

```
L  A  C  R  I  M  A  L  A  P  P  A  R  A  T  U  S  C  I  N  U  T
L  S  E  B  U  T  N  A  I  H  C  A  T  S  U  E  U  A  T  L  A  Y
E  E  Q  U  I  L  I  B  R  I  U  M  L  A  V  O  O  V  H  O  E  M
M  I  E  O  T  O  N  O  I  T  A  T  P  A  D  A  E  I  G  B  L  P
S  T  L  O  C  I  L  I  A  R  Y  B  O  D  Y  E  U  T  I  E  H  A
L  R  D  T  E  E  N  O  I  T  A  S  N  E  S  T  Q  Y  S  S  C  H
A  O  D  O  A  H  A  M  M  E  R  D  U  C  T  S  A  A  S  I  O  I
N  C  I  H  R  L  A  N  R  E  T  X  E  N  N  A  L  D  N  S  C  C
A  F  M  P  S  S  W  E  E  T  S  P  N  S  O  T  O  N  J  F  X  M
C  O  W  C  H  C  O  N  E  S  R  A  O  M  I  R  E  C  O  E  S  E
R  N  I  H  E  U  S  E  Y  E  E  I  I  A  T  R  N  C  V  T  O  M
A  A  N  S  T  R  M  E  S  S  B  N  T  C  A  I  U  M  A  P  S  B
L  G  D  D  T  N  U  O  I  N  M  S  C  U  D  S  O  P  T  S  E  R
U  R  O  S  I  I  I  M  R  E  A  R  A  L  O  C  E  I  S  U  V  A
C  O  W  D  C  O  R  R  I  L  H  A  R  A  M  S  C  E  U  O  A  N
R  S  S  S  N  L  R  R  Y  N  C  E  F  L  M  S  A  L  E  E  W  E
I  S  L  U  V  U  E  O  V  B  O  T  E  U  O  H  N  C  L  R  D  V
C  I  I  O  I  L  O  R  H  P  A  U  R  T  C  C  I  I  L  T  N  A
I  C  P  E  S  I  S  R  A  C  S  L  S  E  C  U  T  R  A  I  U  C
M  L  U  S  I  V  O  P  H  T  H  A  L  A  A  O  E  U  M  V  O  N
E  E  P  S  O  N  U  F  O  V  E  A  C  E  N  T  R  A  L  I  S  O
S  S  U  O  N  A  R  B  M  E  M  V  I  T  C  N  U  J  N  O  C  A
```

WORDS TO LOOK FOR IN THE WORD PUZZLE

1. accommodation
2. adaptation
3. anvil
4. aqueous
5. auricle
6. cavity
7. ceruminous
8. chambers
9. choroid
10. ciliary body
11. cochlea
12. concave
13. cones
14. conjunctiva
15. convex
16. ducts
17. ears
18. equilibrium
19. eustachian tube

20. external
21. eyes
22. focus
23. fovea centralis
24. hammer
25. humor
26. incus
27. inner
28. iris
29. labyrinth
30. lacrimal apparatus
31. lens
32. lobes
33. macula lutea
34. malleus
35. membranous
36. middle
37. ophthal-
38. optic

39. organ of Corti
40. osseous
41. ossicles
42. oto
43. oval
44. pain
45. photo
46. pupils
47. refraction
48. retina
49. rods
50. round
51. salt
52. sclera
53. semicircular canals
54. sensation
55. sight
56. smell
57. sound waves

58. sour
59. stapes
60. stirrups
61. sweet
62. taste
63. tears
64. touch
65. tunics
66. tympanic membrane
67. vision
68. vitreous
69. windows
SENSES

CHAPTER 19 — Endocrine System

OBJECTIVES

After completing this chapter and the exercises, the student should be able to:

1. Locate and name the endocrine glands and list the hormones produced by each gland.
2. Describe the major function(s) of each of the endocrine glands.
3. Build and define medical words related to the endocrine system.
4. Define and explain various pathological conditions of the endocrine system.
5. Differentiate between diabetes mellitus, diabetes insipidus, and gestational diabetes.
6. Identify laboratory tests and clinical procedures related to endocrinology.
7. Identify and define abbreviations related to endocrinology.

OVERVIEW

The endocrine system interacts with the nervous system to regulate and coordinate body activities (see Plate 9). *Endocrine glands* have no ducts. They secrete hormones directly into the tissue fluid that surrounds their cells. In contrast, *exocrine* glands, such as salivary glands, secrete their products into ducts. Endocrine control is regulated by chemical messengers (hormones). The word *hormone* comes from the Greek *hormon*, which means to excite or stimulate. A *hormone* is a chemical product produced and released by the endocrine glands and transported by the blood to cells and organs of the body on which it has a specific regulatory effect. Hormones produce their effects by binding to receptors that are recognition sites in the various target cells. The target cells are very selective and respond only to specific hormones. They usually secrete more than one hormone. The parathyroid gland is the exception, secreting only parathyroid hormone.

Glands of the endocrine system include the following:

1. Anterior and posterior pituitary gland
2. Thyroid gland
3. Four parathyroid glands
4. Two adrenal glands
5. Islets of Langerhans in the pancreas
6. Two ovaries
7. Two testes
8. Pineal gland
9. Thymus gland.

Many activities are regulated or influenced by the endocrine glands, including (1) reproduction and lactation; (2) immune system; (3) acid-base balance; (4) fluid intake and fluid balance; (5) carbohydrate, protein, lipid, and nucleic acid metabolism; (6) digestion, absorption, and nutrient distribution; (7) blood pressure; (8) stress resistance; and (9) adaptation to environmental change. The specific function of each of the glands can be found in anatomy and physiology texts, because space limits that discussion in this chapter. The glands are defined and classified in Lesson One (also see Plate 9).

The endocrine system is cyclical in nature. Cycles occur over hours or days rather than seconds or minutes. Integration of nervous and endocrine influences on the body occurs in the *hypothalamus,* a structure of the central nervous system (CNS).

Endocrinology is the study of the endocrine system and the disorders and diseases that affect the system. An *endocrinologist* is a physician who specializes in the medical practice of endocrinology.

LESSON ONE   MATERIALS TO BE LEARNED

The endocrine system is a unique body system that uses hormones to help regulate practically all facets of body activity. Glands are body structures (organs) and are divided into two types. A gland may or may not have a duct. A ducted gland secretes its materials by way of the duct into the bloodstream. In this case, the gland is an *exocrine gland.* The exocrine system is made up of all such glands. A ductless gland has no duct and secretes its materials directly into the bloodstream. Thus, the gland is an *endocrine gland*, and the endocrine system is made up of all such glands. Endocrine glands secrete important hormones. Occasionally, a gland contains an endocrine section and an exocrine section.

Refer to Figure 19–1 when you study the classification of the endocrine system.

CLASSIFICATION AND FUNCTION OF THE ENDOCRINE SYSTEM

Table 19–1

Gland	Pronunciation	Definition
pituitary gland	pe-<u>tu-i-tar</u>'-ee	also known as the hypophysis, the pituitary gland is about the size of a pea. It is located on the underside of the brain in a depression at the base of the skull called the *sella turcica*, and is protected by the brain above it and the nasal cavities below it. It is connected by a thin stalklike projection to the hypothalamus. The pituitary is a very complex gland that secretes many hormones that affect body functions. It is often referred to as the master gland. It contains two major parts, the anterior pituitary and the posterior pituitary lobes
thyroid	thi-royd	consisting of a right and left lobe, the thyroid gland is a U- or H-shaped gland located in front of the neck just below the larynx. The lobes are connected by a narrow piece of thyroid cartilage that produces the prominence on the neck known as the Adams apple. The thyroid gland produces three hormones: 1. Thyroxin (T4) helps maintain normal body metabolism. 2. Triiodthyronine (T3), a chemically similar compound, helps regulate growth and development and control metabolism and body temperature. 3. Calcitonin regulates the level of calcium in the blood. It lowers the blood calcium level by inhibiting the release of calcium from the bones by a negative feedback loop when blood calcium levels are high
parathyroid	par'-ah-<u>thi</u>'-royd	the parathyroid glands are four small nodules of tissue embedded in the back side of the thyroid glands. They secrete a hormone known as parathyroid hormone or parathormone (PTH), which increases blood calcium levels

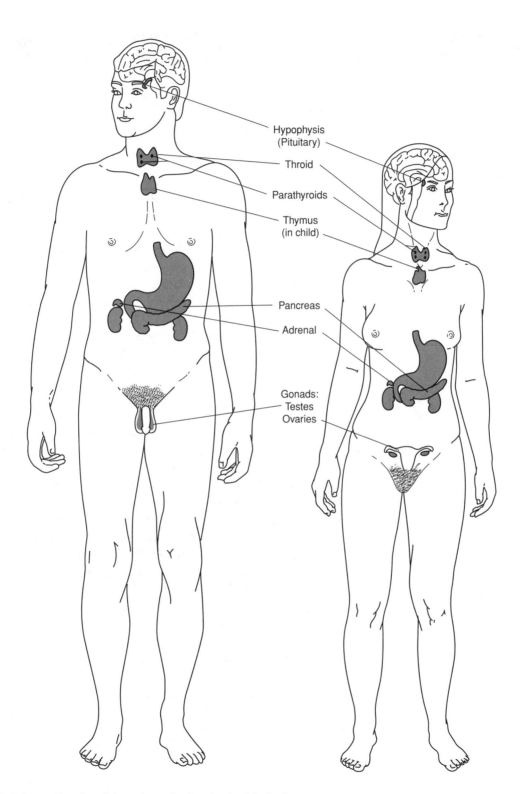

FIGURE 19–1 General location of the major endocrine glands of the body.

Gland	Pronunciation	Definition
adrenal	ah′-<u>dre</u>-nal	also called suprarenal glands, the two adrenal glands sit one atop each kidney. Each consists of two portions, the central region, or adrenal medulla, and the outer region, or adrenal cortex. The adrenal cortex is the largest portion of the gland. It secretes three types of steroid hormones called corticosteroids. Each has different functions. 1. Glucocorticoids affect glucose metabolism and maintain blood glucose levels. 2. Mineralocorticoids are involved in electrolyte balance. The most important is aldosterone, whose main function is to control sodium and potassium ion concentration in the kidney. 3. Gonadocorticoids are sex hormones released from the adrenal cortex instead of the gonads, but the small amounts secreted by the adrenal cortex contribute to the secondary sex characteristics, such as breast and beard development, and are necessary for reproduction. The adrenal medulla, the inner portion of the adrenal gland, secretes two nonsteroid hormones called catecholamines. The two hormones, adrenaline (epinephrine) and noradrenaline (norepinephrine), are the stress hormones that exert physiological changes during times of stress (the fight or flight response)
pancreas	<u>pan</u>′-kree-as	an elongated structure located behind the stomach in the left upper quadrant. The specialized cells that produce hormones are called the islets of Langerhans. These cells produce two hormones, insulin and glucagon. Both play a role in glucose levels in the body. The islets of Langerhans carry on the endocrine functions of the pancreas; other cells within the organ carry on its exocrine functions • Insulin, produced in the beta cells of the pancreas, is necessary for glucose to pass from the blood into the cells and be used for energy. Skeletal muscles are virtually impermeable to glucose in the absence of insulin. Insulin also promotes the conversion of glucose into glycogen for storage (glycogenesis) in the liver. When blood sugar is high (hyperglycemia), the pancreas is stimulated to release insulin and convert the excess glucose into glycogen. • Glucagon, produced in the alpha cells, increases blood levels of glucose by stimulating the breakdown of glycogen stored in the liver cells. Glycogen is the major carbohydrate in the body. This process, called glycogenolysis, helps maintain blood glucose levels between meals. It also helps synthesize glucose from amino acids and glycerol derived from triglycerides (gluconeogenesis), and elevates blood glucose levels

Gland	Pronunciation	Definition
ovaries	<u>oh</u>-vah-reez	two small glands located in the upper pelvic cavity, on either side of the uterine wall, near the fallopian tubes of the female. Each of the pair is almond-shaped and held in place by ligaments. Ovaries are the female sex glands, also known as female gonads. They produce mature ova as well as two hormones responsible for female sex characteristics and regulation of the menstrual cycle. The hormones are estrogen and progesterone. • Estrogen promotes maturation of the ova in the ovary and prepares the uterine lining for implantation of a fertilized egg, should fertilization occur. It is also responsible for the development and maintenance of secondary female characteristics that occur in puberty, such as breast development, growth of pubic and axillary hair, widened pelvis, general growth spurt, and onset of menstruation • Progesterone is responsible for preparation and maintenance of the uterus in pregnancy, and for the development of the placenta after implantation of a fertilized ovum
testes	<u>tes</u>-teez	male gonads, also known as testicles, are two small ovoid glands suspended from the inguinal region of the male by the spermatic cord and surrounded by the scrotal sac. After descending from high in the abdominal cavity during fetal growth, they descend shortly before birth into the scrotum and remain there. Testes are the primary organs of the male reproductive system. The testes produce male sperm cells and secrete *androgens*, the male steroid hormone. They also produce *testosterone*, the male hormone necessary for secondary sex characteristics that appear in the male during puberty, such as growth of the beard and pubic hair, growth of skeletal muscles, deepening of the voice, and enlargement of the testicles, penis, and scrotum. Testosterone is also responsible for sperm maturation
pineal	<u>pin</u>-e-al	the pineal gland is a cone-shaped structure attached by a stalk to the posterior wall of the cerebrum. Its exact function is unclear, but it is thought to function as a light receptor and to play a part in regulation of the "biological clock" (patterns of sleeping, eating, and reproduction). It secretes melatonin, the hormone believed to induce sleep
thymus	thi-mus	a single gland located behind the sternum in the mediastinum. It resembles a lymph gland in structure, as it is part of the lymphatic system, but it is also a hormone-secreting endocrine gland. The thymus is large in children, but shrinks with age until there is only a trace of active tissue in older adults. The gland secretes thymosin and thymopoitin, which stimulate the production of T cells, the specialized lymphocytes involved in the immune response

DISORDERS OF THE ENDOCRINE SYSTEM

Table 19–2

Clinical Condition	Pronunciation	Definition
acromegaly	ak'ro-meg-ah-le	abnormal enlargement of the extremities of the skeleton, nose, jaws, fingers, and toes; caused by hypersecretion of the pituitary growth hormone after maturity
Addison's disease	ad-i-sonz di-zez	bronzelike pigmentation of the skin, severe prostration, progressive anemia, low blood pressure, diarrhea, and digestive disturbance, caused by adrenal hypofunction
adrenalectomy	ah-dre-nal-ect-omy	surgical excision of the adrenal gland
adrenogenital syndrome	ah-dre-no-jen'-i-tal sin-drom	group of symptoms associated with alterations in sex characteristics due to abnormally increased production of androgens
adrenomegaly	ah-dre-no-meg-ah-le	enlargement of adrenal gland
cretinism	kre-ti-nizm	arrested physical and mental development owing to congenital lack of thyroid secretion
Cushing's disease	Koosh-ingz di-zez	obesity, weakness, moon face, edema, and high blood pressure; caused by hyperfunction of the adrenals
diabetes insipidus	dye-ah-bee-tez in-sip-ih-dus	a condition caused by insufficient excretion of antidiuretic hormone (ADH) (vasopressin) by the posterior pituitary gland. Deficient ADH causes the kidney tubules to fail to reabsorb needed water and salts. Clinical symptoms include polyuria (increased urination) and polydipsia (increased thirst). The person will complain of excessive thirst and drink large volumes of water. The urine will be very dilute with a low specific gravity. Synthetic preparations of ADH are administered as treatment for diabetes insipidus
diabetes mellitus	dye-ah-bee-tez mel-li-tus	inability to metabolize sugar because of abnormal insulin function; high blood sugar, excessive urination, thirst, hunger, emaciation, and weakness are cardinal symptoms of the most severe type (type 1)

Clinical Condition	Pronunciation	Definition
exophthalmic goiter	ek'sof-<u>thal</u>-mic <u>goi</u>-ter	toxic goiter; Graves' disease; protrusion of the eyeballs, swollen neck, weight loss, shaking, and mental deterioration are symptoms
gestational diabetes	jes-tay'-shun-al <u>dye</u>-ah-<u>bee</u>-tez	a condition in which pregnant women sometimes show abnormal glucose levels during the course of pregnancy (hyperglycemia)
goiter (simple)	<u>goi</u>-ter	enlargement of the thyroid gland; swelling in the front part of the neck, mostly caused by dietary deficiency of iodine
Hashimoto's disease	hash'i-<u>mo</u>-toz di-<u>zez</u>	a progressive disease of the thyroid gland with degeneration of its epithelium and replacement by lymphoid and fibrous tissue
hyperglycemia	hi-per-gli-<u>se</u>-me-ah	blood sugar (glucose) level above normal
hyperthyroidism	hi-per-<u>thi</u>-roi-dizm	excessive activity of the thyroid gland
hypothyroidism	<u>high</u>-poh-thigh-royd-ism	underactivity of the thyroid gland. Shortage of thyroid hormones causes a low body metabolism because of the body's reduced use of oxygen. Any one of several conditions can produce hypothyroidism, such as endemic goiter, thyroidectomy, faulty hormone synthesis, and congenital thyroid defects, a condition that is called cretinism, and which results in a child lacking normal mental and physical growth
myxedema	mik'se-<u>de</u>-mah	a dry, waxy type of swelling with deposits of mucin in the skin, swollen lips, and thickened nose. Myxedema is the advanced form of hypothyroidism in adults
ovariorrhexis	o-va're-o-<u>rek</u>-sis	rupture of an ovary
pancreaticogastrostomy	pan-kre-at'i-ko-gas-<u>tros</u>-to-me	anastomosis of the pancreatic duct to the stomach
pancreatitis	pan'kre-ah-<u>ti</u>-tus	inflammation of the pancreas due to autodigestion of pancreatic tissue by its own enzymes
pheochromocytoma	fe'o-kro'mo-si-<u>to</u>-mah	"pheochromo" means dusky color; tumor of the medulla characterized by hypertension, weight loss, and personality changes

Clinical Condition	Pronunciation	Definition
Simmonds' disease (panhypopituitarism)	<u>sim</u>-ondz di-<u>zez</u> (pan-hi'po-pi-<u>tu</u>-i-tar-izm)	generalized hypopituitarism owing to absence or damage of the pituitary gland; exhaustion, emaciation, and cachexia are symptoms
tetany	<u>tet</u>-ah-ne	sharp flexion of the wrist and ankle joints, muscle twitching, cramps, and convulsion; caused by abnormal calcium metabolism
thyroidectomy	thi-roi-<u>dek</u>-to-me	surgical excision of the thyroid gland
thyrotherapy	thi-ro-<u>ther</u>-ah-pe	treatment with thyroid preparations
thyrotomy	thi-<u>rot</u>-o-me	surgical division of thyroid cartilage

MISCELLANEOUS TERMS

Table 19–3

Term	Definition	Pronunciation
acidosis	as'i-<u>do</u>-sis	a pathologic condition caused by accumulation of acid in, or loss of base from, the body
anorexia	an'o-<u>rek</u>-se-ah	lack or loss of appetite for food
cachexia	kah-<u>kek</u>-se-ah	malnutrition, wasting, and emaciation
cataract	<u>kat</u>-ah-rakt	clouding of the eye lens
convulsions	kon-<u>vul</u>-shunz	involuntary muscular contractions
diaphoresis	di'ah-fo-<u>re</u>-sis	profuse perspiration
emaciation	e-ma'se-<u>a</u>-shun	excessive leanness; a wasted condition
endocrine	<u>en</u>-do-krin	ductless gland that secretes directly into the bloodstream
exocrine	<u>eks</u>-oh-krin	a ducted gland that secretes into various organs
gangrene	<u>gang</u>-grēn	death of tissue from lack of circulation and consequent loss of nutrients
gland	gland	an organ that secretes a metabolic substance. May be endocrine or exocrine

Term	Definition Pronunciation	
hypoglycemia	hi'po-gli-<u>se</u>-me-ah	blood sugar (glucose) level is below normal
hypoglycemic agent	hi'po-gli-<u>se</u>-mik	drug for the diabetic to decrease the amount of glucose in the blood
hypophysectomy	hi-pof'i-<u>sek</u>-to-me	excision of the pituitary gland (hypophysis)
insulin	<u>in</u>-su-lin	a protein hormone produced by the pancreatic islets of Langerhans. It is secreted into the blood in response to a rise in concentration of blood glucose. Insulin promotes the entrance of glucose from the blood into cells. A diabetic patient is deficient in insulin or insulin receptors leading to a rise in blood glucose
ketosis	ke-<u>to</u>-sis	accumulation of excessive amounts of ketone bodies in body tissues and fluids; a complication in some diabetic patients
ketoacidosis	ke-to-as-i-<u>do</u>-sis	accumulation of ketone bodies in the blood that results in metabolic acidosis (ketosis and ketoacidosis are often used interchangeably)
neuropathy	nu-<u>rop</u>-ah-the	any functional disturbances and/or pathologic changes in the peripheral nervous system; a complication in some diabetic patients

LESSON TWO   PROGRESS CHECK

■ MULTIPLE CHOICE

Circle the letter of the correct answer:

1. Which of the following statements *best* describes the endocrine glands?
   a. They are small bodies in the region of the neck.
   b. They secrete hormones that regulate the body's activity.
   c. They secrete materials into the gastrointestinal tract to help digest food.
   d. They prevent chronic degenerative diseases.

2. Glands are body structures that
   a. are classified as endocrine or exocrine
   b. are not organs, but are attached to them
   c. are classified as exogenous or endogenous
   d. exert little influence over other body systems

3. A gland that secretes its fluids into a duct and then into the bloodstream is a (an) _____ gland.
   a. endogenous
   b. exogenous
   c. endocrine
   d. exocrine

4. The endocrine system is composed of
   a. the adrenal and thyroid glands
   b. ducted and ductless glands
   c. glands that secrete to the outside of the body
   d. ductless glands

5. The endocrine gland at the base of the brain is the
   a. pituitary
   b. parathyroid
   c. pineal
   d. pancreas

6. The endocrine gland with a lobe on each side of the trachea is the
   a. pituitary
   b. pancreas
   c. thyroid
   d. adrenal

7. The two small glands atop the kidneys are the
   a. pituitary
   b. adrenal
   c. thyroid
   d. thymus

8. The large organ situated transversely behind the stomach is the
   a. adrenal
   b. thymus
   c. sex
   d. pancreas

9. The organ situated in the pleural cavity that is believed to be part of the body's immune system is the
   a. pancreas
   b. pituitary
   c. thymus
   d. thyroid

10. The islets (islands) of Langerhans refer to
   a. small bodies in the pituitary gland
   b. the endocrine part of the pancreas
   c. the testes and ovaries
   d. the exocrine part of the adrenals

■ MATCHING

Match the disease with the malfunctioning gland that causes it (answers may be used more than once):

1.	acromegaly	**a.**	parathyroid
2.	Addison's disease	**b.**	pituitary
3.	cretinism	**c.**	adrenal
4.	Cushing's disease	**d.**	thyroid
5.	goiter (simple)	**e.**	pancreas
6.	Graves' disease		
7.	diabetes mellitus		
8.	Simmonds' disease		
9.	tetany		

■ FILL-IN

From the word pool, fill in the correct phrase(s) to make a true sentence:

WORD POOL

cretinism, Cushing's disease, diabetes mellitus, Graves' disease, myxedema, pheochromocytoma, tetany

1. Inability to metabolize sugar due to lack of insulin leads to _____ .

2. Arrested mental and physical growth is a sign of _____ caused by congenital lack of thyroxine.

3. Swollen neck, weight loss, shaking, and mental deterioration are symptoms of _____ .

4. _____ is characterized by hypertension, weight loss, and personality changes.

5. _____ is characterized by muscle twitching, cramps, and convulsions.

6. A dry, waxy swelling with swollen lips and thickened nose is diagnosed as _____ .

7. Obesity, weakness, moon face, edema, and high blood pressure characterize _____ .

■ DEFINITIONS

Define the following terms:

1. convulsion _____

2. diaphoresis _____

3. emaciation _____

4. insulin _____

5. ketosis _____

6. neuropathy _____

7. hypoglycemic agent _____

■ COMPARE AND CONTRAST

Explain the *differences* in the following terms:

1. acidosis/anorexia _____

2. cachexia/cataract _____

3. gangrene/gland _____

4. hypoglycemia/hypophysectomy _____

■ WORD PUZZLE ON THE ENDOCRINE SYSTEM

Find the 50 words related to the endocrine system by reading forward, backward, up, down, or diagonally. When the 50 listed words have been circled, the remaining letters (from left to right) spell TO ALWAYS MAINTAIN HOMEOSTASIS.

```
A  L  L  U  D  E  M  T  P  I  T  C  O  R  T  I  S  O  N  E
C  D  T  E  S  T  E  S  N  I  T  C  A  L  O  R  P  O  N  N
T  L  R  A  L  P  H  A  C  E  L  L  S  P  T  H  R  D  A  O
H  A  L  E  N  O  M  R  O  H  H  T  W  O  R  G  O  W  C  R
K  E  P  I  N  E  P  H  R  I  N  E  A  T  E  C  G  B  I  E
C  S  A  N  I  O  V  A  R  Y  A  D  H  N  R  A  E  E  T  T
A  Y  D  S  O  Y  C  S  R  N  I  Y  O  I  M  L  S  T  E  S
B  H  R  U  D  A  I  O  D  O  R  R  N  N  G  C  T  A  R  O
D  P  E  L  I  T  I  R  R  O  E  E  R  N  M  I  E  C  U  D
E  O  N  I  N  R  O  Y  I  T  S  O  I  U  M  T  R  E  I  L
E  P  A  N  E  G  H  D  S  Y  I  Z  I  C  A  O  O  L  D  A
F  Y  L  T  E  T  A  O  S  R  I  C  I  H  S  N  N  L  I  F
E  H  N  N  A  S  T  T  E  N  L  N  O  O  T  I  E  S  T  O
V  A  S  R  D  S  E  T  I  A  H  L  H  T  E  N  O  M  N  L
I  E  A  A  E  M  S  E  C  G  L  A  N  D  R  A  D  H  A  L
T  P  N  T  O  O  T  S  U  M  A  L  A  H  T  O  P  Y  H  I
A  O  H  S  P  U  G  H  S  A  E  R  C  N  A  P  P  T  A  C
G  F  S  H  L  D  U  C  T  L  S  F  E  M  A  L  E  I  I  L
E  S  T  R  O  G  E  N  S  E  S  O  X  Y  T  O  C  I  N  E
N  S  E  B  O  L  D  N  A  L  G  Y  R  A  T  I  U  T  I  P
```

WORDS TO LOOK FOR IN THE WORD PUZZLE

1. ACTH
2. ADH
3. adrenal
4. adrenocorticotropin
5. aldosterone
6. alpha cells
7. androgens
8. anterior
9. antidiuretic
10. beta cells
11. calcitonin
12. calcium
13. CHO
14. cortisone
15. duct
16. endocrine system
17. epinephrine
18. estrogens
19. female
20. follicle
21. FSH
22. GH
23. gland
24. gonads
25. growth hormone
26. hypophyseal
27. hypothalamus
28. insulin
29. iodine
30. LH
31. lobes
32. luteinizing
33. male
34. master
35. medulla
36. negative feedback
37. ovary
38. oxytocin
39. pancreas
40. parathyroid
41. pit
42. pituitary gland
43. posterior
44. progesterone
45. prolactin
46. PTH
47. testes
48. testosterone
49. thyroid
50. TSH

TO ALWAYS MAINTAIN HOMEOSTASIS

CHAPTER 20 Cancer Medicine

OBJECTIVES

After completing this chapter and the exercises, the student should be able to:

1. Define cancer.
2. Classify cancer.
3. Identify rules and exceptions in naming cancer.
4. Describe the types of cancer normally affecting men and women.
5. Explain the two major clinical phases in cancer medicine: diagnosis and treatment.
6. Describe the details of screening, detection, and diagnosis of cancer.
7. Present the methods of treating cancer.

OVERVIEW

Cancer is the second leading cause of death from disease in the United States. Skin cancer is the most common type of cancer; however, lung cancer is the leading cause of death from cancer, followed by colon cancer in men and breast cancer in women. Brain cancer and leukemia are the most common cancers in children and young adults. Refer to Table 20–1.

2006 ESTIMATED U.S. CANCER DEATHS (ALL RACES)

Table 20–1

Site	%	Men 291,270	Women 273,560	%	Site
Lung and bronchus	31			26	Lung and bronchus
Colon and rectum	10			15	Breast
Prostate	9			10	Colon and rectum
Pancreas	6			6	Pancreas
Leukemia	4			6	Ovary
Liver and intrahepatic bile duct	4			4	Leukemia
Esophagus	4			3	Non-Hodgkin's lymphoma
Non-Hodgkin's lymphoma	3			3	Uterine corpus
Urinary bladder	3			2	Multiple myeloma
Kidney	3			2	Brain/CNS
All other sites	33			23	All other sites

Source: American Cancer Society, 2006.

Normally, cells divide to produce more cells only when the body needs them. Normal life processes are characterized by continuous growth and maturation of cells that are subject to control mechanisms that regulate growth. This ongoing growth process serves the purpose of replacing cells that have been injured or have undergone degenerative changes. If cells keep dividing when new cells are not needed, a tumor or neoplasm is formed. A neoplasm (neo = new + plasm = growth) is an overgrowth of cells that serves no useful purpose. Neoplasms appear not to be subject to the control mechanisms that normally regulate cell growth and differentiation. The terms *neoplasm* and *tumor* have essentially the same meaning and may be used interchangeably.

A malignant neoplasm is composed of less well differentiated cells that grow rapidly and infiltrate surrounding tissues. The process by which a tumor spreads (meta = change) and the secondary deposits (+ stasis = standing) are called metastatic tumors, as illustrated by various tumors in Figure 20–1.

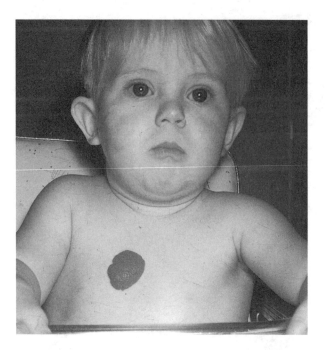

FIGURE 20–1 A Benign tumor of the skin.

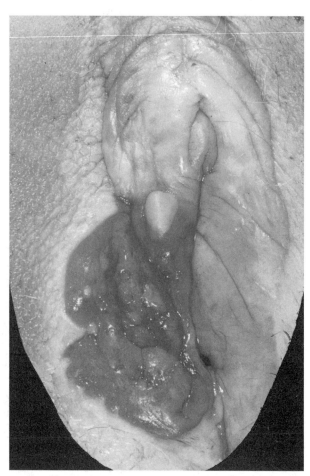

FIGURE 20–1 C Metastasis of tumor of the vulva.

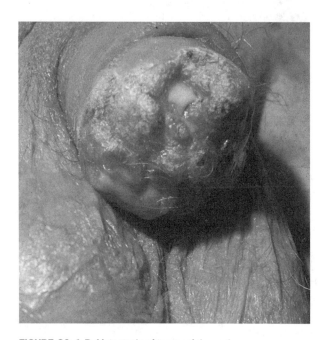

FIGURE 20–1 B Metastasis of tumor of the penis.

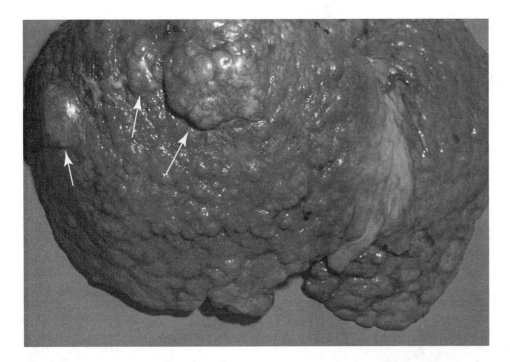

FIGURE 20–1 D Metastasis of liver tumor.

LESSON ONE   MATERIALS TO BE LEARNED

MEDICAL TERMS IN CANCER MEDICINE

The medical terms associated with cancer medicine are grouped as follows:

1. Those associated with the word *cancer*.
2. Those associated with the cancer site (organ or tissue).
3. Those associated with the diagnosis.
4. Those associated with the treatment.

CANCER: CLASSIFICATION, TERMINOLOGY, AND TYPES

Basic Classification

There are two large classes of neoplasms, benign and malignant, with characteristics of each described in Table 20–2.

Comparison of Benign and Malignant Tumors

Table 20–2

	Benign Tumor	Malignant
Growth rate	slow	rapid
Character of growth	expansion	infiltration
Tumor spread	remains localized	metastasis by bloodstream and lymphatics
Cell differentiation	well differentiated	poorly differentiated

A benign tumor that projects from an epithelial surface is usually called a polyp or papilloma, as shown in Figure 20–2 and listed in Table 20–3.

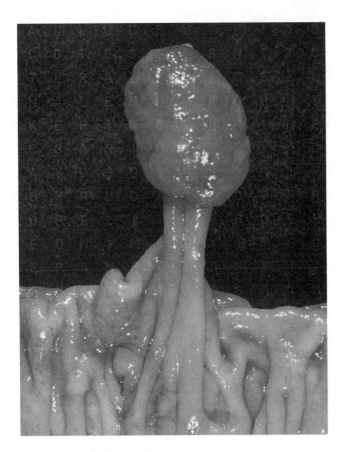

FIGURE 20–2 Benign polyp of colon.

General Principles of Naming Tumors

Table 20–3

General Term	Meaning
polyp, papilloma	any benign tumor projecting from surface epithelium
root word + oma (suffix)	a benign tumor. Root word designates primary tissue of origin
carcinoma	malignant tumor arising from surface, glandular, or parenchymal epithelium (but not endothelium or mesothelium)
sarcoma	malignant tumor of any primary tissue other than surface, glandular, and parenchymal epithelium
leukemia	neoplasm of blood cells

Most benign tumors are named by adding the suffix "-oma" to the prefix that designates the cell of origin, as shown in Table 20–4. For example, a benign tumor arising from glandular epithelium is called an adenoma. A benign tumor of blood vessels is an angioma, and one arising from cartilage is designated a chondroma.

Using Root Words to Name Tumors

Table 20–4

Combining Form	Meaning
aden/o	gland
angi/o	vessels (type not specified)
chondr/o	cartilage
fibr/o	fibrous tissue
hemangi/o	blood vessels
lymphangi/o	lymph vessels
lip/o	fat
my/o	muscle
neur/o	nerve
oste/o	bone

There are many types of malignant tumors, but all can be classified into three groups according to the cancer site and tissue type: (1) *carcinomas*,

(2) *sarcomas*, and (3) *leukemias*. The term *cancer* is a word used to indicate any type of malignant tumor.

A carcinoma is any malignant tumor arising from surface, glandular, or parenchymal epithelium and is classified further by designating the type of epithelium from which it arose. For example, a carcinoma arising from the glandular epithelium of the pancreas is termed an adenocarcinoma of the pancreas (aden = gland).

Sarcoma is a general term referring to a malignant tumor arising from primary tissues other than surface, glandular, or parenchymal epithelium. The exact type of sarcoma is specified by using the prefix that designates the cell of origin. For example, a malignant tumor of bone is designated as an osteosarcoma.

The term *leukemia* is applied to any neoplasm of blood-forming tissues. Neoplasms arising from the precursors of white blood cells usually do not form solid tumors but, instead, the abnormal cells proliferate within the bone marrow where they overgrow and crowd out the normal blood-forming cells. The abnormal cells also "spill over" into the bloodstream, and large numbers of abnormal cells circulate in the blood.

Tumors are named and classified according to the cells and tissues from which they originate. However, when cancer spreads, the new tumor has the same kind of abnormal cells and the same name as the primary tumor. For example, if lung cancer spreads to the liver, the cancer cells in the liver are lung cancer cells. The disease is called metastatic lung cancer (not liver cancer).

Cancer with Specific Names

The following will explore some tumors with specific names. They do not follow the "rules" discussed above.

Table 20–5

Tumor	Explanation for Nomenclature
lymphoid tumors	all neoplasms of lymphoid tissue are called lymphomas and are malignant: Hodgkin's disease and non-Hodgkin's lymphomas

skin tumors	*pigment-producing cells of the epidermis*
	benign:
	    nervus, a Latin word that means "birthmark"
	malignant:
	    melanoma or malignant melanoma
	keratinocytes
	benign:
	    basal cell carcinoma
	malignant:
	    squamous cell carcinoma (sometimes metastasizes)

Tumor	Explanation for Nomenclature
teratoma tumors (of mixed components)	derived from cells that have the potential to differentiate into different types of tissue (bone, muscle, glands, epithelium, brain tissue, hair) and may be either benign or malignant. A common type of cystic benign teratoma arising in the ovary is usually called a dream cyst
embryonic tumors	derived from persisting groups of embryonic cells of the brain, retina, adrenal gland, kidney, liver, or genital tract. Named from the site of origin, with the suffix "-blastoma" added (blast = a primitive cell + oma = tumor); medulloblastoma: medulla of the brain; retinoblastoma: retina of the eye; hepatoblastoma: liver; Wilm's tumor: kidney, exception in naming (nephroblastoma not used)
noninfiltrating (in situ) carcinoma	noninfiltrating tumors are common in many locations, including the breast, cervix, colon, skin, and urinary tract. In situ carcinoma can be completely cured by surgical excision

precancerous conditions	refers to conditions that have a high likelihood of developing into cancer:
	 skin cancer
	     actinic keratoses ("actinic" refers to sun rays)
	     lentigo maligna (a latin term meaning "malignant freckle")
	 oral cancer
	     leukoplakis (leuko = white + plakia = patch) may develop in the mucous membranes of the mouth as a result of exposure to tobacco tars from smoking or use of smokeless tobacco
	 colon polyps

SCREENING AND EARLY DETECTION

The early detection of cancers relies on two conditions: The existence of a premalignant, or detectable, preclinical phase, and the availability of appropriate tests that can detect the tumor during the preclinical phase. On an individual basis, the standard history and physical examination provides a comprehensive format for early detection of cancer. Refer to Figures 20–3, 20–4, and 20–5 for physical signs of cancer. Emphasis is placed on the following areas:

1. History and physical examination, including family history of cancer, personal habits—smoking, alcohol use, and sexual history—and occupational exposure to chemicals or radiation.
2. Signs and symptoms related to specific organ systems:

    a. Bladder: hematuria, dysuria
    b. Breast: nipple discharge, mass
    c. Gastrointestinal: change in bowel habits, bleeding
    d. Gynecological: abnormal vaginal bleeding or discharge, dyspareunia

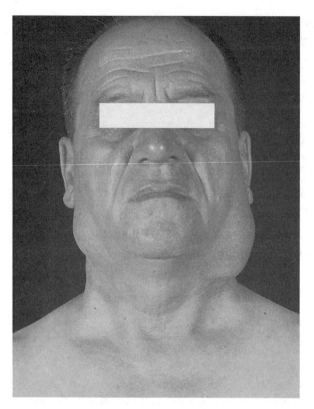

FIGURE 20–3 Marked enlargement of cervical lymph nodes as a result of malignant lymphoma.

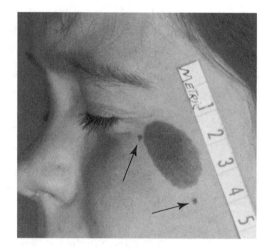

FIGURE 20–4 Benign nevi of skin. Large nevus near eye and two smaller adjacent nevi.

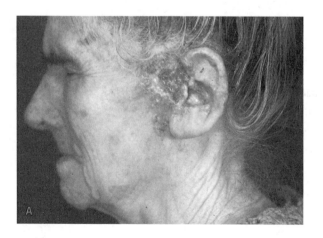

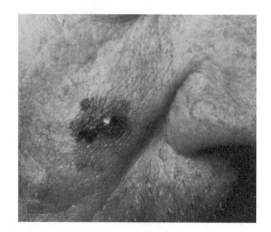

FIGURE 20–5 A and **B** Common skin cancers caused by excessive sun exposure.

   e.   Lymphadenopathy: abnormal size or number of lymph nodes
   f.   Oropharynx: hoarseness for >1 week, abnormal bleeding, pain
   g.   Prostrate cancer: hematuria, dysuria
   h.   Pulmonary: cough, pain, dyspnea, hemoptysis
   i.   Skin: slow-healing sore, changing mole

The most common detection and diagnostic tools or tests are described in Table 20–6.

MEDICAL TERMS RELATED TO THE DIAGNOSIS OF CANCER

Table 20–6

Term	Pronounciation	Definition
aspirate	<u>as</u>-pi-rit	withdrawl of fluid from a lump, often a cyst
biopsy	<u>by</u>-ahp-see	removal of cells or tissues for examination under a microscope
Scope		a procedure in which a thin, lighted tube is inserted into the body part being examined and a tissue sample (biopsy) is taken to examine under a microscope to determine if cancer cells are present
bronchoscopy	bron-<u>kos</u>-ko-pee	scope inserted through the nose or mouth to examine the inside of the trachea, bronchi, and lung
colonoscopy	ko-lun-<u>ahs</u>-ko-pee	scope inserted into the rectum to examine the colon
cystoscopy	sist-<u>ahs</u>-ko-pee	scope inserted into the urethra to examine the bladder
laryngoscopy	lair-in-<u>gos</u>-ko-pee	examination of the larynx (voice box) with a mirror (indirect laryngoscopy) or with a laryngoscope (direct laryngoscopy)
sigmoidoscopy	sig-moid-<u>oss</u>-ko-pee	scope inserted into the sigmoid part of the colon. Also called proctosigmoidoscopy

SPECIAL CANCER DIAGNOSTIC TESTS

Table 20–7

Test	Purpose	Comments
Tumor markers		obtained from blood sample
acid phosphatase	cancer of the prostate	may be used to monitor response to treatment or recurrence

Test	Purpose	Comments
AFP	hepatocellular carcinoma germ cell tumors	used to monitor treatment response
CA 19-9	cancers of the pancreas, colon, cervix, and ovary	a relatively specific tumor-associated antigen
CA 125	epithelial ovarian cancer	a tumor-associated antigen that might be used in conjunction with vaginal ultrasound for screening
CEA	cancers of the pancreas, colon, breast, lung, stomach, ovary	high levels correlate with high tumor burden
HCG/AFP	malignant germ cell tumors originating from ovaries or sperm; ovarian or uterine cancer in women and testicular cancer in men	return to normal indicates cure
monoclonal immunoglobulins	multiple myeloma	malignant clone can be IgG, IgM, or IgA
PSA	cancer of the prostate	used particularly to monitor response to treatment
Imaging		x-ray or computerized view with or without a contrast dye or radioactive substance
barium enema	cancer of the colon	series of x-rays of the colon taken after the person is given an enema that contains barium. Barium outlines the intestines on the x-rays
computed axial tomography (CAT, CT, ACTA)	cross-section images of internal structures	x-ray ± contrast dye with the creation of pictures by a computer linked to an x-ray machine; high specificity, especially brain tumors
intravenous pyelogram or intravenous pyelography (IVP)	cancer of the kidneys, ureters, and bladder	dye is injected into a blood vessel and concentrated in the urine to visualize the kidneys, ureters, and bladder
lymphangiography	lymph node involvement, especially Hodgkin's disease, lymphoma, cancer of testes	blue dye, injected into lymphatic channel, visualizes abdominal lymph nodes

Test	Purpose	Comments
radionuclide scan	shows function and size of specific organ (brain, bone, liver, spleen, kidney)	used for staging because of specificity; radioactive material is injected or swallowed and radioactivity measured with a scanner
ultrasound	visualizes structural changes, mass (stomach, pancreas, kidney, uterus, ovary)	uses high-frequency sound waves
Microscopic examination		obtained from a tissue sample
bone-marrow aspirate	tumor involvement, especially by leukemia or lymphoma	needle aspirate of marrow from iliac crest or sternum
estrogen/progesterone receptors	cancer of the breast	cells taken from breast tissue; defines certain tumors that may be more responsive to hormonal therapy
Pap smear	cancer of the cervix or uterus	cells obtained by swab of vagina, endocervical canal, and exocervix
sentinel lymph node biopsy	tumor metastasis, for example, breast cancer	dye or radioactive substance injected near a tumor flows into the sentinel lymph node(s)—the first lymph node(s); that cancer is likely to spread from the primary tumor
sputum cytology	bronchogenic cancer	examination of mucus coughed up from the lungs; used to detect abnormal lung cells
Other		
stool guaiac	cancer of the colon/rectum	a test to check for blood in stool (fecal refers to stool, occult means hidden)

AFP, alpha-fetoprotein; CEA, carcinoembryonic antigen; HCG, human chorionic gonadotropin; PSA, prostate specific antigen. CA 125 and CA 19-9: special antigens.

METHODS OF CANCER TREATMENT

Cancer Treatment

Cancer is treated with surgery, radiation therapy, chemotherapy, hormone therapy, or biological therapy, or a combination of these treatments. Treatment may be prophylactic for precancerous lesions, palliative to reduce the size of a tumor when the tumor has metastasized, or reconstructive after a mastectomy for breast cancer. Patients with cancer are often treated by a team of specialists, which may include a medical oncologist (specialist in cancer treatment), a surgeon, a radiation oncologist (specialist in radiation therapy), and others. The choice of treatment depends on the type and location of the cancer, the stage of the disease, the patient's age and general health, and other factors.

MEDICAL TERMS RELATED TO THE TREATMENT OF CANCER

Table 20–8

Term	Pronunciation	Definition
Biological		treatment to stimulate or restore the ability of the immune system to fight infection and disease [also, immunotherapy or biological response modifier (BRM) therapy]
autologous bone marrow transplantation	aw-<u>tahl</u>-o-gus	a procedure in which bone marrow is removed from a person, stored, and then given back to the person following intensive treatment
BCG vaccine		an anticancer drug, bacille calmette-Guerin (BCG), that activates the immune system
colony-stimulating factors		substances that stimulate the production of blood cells; granulocyte colony-stimulating factors (G-CSF); granulocyte-macrophage colony-stimulating factors (GM-CSF)
peripheral stem cell transplantation	per-<u>if</u>-er-al	replacing blood-forming cells destroyed by cancer treatment. Immature blood cells (stem cells) are given after treatment to help the bone marrow recover and produce healthy blood cells. Sources of stem cells are bone marrow and are allogeneic, autologous, or syngeneic
allogeneic	<u>al</u>-o-jen-<u>ay</u>-ik	stem cells donated by someone else
autologous	aw-<u>tahl</u>-o-gus	stem cells removed from a person, stored, and then given back to the person following intensive treatment
syngeneic	<u>sin</u>-juh-<u>nay</u>-ik	stem cells donated by an identical twin
Chemotherapy	kee-mo-<u>ther</u>-a-pee	treatment with anticancer drugs to destroy cancer cells by stopping them from growing or multiplying
Radiation therapy	ray-dee-<u>ay</u>-shun	radiotherapy uses high-energy radiation from x-rays, neutrons, and other sources to kill cancer cells and shrink tumors
external		uses a machine to aim high-energy rays at the cancer

Term	Pronunciation	Definition
internal		given internally by placing radioactive material that is sealed in needles, seeds, wires, or catheters directly into or near the tumor
systemic radiation therapy		giving a radioactive substance, such as a radiolabeled monoclonal antibody, that circulates throughout the body
Surgery		a procedure to remove a part of the body because of the presence of cancer
cystectomy	sis-<u>tek</u>-toe-mee	surgical removal of the bladder
cryosurgery	<u>kyre</u>-o-<u>sir</u>-jer-ee	treatment performed with an instrument that freezes and destroys abnormal tissues
fulguration	ful-gyoor-<u>ay</u>-shun	destroying tissue using an electric current
hysterectomy	hiss-ter-<u>ek</u>-toe-mee	surgical removal of the uterus
laryngectomy	lair-in-<u>jek</u>-toe-mee	an operation to remove all or part of the larynx (voice box)
laser	<u>lay</u>-zer	a device that concentrates light into an intense, narrow beam used to cut or destroy tissue. It is used in microsurgery, photodynamic therapy, and for a variety of diagnostic purposes
lumpectomy	lump-<u>ek</u>-toe-mee	surgery to remove the tumor and a small amount of normal tissue around it
mastectomy	mas-<u>tek</u>-toe-mee	surgery to remove the breast (or as much of the breast tissue as possible)
modified radical mastectomy		surgical procedure in which the breast, some of the lymph nodes in the armpit, and the lining over the chest muscles are removed
orchiectomy	or-kee-<u>ek</u>-toe-mee	surgical removal of one or both testicles
pneumonectomy	noo-mo-<u>nek</u>-toe-mee	surgical removal of an entire lung
prostatectomy	pros-ta-<u>tek</u>-toe-mee	surgical removal of part or all of the prostate
salpingo-oophorectomy	sal-<u>pin</u>-go o-o-for-<u>ek</u>-toe-mee	surgical removal of the fallopian tubes and ovaries
Hormone therapy		treatment of cancer by removing, blocking, or adding hormones. Also called endocrine therapy
antiandrogens	an-tee-<u>an</u>-dro-jens	drugs used to block the production or interfere with the action of male sex hormones

Term	Pronunciation	Definition
luteinizing hormone-releasing hormone agonist	loo-tin-eye-zing ag-o-nist	a substance that closely resembles luteinizing hormone-releasing hormone (LH-RH), which controls the secretion of sex hormones; given to decrease secretion of sex hormones

DIFFERENT SURGICAL PROCEDURES USED TO TREAT CANCER

Table 20–9

Approach	Example
palliative	cytoreduction; oncologic emergencies; neurosurgical procedures/pain control; nutritional support
prophylactic	excision of premalignant lesions
primary/definitive	local excision; en bloc dissection
rehabilitative	cosmetic and functional restoration
resection of metastases	lung; liver
supportive	insertion of access devices such as a porta catheter for infusion of drugs for chemotherapy; radiation implants

BREAST CANCER AND MEDICAL ILLUSTRATIONS

This chapter is unable to discuss medical terms associated with each type of cancer. Figure 20–6 (A–E) provides the progressive development of cells from normal to benign to malignant breast cancer with metastases. Each picture is from a different patient as illustrated in Figure 20–6 A: normal mammogram, Figure 20–6 B: benign cyst of breast, Figure 20–6 C: benign tumor of breast, Figure 20–6 D: breast cancer biopsy and mammogram, and Figure 20–6 E: advanced breast cancer.

Figure 20–7 illustrates the classic failure of the lymphatic system in a person with breast cancer.

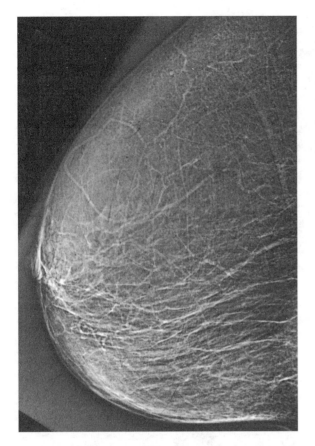

FIGURE 20–6 A Normal mammogram.

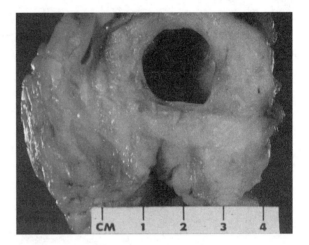

FIGURE 20–6 B Benign cyst of breast.

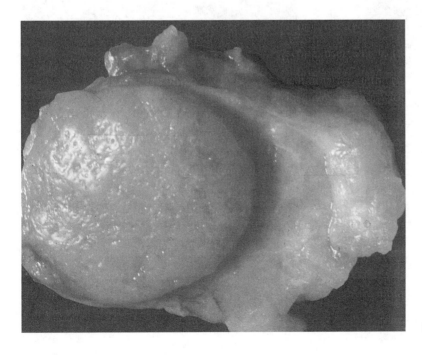

FIGURE 20–6 C Benign tumor of breast.

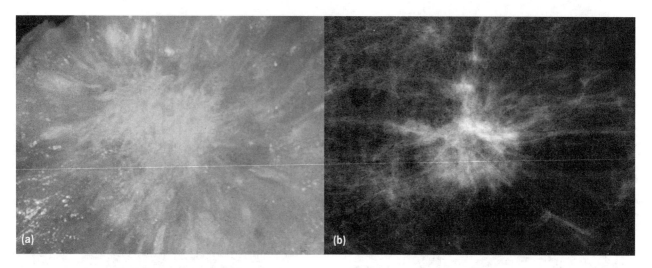

FIGURE 20–6 D (a) Breast cancer biopsy and (b) mammogram.

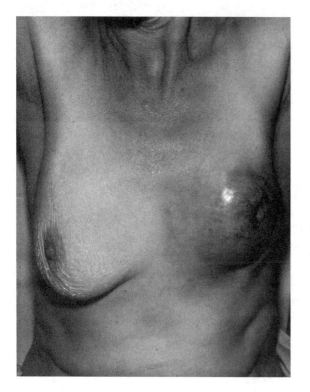

FIGURE 20–6 E Advanced breast cancer.

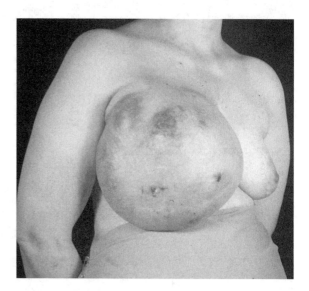

FIGURE 20–7 Large sarcoma of the breast.

MEDICAL TERMS RELATED TO TYPES OF CANCER

Table 20–10

Term	Pronounciation	Definition
adenocarcinoma	<u>ad</u>-in-o-kar-sin-<u>o</u>-ma	cancer that begins in cells that line certain internal organs
atypical hyperplasia	hy-per-<u>play</u>-zha	benign (noncancerous) condition in which cells have abnormal features and are increased in number
benign	beh-<u>nine</u>	not cancerous; does not invade nearby tissue or spread to other parts of the body
cancer		a term for diseases in which abnormal cells divide without control. Cancer cells can invade nearby tissues and spread through the bloodstream and lymphatic system to other parts of the body
carcinogen	kar-<u>sin</u>-o-jin	any substance that causes cancer
carcinoma	kahr-suh-<u>noh</u>-muh	cancer that begins in the skin or in tissues that line or cover internal organs
cyst	sist	a sac or capsule filled with fluid
ductal carcinoma in situ	<u>duk</u>-tal kahr-suh-<u>noh</u>-muh in <u>sye</u>-too	abnormal cells that involve only the lining of a duct. The cells have not spread outside the duct to other tissues in the breast
epidermoid carcinoma	ep-i-<u>der</u>-moyd kahr-suh-<u>noh</u>-muh	a type of cancer in which the cells are flat and look like fish scales. Also called squamous cell carcinoma
familial polyposis	pah-li-<u>po</u>-sis	an inherited condition in which numerous polyps (tissue masses) develop on the inside walls of the colon and rectum. It increases the risk for colon cancer
fibroid	<u>fye</u>-broyd	a benign smooth muscle tumor, usually in the uterus or gastrointestinal tract. Also called leiomyoma
hyperplasia	hye-per-<u>play</u>-zha	an abnormal increase in the number of cells in an organ or tissue
large cell carcinomas	kahr-suh-<u>noh</u>-muhs	a group of lung cancers in which cells are large and look abnormal when viewed under a microscope
lobular carcinoma in situ	<u>lob</u>-yoo-lar kahr-suh-<u>noh</u>-muh in <u>sye</u>-too	abnormal cells found in the lobules of the breast. This condition seldom becomes invasive cancer. However, having lobular carcinoma in situ increases one's risk of developing breast cancer in either breast

Term	Pronounciation	Definition
malignant	ma-<u>lig</u>-nant	cancerous; a growth with a tendency to invade and destroy nearby tissue and spread to other parts of the body
nonsmall cell lung cancer		a group of lung cancers that includes squamous cell carcinoma, adenocarcinoma, and large cell carcinoma
oat cell cancer		a type of lung cancer in which the cells look like oats when viewed under a microscope. Also called small cell lung cancer
polyp	<u>pol</u>-ip	a growth that protrudes from a mucous membrane
sarcoma		a cancer of the bone, cartilage, fat, muscle, blood vessels, or other connective or supportive tissue
small cell lung cancer		a type of lung cancer in which the cells appear small and round when viewed under the microscope. Also called oat cell lung cancer
squamous cell carcinoma	<u>skway</u>-mus. . . kahr-suh-<u>noh</u>-muh	cancer that begins in squamous cells, which are thin, flat cells resembling fish scales. Squamous cells are found in the tissue that forms the surface of the skin, the lining of the hollow organs of the body, and the passages of the respiratory and digestive tracts. Also called epidermoid carcinoma
tumor	<u>too</u>-mer	an abnormal mass of tissue that results from excessive cell division. Tumors may be either benign (not cancerous) or malignant (cancerous)

LESSON TWO   PROGRESS CHECK

The following exercises will permit you to assess your progress in learning medical terms related to cancer.

■ WRITE-IN: TERMINOLOGY

For the type of cancer described, write in the correct term:

1. ~~polyp~~ *Papilloma*   benign cancer of the colon
2. *bone cell* carcinoma   benign skin cancer
3. leukemia   cancer of the blood cells
4. medulla blastoma   embryonic tumor of the brain
5. lymphoma   malignant cancer of the lymph system
6. Chrondosarcoma   malignant tumor of cartilage
7. melanoma   malignant tumor of the skin
8. Osteosarcoma   malignant cancer of the bone
9. fibroid   benign tumor of the uterus
10. oat cell carcinoma   cancer cells appear the size and shape of oats

■ MATCHING: DIAGNOSIS

Match the following diagnostic procedure to its function:

D **1.** biopsy

J **2.** barium enema

H **3.** PSA

G **4.** Pap smear

A **5.** sputum cytology

I **6.** bone marrow aspiration

E **7.** estrogen/progesterone receptors

C **8.** lymphangiography

F **9.** stool guaiac

B **10.** IVP

a. used to detect abnormal lung cells — *sputum cytology*

b. using a dye to visualize kidneys, ureters, and bladder — *IVP*

c. visualization of abdominal lymph nodes — *lymphangiography*

d. tissue sample taken for microscopic examination — *biopsy*

e. tissue sample taken near a breast tumor — *estrogen/progesterone receptors*

f. screen for gastrointestinal bleeding — *stool guaiac*

g. tissue sample taken for diagnosis of uterine cancer — *pap smear*

h. used to detect and monitor treatment of prostate cancer — *PSA*

i. diagnostic tool for detecting cancer of the blood cells — *bone marrow aspiration*

j. outline of the colon on x-ray — *barium enema*

■ MULTIPLE CHOICE: CANCER DIAGNOSIS AND TREATMENT

Circle the letter of the correct answer:

1. A biopsy is not used in the diagnosis of this cancer:
   a. leukemia
   b. breast
   c. lung
   d. bladder

2. Describes radiation therapy with a radioactive substance given intravenously:
   a. external
   b. internal
   c. prophylactic
   d. systemic

3. Surgical removal for treatment of bladder cancer:
   a. orchiectomy
   b. cystectomy
   c. intravenous pyelogram
   d. cystoscopy

4. A procedure that would not be used to diagnose or treat lung cancer:
   a. hormone therapy
   b. bronchoscopy
   c. sputum cytology
   d. pneumonectomy

5. Cancer cells in the liver in someone with metastatic cancer of the colon are described as:
   a. liver cancer
   b. colon cancer
   c. colon and liver cancer
   d. lymph cancer

6. Cryosurgery is a method of surgery using:
   a. electricity
   b. light
   c. freezing
   d. radioisotopes

7. Carcinoma of the breast would be treated by any of the following except:
   a. computed axial tomography
   b. hormone therapy
   c. radiation therapy
   d. modified radical mastectomy

8. Surgical excision of basal cell carcinoma of the skin is a type of treatment described as:
   a. definitive
   b. palliative
   c. prophylactic
   d. resection

9. Used to monitor treatment of cancer of the prostate:
   a. AFP
   b. CEA
   c. HCG
   (d.) PSA

10. Stem cell transplantation when the source of the cells is oneself:
    a. allogeneic
    (b.) autologous
    c. syngeneic
    d. internal

11. Bone marrow aspiration is a diagnostic tool for
    a. leukemia
    b. lymphoma
    (c.) leukemia and lymphoma
    d. neither leukemia nor lymphoma

12. A common symptom of cancer of the bladder or prostrate is
    a. hemoptysis
    b. dyspnea
    c. lymphadenopathy
    (d.) hematuria

Answer Keys

UNIT I: WORD PARTS AND MEDICAL TERMINOLOGY

Answer Key to Chapter 2: Word Parts

PROGRESS CHECK PART A

■ **MATCHING**

1. f
2. d
3. a
4. g
5. b
6. h
7. c
8. e

■ **SPELLING AND DEFINITION**

1. (a) ovary
2. (b) rectum or anus
3. (c) kidney
4. (b) nose
5. (a) testicle
6. (c) sacrum
7. (b) fallopian tube
8. (a) eardrum
9. (b) pharynx
10. (c) vertebra
11. (c) ureter
12. (a) cartilage
13. (b) rib
14. (b) vessel
15. (a) vein

■ **DEFINING MEDICAL WORD ELEMENTS**

1. andr/o
2. gyne
3. cardi/o
4. cephal/o
5. steth/o
6. dent/o or odont/o
7. encephal/o
8. gastr/o
9. hepat/o or hep/a
10. cholecyst/o
11. stomat/o
12. lingua
13. mast/o or mamm/o
14. my/o or myos
15. neur/o

■ **BUILDING MEDICAL WORDS**

1. tendinitis
2. thyroidectomy
3. tracheotomy
4. enteropathy
5. neuralgia
6. cystitis
7. arthritis
8. splenectomy
9. ophthalmologist
10. angiogram
11. cholelithiasis
12. arteriosclerosis
13. pneumonectomy
14. myelogram
15. otoscope
16. phlebotomy
17. prostatectomy
18. cerebrovascular accident
19. esophagitis
20. thoracotomy

PROGRESS CHECK PART B

■ **MATCHING**

1. i
2. j
3. g
4. h
5. f
6. e
7. c

8. d
9. a
10. b

■ SPELLING AND DEFINITION

1. (a) centesis: surgical puncture
2. (b) clasis: to break down; refracture
3. (c) ectasis: to expand, dilate
4. (d) malacia: softening
5. (a) plegia: paralysis (stroke)
6. (b) ptosis: prolapse, falling, drooping
7. (c) sclerosis: hardening
8. (d) megaly: enlargement
9. (a) cele: hernia, swelling
10. (b) iasis: abnormal condition: presence of, formation of

■ BUILDING MEDICAL WORDS

1. cephalgia or cephalodynia
2. roentgenography
3. gastritis
4. cholelithiasis
5. polycythemia
6. osteomalacia
7. arthrocentesis
8. phlebotomy
9. rhinoplasty
10. biology
11. hepatomegaly
12. dermatosis
13. appendectomy
14. psychiatry
15. encephalotomy
16. chemotherapy
17. hemostasis
18. carcinogen
19. nephropathy
20. aphasia

■ DEFINING MEDICAL TERMS

1. surgical fracture or refracture of a bone
2. surgical separation of intestinal adhesions
3. crushing of a stone in the bladder and washing out the fragments
4. death of cells or tissue
5. removal of the foreskin from the penis
6. a gland tumor
7. difficulty in swallowing
8. reduced number of white blood cells
9. paralyzed on one side of the body
10. morbid fear of heights

UNIT II: ROOT WORDS, MEDICAL TERMINOLOGY, AND PATIENT CARE

Answer Key to Chapter 3: Bacteria, Color, and Some Medical Terms

■ **MULTIPLE CHOICE**
1. c
2. c
3. b
4. d
5. b
6. a

■ **MATCHING**
1. h
2. e
3. j
4. i
5. f
6. g
7. a
8. h
9. c
10. d
11. h
12. b
13. a

■ **WRITE IN THE PREFIX**
1. acro-
2. aniso-
3. hetero-
4. dys-
5. homo-
6. iso-
7. mal-
8. megaly
9. pan-
10. post-
11. hemo-

■ **DEFINE THE PREFIX**
1. bad, poor
2. bad, painful, difficult
3. enlarged, large
4. excessive, beyond, above normal
5. fast
6. under, below normal
7. slow

8. take away, remove
9. put back
10. water
11. beside
12. around
13. many
14. before
15. before, preceding
16. through
17. together, united
18. night
19. night
20. through

Answer Key to Chapter 4: Body Openings and Plural Endings

■ **SPELLING AND DEFINITION**

1. (c) aperture: opening (orifice)
2. (a) constriction: closed, narrowed
3. (b) foramen: a natural opening or passage
4. (d) hiatus: a gap, cleft, or opening
5. (a) orifice: any opening (aperture)
6. (b) introitus: vaginal cavity (opening)
7. (c) ventricle: a small cavity or chamber (especially in the brain or heart)
8. (b) lumen: opening within a hollow tube or organ

■ **WORD CONSTRUCTION**

1. ae
2. aces
3. ina
4. es (or) a
5. ices
6. inges
7. ges
8. a
9. a
10. i
11. ora
12. ies
13. vertebra
14. thorax
15. lumen
16. crisis
17. ovary
18. artery
19. diverticulum

20. nucleus
21. meninx
22. diagnosis
23. spermatozoon
24. femur
25. appendix
26. ovum
27. thrombus

■ BUILDING MEDICAL TERMS

1. cavity
2. dilated
3. foramen
4. lumen
5. stoma
6. ventricle
7. patent
8. vaginal canal
9. alimentary canal
10. hiatus (hernia)

■ DEFINITIONS

1. thigh bone
2. a membrane covering the brain
3. chest
4. small cavity that prevents friction between tissues
5. any bone of the finger or toe
6. blood vessel
7. cavity (orifice) in the body
8. female gonad
9. slender outgrowth from the small intestine
10. male seed (germ) (semen)
11. red blood cell
12. outgrowth (pouch) on large intestine (colon)
13. mouth (oral cavity)
14. general term for the entrance to a cavity or space, e.g., vaginal cavity

Answer Key to Chapter 5: Numbers, Positions, and Directions

■ COMPARE AND CONTRAST

1. circum—around/contra —against
2. ecto—outside/endo—inside
3. infra—below/ipsi—same
4. para—near/peri—about (around)
5. uni—one/bi—two/tri—three
6. prima—first/multi—many
7. semi—half/hemi—one-sided (half)

8. ambi—both (sides)/quadri—four
9. meso—middle/meta—after (beyond)
10. retro—behind (backward)/trans—across (through)

■ IDENTIFY THE LOCATION

1. anterior
2. posterior
3. cephalic
4. caudal
5. supine or prone
6. eversion
7. extension
8. oblique
9. medial
10. adjacent

■ MATCHING: POSITIONS

1. m
2. o
3. n
4. j
5. a
6. l
7. b
8. c
9. k
10. d
11. i
12. e
13. f
14. h
15. g

■ DEFINE THE TERM

1. System for weighing and measuring drugs and solutions, precious metals, and precious stones
2. English system of weights and measures for all commodities except drugs, stones, metals
3. System of measures and weights based on the meter and based on multiples of ten
4. Monster
5. Small
6. Degree of heat or cold based on a specific scale
7. A temperature scale where H_2O boils at 100° and freezes at 0°
8. A temperature scale where H_2O boils at 212° and freezes at 32°
9. Change from one scale or system to another
10. Conversions that are equal to each other

■ **MATCHING: METRIC UNITS**

1. d
2. c
3. g
4. e
5. f
6. a
7. b

■ **SHORT ANSWER**

1. 1000
2. 1000
3. 100
4. 10
5. 100
6. 1000
7. 1000
8. one
9. 2.2
10. 2.5
11. 1000; 1000
12. 9, 5, 32
13. 32, 9, 5
14. 4.18
15. 3
16. 30
17. 240
18. 4.2

■ **FILL-IN**

1. milligram
2. microgram
3. kilogram
4. drops
5. dram
6. ounce
7. giga
8. liter
9. joule
10. tera
11. degrees Celsius
12. gram
13. elevated, high
14. take; prescription
15. without
16. with
17. infinity
18. before

19. after
20. male

Answer Key to Chapter 6: Medical and Health Professions

■ **MULTIPLE CHOICE: SCIENTIFIC STUDIES**

1. d
2. b
3. c
4. a
5. c
6. d
7. c

■ **MATCHING**

1. h
2. d
3. e
4. i
5. f
6. g
7. j
8. c
9. b
10. a

■ **SHORT ANSWER**

1. Care and treatment of the teeth and related structures. Dentist (D.M.D.) (D.D.S.)
2. Use of diet in promotion of health, and disease prevention and its treatment. Registered Dietitian (R.D.)
3. Care and treatment of the foot. Podiatrist (D.M.P.)
4. Care of women throughout pregnancy, delivery, and postpartum. Registered Nurse, Midwife (R.N.)
5. Routine care for persons in acute and chronic institutional facilities or community settings. Licensed Practical Nurse or Licensed Vocational Nurse (L.P.N. or L.V.N.)
6. Use of a variety of techniques with persons who have disturbed mental faculties and/or behavior problems. Psychologist (title depends on degree; usually M.S. or Ph.D.)
7. Interpretation and dispensing of drugs. Pharmacist (R.Ph.)
8. Direct care of ill persons in a variety of settings under the supervision of a physician. May also function independently. Registered Nurse (R.N.) or Public Health Nurse (P.H.N.)
9. The practice of medicine and/or surgery as well as research on animals. Veterinarian (D.V.M.)

■ **COMPLETION**

1. oral surgeon
2. periodontist
3. dental hygienist
4. dietetic technician
5. podiatrist
6. medical technician
7. physical therapist
8. psychologist
9. pharmacist
10. optometrist

■ **MULTIPLE CHOICE: PROFESSIONS**

1. a, b, c, d
2. a, b, c, d
3. a, b, c, d
4. Although 44 states and the District of Columbia require licensing, it is not required everywhere; therefore, no regulations apply universally.

■ **ABBREVIATIONS**

1. O.T.R
2. R.P.T.
3. P.H.N.
4. R.D.
5. L.P.N./L.V.N.
6. R.N. or P.H.N.
7. R.M.T.
8. R.T.
9. D.D.S./D.M.D.
10. D.V.M.
11. O.D.
12. M.D.
13. M.S./Ph.D.
14. M.D.
15. R.Ph.
16. A.R.R.T.
17. D.O.
18. M.D.

■ **DESCRIBE THE SPECIALTY**

1. Administration of medications to kill pain sensation
2. Study of the endocrine gland functions and illness
3. Study of the blood and blood-forming tissue
4. The use of x-ray and radioactive substances to diagnose disease
5. Study of body tissues for diagnosis of all diseases, and the nature of disease
6. Study of bacteria, especially disease-producing bacteria (pathogens)
7. Study of living organisms
8. Study of the care of the aging and elderly

9. Study of the care of children
10. Care of the foot
11. Promotion of health, and disease prevention and treatment as related to nutrition
12. Care of the pregnant woman through delivery

UNIT III: ABBREVIATIONS

Answer Key to Chapter 7: Medical Abbreviations

■ **IDENTIFY THE DEPARTMENT**

1. Admitting and Discharge
2. Central Service
3. Operating Room
4. Physical Medicine and Rehabilitation
5. Radiology
6. Laboratory
7. Obstetrics
8. Pediatrics
9. Outpatient Department
10. Emergency Room
11. Social Service
12. Intensive Care Unit
13. Food Service

■ **IDENTIFY THE PRESCRIPTION**

1. 2 grams by mouth three times a day
2. 60 milliequivalents by rectal suppository at bedtime
3. 6 drops under the tongue every 4 hours
4. 2 liters intravenously every day
5. 30 units intramuscularly before meals
6. 10 milliliters under the skin as needed
7. 2 grains in 10 cubic centimeters of normal saline by needle under the skin once a day
8. one half of a 5-milligram tablet by mouth after meals

■ **IDENTIFY THE DIET ORDER**

1. nothing by mouth
2. diet as tolerated
3. Carbohydrate or consistent carbohydrate diet
4. 2 g sodium medical soft
5. mechanical soft
6. clear liquid
7. regular high fiber, force fluids
8. full liquid with interval nourishment at 10 AM to 2 PM and at bedtime. Intake and output recorded

■ **MATCHING**

1. f
2. d
3. g
4. h
5. c
6. e
7. b
8. a

■ **SPELL OUT THE ABBREVIATION**

1. prepare preoperatively
2. dead on arrival
3. with; without; temperature, pulse, respiration
4. cardiopulmonary resuscitation
5. blood pressure; millimeters; mercury
6. tender loving care
7. discontinue; intravenous (line); as soon as possible
8. carbon dioxide and water
9. treatment; symptoms
10. sodium; potassium
11. diagnosis; iron

Answer Key to Chapter 8: Diagnostic and Laboratory Abbreviations

■ **IDENTIFY THE DISEASE**

1. arteriosclerotic heart disease
2. coronary heart disease
3. congestive heart failure
4. cardiovascular disease
5. cerebrovascular accident
6. chronic brain syndrome
7. chronic obstructive pulmonary disease
8. myocardial infarction
9. rheumatoid arthritis
10. transient ischemic attack

■ **SHORT ANSWER**

1. auscultation and percussion
2. pupils equal, round, react to light and accommodation
3. percussion and auscultation
4. rule out
5. systems review
6. tonsillectomy and adenoidectomy
7. physical examination
8. prescription
9. head, eyes, ears, nose, throat
10. diagnosis

■ MATCHING

1. c
2. h
3. f
4. b
5. a
6. e
7. g
8. d
9. m
10. p
11. q
12. o
13. n
14. j
15. r
16. l
17. i
18. k

■ DEFINE THE ABBREVIATION

1. chief complaint
2. complains of
3. family history
4. fever of undetermined origin
5. history
6. short of breath
7. upper respiratory infection
8. urinary tract infection
9. murmur
10. present illness
11. symptoms
12. past history

UNIT IV: REVIEW

Answer Key to Chapter 9: Review of Root Words

■ COMPARE AND CONTRAST

1. lipo: a term for fat; litho: stone
2. para: to bear; pathy: any disease
3. phagia: swallowing; phasia: speech; phonia: voice
4. schizo: split; sclero: hardening
5. thrombo: clot; thermo: heat; trauma: injury
6. abscess: pus; adnexa: accessory structure
7. axilla: armpit; anomaly: defect
8. cervical: neck; coccyx: tailbone
9. edema: excess fluid; embolus: clot in a vessel

10. emesis: vomiting; enema: fluid injected into rectum
11. icterus: jaundice; ischemia: lack of blood to a part
12. palpable: felt by touch; parietal: walls of a cavity
13. prolapse: falling downward; prophylaxis: preventive treatment
14. suture: stitch; sputum: expectorate
15. viscera: interior organ; virus: infectious agent

■ BUILDING MEDICAL TERMS: INFLAMMATION OF A BODY PART

1. chondritis
2. colpitis or vaginitis
3. laryngitis
4. paronychia
5. pancreatitis
6. phlebitis
7. salpingitis
8. otitis
9. pleurisy (pleuritis)
10. spondylitis
11. stomatitis
12. ureteritis
13. urethritis
14. esophagitis
15. neuritis

■ BUILDING MEDICAL TERMS: GENERAL

16. aphasia
17. dysphagia
18. carcinoma
19. necrosis
20. lipid
21. scleroderma
22. hemostasis
23. trauma
24. acute
25. anomaly
26. chronic
27. embolus
28. emesis
29. voiding
30. edema
31. coccyx
32. cervical vertebrae
33. excreting
34. exacerbation
35. incontinence
36. inflammation
37. ischemia

38. hemorrhage
39. metastasis
40. obesity
41. palpable
42. prophylaxis
43. sputum
44. virus
45. suture

■ FILL-IN

1. metacarpals
2. laparotomy (celiotomy)
3. oophorectomy (or) ovariectomy
4. podiatry
5. rhinoplasty
6. metatarsals
7. thoracentesis
8. cryptorchidism
9. primigravida
10. multipara

■ DEFINE THE TERM

1. Expulsion of the fetus from the uterus before it is viable
2. Listening for sounds within the body
3. Strand of collagen from a mammal, used to suture
4. A flexible tube to be passed into body channels
5. Stretching; expanding
6. A clot or other plug taken by the blood to a smaller vessel
7. Increase in severity of a disease or symptoms
8. Deep band of fibrous tissue
9. Transfer of disease from one organ or body to another area not connected directly
10. Striking a part with short, sharp blows

■ MATCHING

1. e
2. d
3. a
4. h
5. j
6. i
7. b
8. c
9. f
10. g

■ **SHORT ANSWER: ROOT WORDS**

1. carp/o
2. cervic/o
3. dent/o, odont
4. esophag/o
5. lapar/o, celi/o
6. onych/o
7. ophthalm/o
8. pancreat/o
9. soma
10. pod/o
11. pubis
12. rhin/o
13. stomat/o
14. tarslo
15. thorac/o

■ **SHORT ANSWER: BODY PARTS**

1. vagina
2. vein
3. pleura
4. vertebra
5. mouth

UNIT V: MEDICAL TERMINOLOGY AND BODY SYSTEMS

Answer Key to Chapter 10: Body Organs and Parts

■ **SPELLING AND DEFINITION**

1. Integumentary; skin, nails, hair, oil and sweat glands
2. Cardiovascular; heart and blood vessels
3. Musculoskeletal; bones, joints, ligaments, cartilage, and muscles
4. Gastrointestinal; mouth, esophagus, stomach, intestines, and accessory organs
5. Respiratory; nose, pharynx, larynx, trachea, bronchi, and lungs
6. Genitourinary; kidneys, bladder, ureters, urethra, gonads, genitalia, and internal organs
7. Endocrine; ductless glands and supporting structures
8. Nervous; brain, spinal cord, cranial and spinal nerves

■ **FILL-IN**

1. cell
2. genetic
3. mitosis
4. multiplying
5. membrane
6. tissues
7. epithelial tissue
8. connective tissue

9. muscle tissue
10. nerve tissue
11. organ
12. systems
13. cavity
14. planes
15. diaphragm

■ **DEFINITIONS**

1. Sum of physical and chemical processes that convert food into elements for growth, repair, and energy as well as recycling and excretion.
2. When the body systems maintain a balance optimal for survival: a steady state.

■ **SHORT ANSWER**

1. epithelial
2. protects, absorbs, secretes
3. connective
4. binds all tissue together
5. muscle
6. contracts and relaxes
7. nerve
8. controls and coordinates body activity
9. serves as the wall or outer covering; allows some substances to go into the cell, but keeps others out
10. contains genes and chromosomes for reproduction

Answer Key to Chapter 11: Integumentary System

■ **SPELLING AND DEFINITION**

1. (a) epidermis: the outermost nonvascular layer of skin
2. (d) subcutaneous: beneath the skin
3. (b) biopsy: removal of tissue from the body for examination
4. (c) debridement: removal of devitalized tissue
5. (a) escharotomy: removal of burn scar tissue
6. (b) keratosis: any horny growth
7. (c) steatoma: a fatty mass within an oil gland
8. (d) verruca: a wart
9. (b) impetigo: a staphylococcal or streptococcal skin infection marked by vesicles that become pustular
10. (a) pediculosis: infestation with lice
11. (c) eczema: redness in the skin
12. (b) psoriasis: chronic, hereditary, recurrent dermatosis
13. (d) erysipelas: a contagious skin disease
14. (a) varicella: chickenpox
15. (b) actinic: referring to ultraviolet rays reacting on the skin

■ **WRITE-IN**

1. albinism
2. alopecia
3. dermatology
4. erythema
5. eschar
6. nummular
7. papule
8. urticaria
9. pustule
10. cicatrix

■ **MATCHING: SKIN TERMS**

1. h
2. g
3. f
4. e
5. d
6. c
7. b
8. a

■ **DEFINITIONS**

1. A test for tuberculosis (TB)
2. A test for scarlet fever
3. A test for diphtheria
4. A test for the presence of cystic fibrosis
5. A test for valley fever
6. A test for systemic fungal disease

■ **MATCHING: SKIN DISEASES**

1. d
2. g
3. e
4. c
5. f
6. b
7. a
8. i
9. h

■ **LIST THE FUNCTIONS**

1. A protective barrier from many things
2. Enables the body to sense heat, cold, or pain
3. Assists in regulating body temperature by insulating
4. Eliminates body wastes through perspiration
5. Synthesizes vitamin D

■ ANSWER TO THE WORD PUZZLE ON THE INTEGUMENTARY SYSTEM

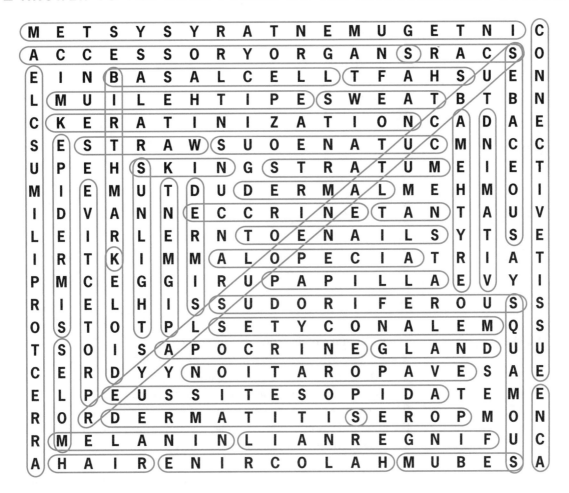

Answer Key to Chapter 12: Gastrointestinal System

■ WRITE-IN

1. adhesions
2. botulism
3. carcinoma
4. cholelithiasis
5. colitis
6. diverticula
7. gastric ulcer
8. gastritis/gastroenteritis
9. glossitis
10. hernia
11. intussusception
12. strangulated

13. hepatitis
14. nausea and vomiting
15. obesity
16. pancreatitis
17. peritonitis
18. pyloric stenosis
19. steatorrhea
20. cirrhosis

■ **MATCHING**

1. c
2. h
3. a
4. g
5. e
6. f
7. d
8. i
9. j
10. b

■ **DEFINITIONS**

1. Chief organ of digestion and absorption
2. An M.D. who specializes in the study of the GI tract
3. Process of converting food into nutrients
4. Process that transfers nutrients to the bloodstream
5. The entire gastrointestinal tract
6. Rhythmic motion of the muscles that move food through the GI tract
7. Slime produced in mucous membranes
8. First 10–12 in. of the small intestine
9. Valve that passes food from the stomach to the intestine in one direction only
10. Opening of the common bile duct into the duodenum
11. Special double-layered tissue that suspends the intestine in the abdominal cavity
12. Veins in the region of the anus
13. Additional covering of the alimentary canal
14. The large intestine, which extends from cecum to rectum
15. The beginning of the large intestine of the GI tract

■ **WORD POOL: STRUCTURE OF THE GI TRACT**

1. mouth or oral cavity
2. small intestine
3. duodenum
4. cecum
5. liver, gallbladder, pancreas
6. deciduous
7. rectum
8. anus

9. greater omentum
10. duodenum, jejunum, ileum
11. palate
12. peridental disease

■ **MATCHING:**
SURGICAL
PROCEDURES

1. g
2. f
3. h
4. j
5. e
6. a
7. b
8. d
9. c
10. i

■ ANSWER TO THE WORD PUZZLE ON THE DIGESTIVE SYSTEM

Answer Key to Chapter 13: Respiratory System

■ **MATCHING**

1. j
2. i
3. e
4. g
5. a
6. b
7. h
8. d
9. c
10. f

■ **MULTIPLE CHOICE**

1. c
2. a
3. b
4. d
5. b
6. b
7. c
8. a
9. c
10. d

■ **DEFINITIONS**

1. The throat; the cavity between nasal passages and mouth; passageway for food and liquid (also airway)
2. Voice box; contains the vocal cords
3. The windpipe; a long tube extending from the trachea to the chest
4. A cluster of air sacs whose walls exchange oxygen and carbon dioxide
5. The main branches conveying air from the trachea to the lungs
6. Between the ribs
7. Pockets (cavities) in the face and skull bones
8. Organs of respiration where blood and air meet and mix
9. Chief muscle of respiration; separates the lungs from the abdomen
10. Sudden infant death syndrome. The dying during sleep of healthy infants, cause unknown; also called crib death
11. Chronic obstructive pulmonary disease (also COLD: chronic obstructive lung disease). A group of chronic, progressively debilitating lung diseases including emphysema, bronchitis, and asthma
12. Inflammation of the pleura, the lining that encases the lungs
13. Hereditary disorder present from birth associated with malfunction of the pancreas and frequent respiratory infections
14. Contagious inflammation of the upper respiratory tract

15. Pus in a body cavity

16. Acute (adult) respiratory distress syndrome. Faulty gaseous exchange leading to shock lung

■ ABBREVIATIONS

1. upper respiratory infection
2. shortness of breath
3. intermittent positive pressure breathing
4. submucous resection
5. complete blood count
6. temperature, pulse, and respiration
7. purified protein derivative (TB test)
8. cardiopulmonary resuscitation
9. endotracheal tube
10. auscultation and percussion

■ NAMING

1. hypercapnia
2. orthopnea
3. dyspnea
4. cyanosis
5. hemoptysis
6. hypoxia
7. pyothorax; empyema
8. stridor
9. dysphonia
10. hemothorax

■ MATCHING

1. f
2. a
3. b
4. e
5. d
6. c

■ **ANSWER TO THE WORD PUZZLE ON THE RESPIRATORY SYSTEM**

```
L O B U L E S A N I R A C I C A R O H T
A M U T P E S L A S A N X O B E C I O V
R T H R O A T X N Y R A H P S T I D A L
Y S C A S Y R A N O M L U P A S S A G E
N I N S P I R A T I O N I N H A L E A B
X N O I T A R I P S E R C I L I A B S R
E E R U S S E R P L A I T R A P T R E O
D S H A L L O W C T R A C H E A I O X N
I A E R A T E I O E V R E S E R V N C C
X H E T A R B R L S U L O E V L A C H H
O C S A A O Y A M U C U S E B O L H A I
I N O N R C H E C N A I L P M O C U N O
D O N E E X P I R A T I O N I O N S G L
N C A N E M G A R H P A I D U C T S E E
O Y T I L I B I S N E T S I D T U B E S
B E E R T L A I H C N O R B O X Y G E N
R V E N T I L A T I O N L A U D I S E R
A I T R A N S P O R T R C E L L U L A R
C A P A C I T Y T I V A C L A R U E L P
G N U L S U R F A C T A N T B R E A T H
```

Answer Key to Chapter 14: Cardiovascular System

■ **DEFINITIONS**

1. X-ray examination of vessels
2. A balloon-type catheter is used to exert pressure on the plaque in a vessel, opening up a blocked area
3. Medication to delay blood clotting
4. Catheter passed into the heart through a vein in the arm and used to detect abnormal blood flow in arteries
5. Cutting of a heart valve that is defective
6. Medication that reduces intravascular blood volume, thus lowering blood pressure
7. Ultrasonic probe that checks blood flow
8. Picture of electrical impulses of the heart
9. Boring out the inner lining of an artery to increase the size of the lumen

10. A battery-powered device implanted to regulate heartbeat
11. Adjunct treatment used to help reduce edema and blood pressure
12. A drug that causes a vessel to dilate
13. A drug that causes a vessel to constrict
14. Puncture of a vein

■ NAMING

1. right lymphatic duct
2. adenoids
3. thymus gland
4. lymph capillaries
5. lymph nodes
6. thoracic duct
7. interstitial fluid
8. spleen

■ MATCHING

1. c
2. g
3. j
4. e
5. b
6. a
7. i
8. h
9. f
10. d

■ MULTIPLE CHOICE

1. a
2. d
3. a
4. c
5. b
6. b
7. a
8. b
9. d
10. c

■ ABBREVIATIONS

1. atrial septal defect
2. blood pressure
3. complete blood count
4. coronary care unit
5. congestive heart failure
6. carbon dioxide
7. cardiopulmonary resuscitation
8. cerebrovascular accident (stroke)

9. electrocardiogram
10. myocardial infarction (heart attack)
11. oxygen
12. premature ventricular contraction
13. red blood cell/red blood cell count
14. transient ischemic attack
15. white blood cell/white blood cell count

■ ANSWER TO THE WORD PUZZLE ON THE HEART

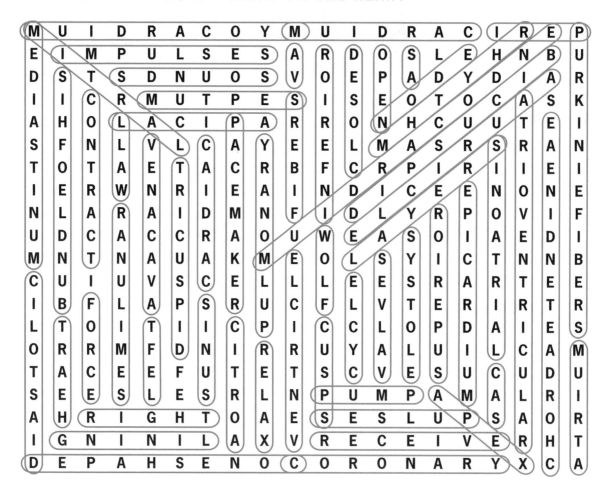

Answer Key to Chapter 15: Nervous System

■ FILL-IN

1. central
2. central
3. autonomic
4. ventricles
5. plexus
6. sulcus

7. limbic
8. ganglion
9. hemisphere
10. encephalon
11. opening in the occipital bone through which the spinal cord passes
12. cauda equina
13. cerebellum
14. dura mater
15. sympathetic

■ MATCHING: NERVES

1. g
2. e
3. a
4. b
5. c
6. f
7. d

■ MATCHING: DISEASES

1. a
2. f
3. e
4. g
5. h
6. d
7. c
8. b

■ TRUE/FALSE

1. T
2. F
3. T
4. F
5. T
6. F
7. F
8. T
9. T
10. F

■ DEFINITIONS

1. Conflicting emotional attitude
2. Complete withdrawal
3. A false personal belief
4. Illusions, excitement, hallucinations (short duration)
5. Automatic repetition of what is said
6. Imaginary illness
7. Belief in one's greatness, power
8. A person abnormally suspicious of others

9. Abnormal dread or fear
10. A group of severe emotional disorders characterized by delirium, delusion, hallucinations, and other bizarre behaviors

■ SPELLING AND DEFINITION

1. (a) cerebrum. The largest portion of the brain; divided into left and right hemispheres; located in the upper part of the cranial cavity
2. (c) meninges. The three membranes covering the brain and spinal cord
3. (b) arachnoid. The delicate membrane between the pia mater and dura mater
4. (d) trochlear. Muscle of the eyes
5. (a) olfactory. Sense of smell
6. (b) hypoglossal. Beneath the tongue
7. (c) anencephaly. Congenital absence of a brain
8. (a) hydrocephalus. Accumulation of cerebrospinal fluid within the skull
9. (d) meningocele. Hernial protrusion of the meninges through a defect in the skull or vertebrae
10. (a) poliomyelitis. An acute viral disease

■ ANSWER TO THE WORD PUZZLE: THE NERVOUS SYSTEM (GENERAL TERMS)

```
A T R E I V N A R F O S E D O N J E R K
C N E S N E U R O G L I A F F E C T O R
T E T E E T A R E N E G E R O T I N O M
I R T N S R O T P E C E R C O N T R O L
O E I S J U N C T I O N O E S P A N Y S
N F M O C N S N P A M M E L O R U E N E
P F S R C H A R G E M U I L U M I T S G
O E N Y D E X I M U S E N S E S S W N N
T S A M Y E L I N S H E A T H C I N O A
E N R O T O M I I T L U S P R T S E I H
N O T R E A C T R A T E A H S P U T C
T R O N E A E A N O H T X D K N A R C T
I U R R T V N I N C H E R E N O C O U C
A E U E R S M O N W L A C N O X E N D E
L N E E M R M A A F W V L D B A S S N T
S R N I E I R Y E A T N E R E F F A O E
T E T T C B S R L T C A F I B E R S C D
I T E F F E C T O R S E T T E T I C X E
N N I O N S L A R T N E C E L L B O D Y
U I I N F O R M A T I O N N A W H C S S
```

Answer Key to Chapter 16: Genitourinary System

■ LISTS

1. a. (two) kidneys
   b. (two) ureters
   c. (one) bladder
   d. (one) urethra
2. a. remove water and wastes, convert to urine, transport, excrete
   b. reabsorb substances the body wants to keep
   c. maintain body system equilibrium by regulation of pH, RBC production, blood pressure, blood glucose
3. perpetuating the species
4. a. (two) ovaries
   b. (two) fallopian tubes
   c. (two) breasts
   d. (one) uterus
   e. (one) vagina
   f. (one) vulva
5. a. (two) testes
   b. (three) glands
   c. (four) ducts
   d. (one) penis
   e. (one) scrotum
   f. (one) urethra

■ MULTIPLE CHOICE

1. b
2. a
3. c
4. d

■ COMPARE AND CONTRAST

1. Albuminuria is the presence of protein (albumin) in the urine; anuria is no (without) urine
2. Enuresis is bed-wetting while asleep; diuresis is increased excretion of urine
3. Incontinence is inability to control bowel or bladder excretion; urinary retention is inability to excrete urine
4. Hydronephrosis is distention of the renal pelvis because of the inability to urinate; nephrolithiasis is kidney (renal) stones
5. Nycturia is excessive night urination; oliguria is diminished urine secretion; and dysuria is painful or difficult urination
6. Pyelitis is inflammation of the renal pelvis; glomerulonephritis is inflammation of the capillary loops in the glomeruli

■ MATCHING:
CLINICAL
PROCEDURES

1. e
2. d
3. f

4. h
5. g
6. c
7. a
8. b

■ **COMPLETION**

1. testis
2. external genitalia
3. vas deferens
4. prostate
5. epididymis
6. seminal duct
7. ovaries
8. fallopian tube
9. uterus
10. vagina

■ **MATCHING: MALE CLINICAL CONDITIONS**

1. c
2. d
3. e
4. b
5. a

■ **MATCHING: FEMALE CLINICAL CONDITIONS**

1. c
2. e
3. d
4. a
5. b

■ **DEFINITIONS**

1. amniocentesis
2. Apgar test
3. cephalopelvic disproportion (CPD)
4. dystocia
5. ectopic or extrauterine
6. gestation
7. gravida
8. neonatal period
9. postpartum
10. placenta

ANSWER TO THE WORD PUZZLE ON THE GENITOURINARY SYSTEM

```
R E D D A L B Y R A N I R U C O R T E X
S E T Y L O R T C E L E D I C A C I R U
U G T R A N S P O R T C I T O M S O E R
T L F R A L U B U T I R E P L U D R I N
A O I B O W M A N S C A P S U L E P B A
E M L A C P A F F E R E N T M O S O S T
M E T R R U E Y E N D I K E N P E L R I
N R A E A R U R E T E R T T N O E G P O
O U T T T E N I R U S S E R O F D N T N
I L E I H A D H T Y V E R R H I I I I O
T U R N I N T S O C C C H H N D O N I
A S I O R A N Y L A N R X P E N G N O T
R R O I A E R U L E S E E E N N D N I
T E N N R A M Y R R I T A N L L N R E T
N N E E L E X Y S U V E Y L E O C E U
E A R F L T U B U L E L C E L L O S T R
C L F I S D I U L F S E T S A W P A I U
N E P P R O X I M A L P D I S T A L I C
O A S T D I M A R Y P M E D U L L A F I
C O N V O L U T E D E M E N O G I R T M
```

Answer Key to Chapter 17: Musuloskeletal System

LIST THE FUNCTION

1. Support and protection—vital organs protected
2. Movement—all body movements
3. Red blood cell turnover—bone marrow is the site
4. Storage—minerals and nutrients

MATCHING: LOCATIONS

1. f
2. g
3. i
4. h
5. j
6. a
7. b

        8. c
        9. d
    10. e

■ **MULTIPLE CHOICE**

        1. b
        2. b
        3. a
        4. c
        5. d
        6. c
        7. b
        8. c
        9. d

■ **NAME THE STRUCTURE**

        1. bursa
        2. fascia
        3. lamina
        4. ligament
        5. aponeurosis
        6. hinges
        7. sutures
        8. ball and socket
        9. tendon
    10. meniscus

■ **MATCHING**

        1. c
        2. d
        3. e
        4. b
        5. a
        6. d
        7. a
        8. b
        9. e
    10. c
    11. g
    12. f
    13. d
    14. e
    15. b
    16. c
    17. a

■ **COMPARE AND CONTRAST**

1. Kyphosis is humpback (or hunchback); lordosis is curvature of the lumbar spine (swayback).
2. Gout is a form of arthritis; rickets is a deficiency of vitamin D.
3. Carpal tunnel syndrome is a painful disorder of the wrist and hand; collagen disease is a disease of connective tissue.
4. Muscular dystrophy is progressive atrophy of the skeleton; myasthenia gravis is lack of muscle strength.
5. Osteomalacia is softening of the bones; osteoporosis is brittle porous bones.
6. Sarcoma is a malignant bone tumor; scoliosis is lateral curvature of the spine.
7. Spina bifida is a congenital defect in the spine; spondylitis is inflammation of the vertebra.

■ **ANSWER TO THE WORD PUZZLE ON THE SKELETAL SYSTEM**

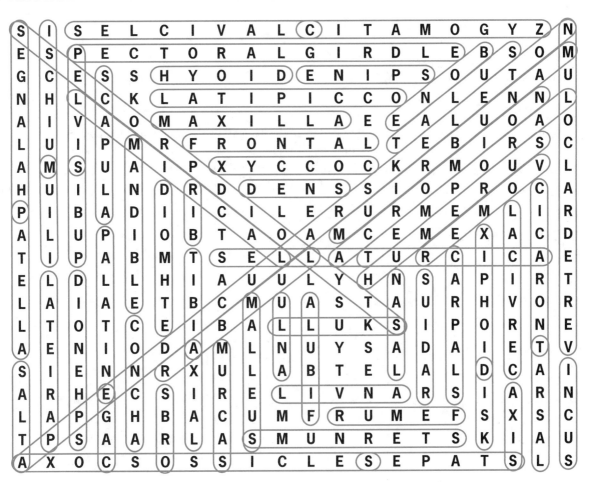

Answer Key to Chapter 18: Eyes and Ears

■ MATCHING: EYE STRUCTURES

1. e
2. f
3. g
4. h
5. i
6. d
7. a
8. b
9. c

■ MULTIPLE CHOICE: EYE

1. c
2. b
3. d
4. c
5. b
6. c
7. a
8. c
9. a

■ EAR STRUCTURES

1. ear canal
2. separated from the external ear by the tympanic membrane
3. membrane labyrinth
4. partition between external and middle ear
5. between the nasopharynx and tympanic cavity
6. earwax in the ear

■ MULTIPLE CHOICE: EAR

1. a
2. b
3. c
4. d
5. a

■ ANSWER TO THE WORD PUZZLE ON THE SENSORY SYSTEM

```
L A C R I M A L A P P A R A T U S  C I N U T
L S E B U T N A I H C A T S U E U  A T L A Y
E E Q U I L I B R I U M L A V O  O V H O E M
M I E O T O N O I T A T P A D A  E U G B L P
S T L O C I L I A R Y B O D Y  E U Y S S A
L R D T E E N O I T A S N E S  T Q A D N C
A F D H A H A M M E R D U C T  N A O N U F X
N O I P R L A N R E T X E N  N O D N S C X
A N M S S W E E T S P N S  I R E C O E S X
C W C H C O N E S R A N M  I R N C V T O
R I H E U S E Y E E I I A  U I U M A P S
A N S T R M E S S N C T  D O S O P T S E
L D D T N U O I N M S  I C E I S U V R
U O S I I I M R E A  F C S A L U E O A
C W D C O R R N C  A M C N C U E W N
R O S N L R R Y B O T R U L A N I R D E
I S U V U E O U A U E A C O I A V U
C L I V U O R H P A R L S C U T R I N
I P S I S R A C S S E A H O E U M V C
M U S O P H T H A L A A C A T E L I U
E U S N U F O V E A C E N T R A L I S O
S S U O N A R B M E M A V I T C N U J N O C
```

Answer Key to Chapter 19: Endocrine System

■ MULTIPLE CHOICE

1. b
2. a
3. d
4. d
5. a
6. c
7. b
8. d
9. c
10. b

■ **MATCHING**

1. b
2. c
3. d
4. c
5. d
6. d
7. e
8. b
9. a

■ **FILL-IN**

1. diabetes mellitus
2. cretinism
3. Graves' disease
4. pheochromocytoma
5. tetany
6. myxedema
7. Cushing's disease

■ **DEFINITIONS**

1. Involuntary muscle contraction
2. Profuse perspiration
3. Wasted condition; excessive leanness
4. Protein hormone produced by the islets of Langerhans
5. Accumulation of excess ketone bodies in tissues and fluids
6. Any functional disturbance or pathologic condition in the nervous system
7. A group of drugs prescribed for the diabetic to reduce circulating glucose

■ **COMPARE AND CONTRAST**

1. Acidosis is a pathologic condition resulting from accumulation of acid or loss of base; anorexia is loss of appetite.
2. Cachexia is extreme wasting of body tissue; cataracts are clouding of the lenses of the eye.
3. Gangrene is death of a tissue from lack of circulation of nutrients; a gland is an organ that secretes.
4. Hypoglycemia is blood sugar that falls below the normal range; hypophysectomy is excision of the pituitary gland.

■ **ANSWER TO THE WORD PUZZLE ON THE ENDOCRINE SYSTEM**

```
A L L U D E M T P I T C O R T I S O N E
C D T E S T E S N I T C A L O R P O N N
T L R A L P H A C E L L S P T H R D A O
H A E N O M R O H H T W O R G O W C I R
K E P I N E P H R I N E A T E C G B I E
C S A N I O V A R Y A D H N R A E E T T
A Y D S O Y C S R N I Y O I M L S B R S
B H R U D A I O D O R R N N G C T A U O
D P E L I T I R R O E E R N M I E C U D
E O N I N R O Y I T S O I U M T R E I L
E P A E G H D S Y I Z I C A O R O L D A
F Y L T E A O S R I C I H S N N L I F
V H N N A S T T E N L N O O I I E S T O
I A S R D S E T I A H L H T E N O M N L
E A A E M S E C G L A N D R A D H A L
P N T O O T S U M A L A H T O P Y H I
A O H S P U G H S A E R C N A P P T A C
G F S H L D U C T L S F E M A L E I I L
E S T R O G E N S E S O X Y T O C I N E
N S E B O L D N A L G Y R A T I U T I P
```

Answer Key to Chapter 20: Cancer Medicine

■ **WRITE-IN**

1. polyp, papilloma
2. basal cell carcinoma
3. leukemia
4. medullablastoma
5. lymphoma
6. chrondosarcoma
7. melanoma
8. osteosarcoma
9. fibroid
10. oat cell carcinoma

■ **MATCHING**
1. d
2. j
3. h
4. g
5. a
6. i
7. e
8. c
9. f
10. b

■ **MULTIPLE CHOICE**
1. a
2. d
3. b
4. a
5. b.
6. c
7. a
8. c
9. d
10. b
11. c
12. d

APPENDIX B   Bibliography

Barton-Burke, Margaret and Wilkes, Gail M. *Cancer Therapies*. Sudbury, MA: Jones & Bartlett, 2006.

Braunwald, Eugene, Zipes, Douglas P., Libby, Peter, Bonow, Robert. *Braunwald's Heart Disease*, 7th ed. Philadelphia: Elsevier, 2005.

Clark, Robert K. *Anatomy and Physiology: Understanding the Human*. Sudbury, MA: Jones & Bartlett, 2005.

Donnersberger, Anne B. *A Laboratory Textbook of Anatomy and Physiology: Fetal Pig Version*, 8th ed. Sudbury, MA: Jones & Bartlett, 2006.

Dorland, W. A. Newman. *Dorland's Medical Dictionary*. Philadelphia: W. B. Saunders, 2004.

Guyton, Arthur C. and Hall, John E. *Textbook of Medical Physiology*, 11th ed. Philadelphia: Elsevier, 2006.

Hay, David W. *Little Black Book of Gastroenterology*, 2nd ed. Sudbury, MA: Jones & Bartlett, 2005.

Mason, Robert J., Broaddus, V. Courtney, Murray, John F., Nadel, Jay A. *Murray and Nadel's Textbook of Respiratory Medicine*, 4th ed. Philadelphia: Elsevier, 2005.

Mosby's Dictionary of Medicine, Nursing & Health Professions, 7th ed. St. Louis: Elsevier, 2006.

Odom, Richard B., James, William D., Berger, Timothy G. *Andrews' Diseases of the Skin: Clinical Dermatology*, 9th ed. Philadelphia: Elsevier, 2005.

Pagana, Kathleen D. and Pagana, Timothy J. *Mosby's Manual of Diagnostic and Laboratory Tests*. St. Louis: Elsevier, 2005.

Ropper, Allan H. and Brown, Robert H. *Adams and Victor's Principles of Neurology*, 8th ed. Columbus, Ohio: McGraw-Hill, 2005.

Stanfield, Peggy S. and Hui, Y. H. *Nutrition and Diet Therapy: Self Instruction Modules*, 4th ed. Sudbury, MA: Jones & Bartlett, 2003.

Thibodeau, Gary A. and Patton, Kevin T. *Anatomy & Physiology*. Philadelphia: Elsevier, 2006.

Weinstein, W. *Clinical Gastroenterology and Hepatology.* St. Louis: Elsevier, 2005.

Wilkes, Gail M. *2005 Oncology Nursing Drug Handbook.* Sudbury, MA: Jones & Bartlett, 2006.

Wu, Alan H. B. *Tietz Clinical Guide to Laboratory Tests,* 4th ed. Philadelphia: Elsevier, 2006.

Yamada, Tadataka, Alpers, David H., Owyang, Chung, et al. *Handbook of Gastroenterology,* 2nd ed. Philadelphia: Lippincott, Williams & Wilkins, 2005.

APPENDIX C | Flash Cards

epithelial tissue ep′-i-<u>the</u>-le-al <u>tish</u>-u Body Organs and Parts	**integumentary system** in-teg′u-<u>men</u>-ter-e <u>sis</u>-tem Body Organs and Parts
musculoskeletal system mus′ku-lo-<u>skel</u>-e-tal <u>sis</u>-tem Body Organs and Parts	**respiratory system** re-<u>spi</u>-rah-to-re <u>sis</u>-tem Body Organs and Parts
genitourinary system jen′i-to-<u>u</u>-ri-ner′e <u>sis</u>-tem Body Organs and Parts	**mediastinum** me′de-ah-<u>sti</u>-num Body Organs and Parts
peritoneal cavity per′i-to-<u>ne</u>-al <u>kav</u>-i-te Body Organs and Parts	**diaphragm** <u>di</u>-ah-fram Body Organs and Parts
midsagittal mid-<u>saj</u>-i-tal Body Organs and Parts	**homeostasis** ho′me-o-<u>sta</u>-sis Body Organs and Parts

skin serves as the external covering of the body. Accessory organs of this system are nails, hair, and oil and sweat glands	the skin and lining surfaces that protect, absorb, and secrete
nose, pharynx, larynx, trachea, bronchi, and lungs. Furnish oxygen, remove carbon dioxide (respiration)	skeleton and muscles: the 206 bones, the joints, cartilage, ligaments, and all of the muscles of the body
the mass of tissues and organs separating the sternum in front and the vertebral column behind, containing the heart and its large vessels	reproductive and urinary organs; also called urogenital system (GU or UG). The urinary organs are the kidneys, ureters, bladder, and urethra. The reproductive organs are the gonads and various external genitalia and internal organs
dome-shaped muscle separating the abdominal and thoracic cavities	the space containing the stomach, intestines, liver, gallbladder, pancreas, spleen, reproductive organs, and urinary bladder
a steady state; the tendency of stability in the normal physiologic systems of the organism to maintain a balance optimal for survival. Body temperature, osmotic pressure, normal cell division rate, and nutrient supply to cells are a few examples	a plane that vertically divides the body, or some part of it, into equal right and left portions (medial)

subcutaneous sub'ku-<u>ta</u>-ne-us Integumentary System	**debridement** da-<u>bred</u>-maw Integumentary System
escharotomy es-kah-<u>rot</u>-omy Integumentary System	**verruca** ve-<u>ru</u>-kah Integumentary System
psoriasis so-<u>ri</u>-ah-sis Integumentary System	**lupus erythematosus** <u>loo</u>-pus er-i-<u>the</u>-ma-to-sus Integumentary System
coccidioidin kok-sid'e-<u>oi</u>-din Integumentary System	**ecchymosis** ek'i-<u>mo</u>-sis Integumentary System
exfoliation eks-fo'le-<u>a</u>-shun Integumentary System	**paronychia** par'o-<u>nik</u>-e-ah Integumentary System

removal of contaminated or devitalized tissue from a traumatic or infected lesion	beneath the skin, containing adipose tissue, connective tissue, vessels, and nerves
a wart	removal of burn scar tissue
a chronic superficial inflammation of the skin; the lesions typically form a butterfly pattern over the bridge of the nose and cheeks	a chronic, hereditary, recurrent dermatosis marked by discrete vivid red macules, papules, or plaques covered with silvery laminated scales
bruise, caused by bleeding under the skin	a sterile preparation injected intracutaneously as a test for valley fever (respiratory fungus disease)
inflammation of the folds of tissue around the fingernail	a falling off in scales or layers

cholelithiasis ko'le-li-<u>thi</u>-ah-sis Gastrointestinal System	**diverticulitis** di'ver-tik'u-<u>li</u>-tis Gastrointestinal System
gastroenteritis <u>gas</u>-tro-en'ter-<u>i</u>-tis Gastrointestinal System	**intussusception** in'tuh-suh-<u>sep</u>-shun Gastrointestinal System
phenylketonuria (PKU) fen-il-ke'to-<u>nu</u>-re-ah Gastrointestinal System	**cheiloplasty** <u>ki</u>-lo-plas'te Gastrointestinal System
cholecystectomy ko'le-sis-<u>tek</u>-to-me Gastrointestinal System	**herniorrhaphy** her'ne-<u>or</u>-ah-fe Gastrointestinal System
esophagogastroduodenoscopy (EGO) e-sof'ah-go-gas'tro-du'o-de-<u>nos</u>-ko-pe Gastrointestinal System	**cachexia** kah-<u>kek</u>-se-ah Gastrointestinal System

inflammation of the large intestine, forming pouches or diverticula	gallstones
prolapse of a part of the intestine into the lumen of an immediately adjacent part	inflammation of the stomach and intestine caused by ingested harmful bacterial toxin, with acute nausea and vomiting, cramps, and diarrhea
surgical repair of a lip defect	a congenital inability to metabolize phenylalanine, a component of protein; may lead to retardation
surgical repair of a hernia, with suturing	excision of the gallbladder
severe malnutrition and wasting; emaciation	using endoscopes to examine esophagus, stomach, and duodenum

asphyxiation as-fik′se-<u>a</u>-shun Respiratory System	**bronchiectasis** brong′ke-<u>ek</u>-tah-sis Respiratory System
coccidioidomycosis kok-sid′e-oi′do-mi-<u>ko</u>-sis Respiratory System	**laryngotracheobronchitis** la-<u>rin</u>-go-tra′ke-o-brong-<u>ki</u>-tis Respiratory System
pneumoconiosis nu′mo-ko′ne-<u>o</u>-sis Respiratory System	**hypercapnia** hi′per-<u>kap</u>-ne-ah Respiratory System
laryngectomy lah-rin-<u>jek</u>-to-me Respiratory System	**parenchyma (lung)** pah-<u>reng</u>-ki-mah Respiratory System
thoracentesis thor′ra h-sen-<u>te</u>-sis Respiratory System	**tracheostomy** tra′ke-<u>os</u>-to-me Respiratory System

chronic dilatation of one or more bronchi	suffocation
inflammation of the larynx, trachea, and bronchi	a respiratory infection caused by spore inhalation of *Coccidioides immitis,* varying in severity from that of a common cold to symptoms resembling those of influenza; also called valley fever
an excess of carbon dioxide in the blood	any lung disease, e.g., anthracosis, silicosis, caused by permanent deposition of substantial amounts of particulate matter in the lungs
the essential elements or "working parts" of an organ, e.g., alveoli in the lung	excision of the larynx
creation of an opening into the trachea through the neck, e.g., insertion of a tube to facilitate ventilation	surgical puncture of the chest wall into the parietal cavity to remove fluid (TB test)

thrombocytes <u>throm</u>-bo-sitz Cardiovascular System	**reticulocytes** re-<u>tik</u>-u-lo-sitz Cardiovascular System
sphygmomanometer sfig′mo-mah-<u>nom</u>-e-ter Cardiovascular System	**arrhythmia** ah-<u>rith</u>-me-ah Cardiovascular System
arteriosclerosis ar-te′re-o-skle-<u>ro</u>-sis Cardiovascular System	**thrombophlebitis** throm′bo-fle-<u>bi</u>-tis Cardiovascular System
bradycardia brad′e-<u>kar</u>-de-ah Cardiovascular System	**endarterectomy** en′dar-ter-<u>ek</u>-to-me Cardiovascular System
percutaneous transluminal coronary angioplasty per′ku-<u>ta</u>-ne-us trans-<u>lum</u>-i-nul <u>kor</u>-o-ner-e <u>an</u>-je-o-plas′te Cardiovascular System	**tachycardia** tak′e-<u>kar</u>-de-ah Cardiovascular System

immature red blood cells, in the bone marrow	blood platelets
variation from the normal rhythm of the heart beat	an instrument for measuring arterial blood pressure
inflammation of a vein associated with thrombus formation	thickening and loss of elasticity of the arterial walls, slowing the flow of blood
excision of thickened areas of the innermost coat of an artery to increase blood flow	slowness of the heart beat, as evidenced by a pulse rate of <60
abnormally rapid heart rate	dilation of a blood vessel by means of a balloon catheter inserted through the skin and into the chosen vessel and then passed through the lumen of the vessel to the site of the lesion, where the balloon is inflated to flatten plaque against the artery wall

meninges men-<u>in</u>-jez Nervous System	**glossopharyngeal** glos'o-fah-<u>rin</u>-je-al Nervous System
amyotrophic lateral sclerosis (AMS) ah'mi-o-<u>troph</u>-ic <u>lat</u>-er-al skle-<u>ro</u>-sis Nervous System	**hydrocephalus** hi'dro-<u>sef</u>-ah-lus Nervous System
meningocele (myelomeningocele) me-<u>ning</u>-go-sel (mi'e-<u>lo</u>-me-<u>ning</u>-go-sel) Nervous System	**pneumoencephalogram (PEG)** nu'mo-en-<u>sef</u>-ah-lo-gram' Nervous System
ventriculography ven-trik'u-<u>log</u>-rah-fe Nervous System	**contrecoup** kon'truh-<u>koo</u> Nervous System
foramen magnum (pl., foramina) fo-<u>rah</u>-men <u>mag</u>-num (fo-<u>ram</u>-i-nah) Nervous System	**syncope** <u>sin</u>-co-pe Nervous System

pertaining to the tongue and pharynx	the three membranes covering the brain and spinal cord: dura mater, arachnoid, and pia mater
"water on the brain"; a congenital or acquired condition marked by dilation of the cerebral ventricles accompanied by an accumulation of cerebrospinal fluid within the skull	progressive degeneration of the upper and lower motor neurons; usually fatal
the radiograph obtained by visualization of the fluid-containing structures of the brain after cerebrospinal fluid is intermittently withdrawn by lumbar puncture and replaced by air, oxygen, or helium	hernial protrusion of the meninges through a defect in the cranium or vertebral column; may be repaired surgically
denoting an injury to the brain, occurring at a site opposite to the point of impact	radiography of the cerebral ventricles after introduction of air or other contrast medium
a faint; temporary loss of consciousness	a large opening in the occipital bone through which the cord passes

glomerulonephritis glo-mer'u-lo-ne-<u>fri</u>-tis Genitourinary System	**epididymis** ep'i-<u>did</u>-i-mis Genitourinary System
cryptorchidism krip'<u>tor</u>-ki-dizm Genitourinary System	**orchiectomy** or'ke-<u>ek</u>-to-me Genitourinary System
hysterosalpingogram his'ter-o-sal'<u>ping</u>-go-gram Genitourinary System	**oophorectomy** o'of-o-<u>rek</u>-to-me Genitourinary System
dystocia dis-<u>to</u>-se-ah Genitourinary System	**meconium** me-<u>ko</u>-ne-um Genitourinary System
multipara mul-<u>tip</u>-ah-rah Genitourinary System	**primipara** pri-<u>mip</u>-ah-rah Genitourinary System

a duct bordering the testes for storage, transit, and maturation of spermatozoa	nephritis with inflammation of the capillary loops in the renal glomeruli
surgical excision of the testicles	undescended testicle(s)
excision of one or both ovaries; female castration	an x-ray film of the uterus and the fallopian tubes to allow visualization of the cavity of the uterus and the passageway of the tubes
dark green mucilaginous material in the intestine of the full-term fetus, expelled as first stool	abnormal labor or childbirth
a woman who has produced one viable child	a woman who has borne more than one viable infant

aponeurosis ap'o-nu-<u>ro</u>-sis Musculoskeletal System	**interphalangeal** in'ter-fah-<u>lan</u>-je-al Musculoskeletal System
acetabulum as'e-<u>tab</u>-u-lum Musculoskeletal System	**foramen** fo-<u>ra</u>-men Musculoskeletal System
malleolus mah-<u>le</u>-o-lus Musculoskeletal System	**supination** su'pi-<u>na</u>-shun Musculoskeletal System
spondylolisthesis span'di-lo-lis-<u>the</u>-sis Musculoskeletal System	**systemic lupus** sis-<u>tem</u>-ik <u>loo</u>-pus Musculoskeletal System
arthrocentesis ar'thro-sen-<u>te</u>-sis Musculoskeletal System	**spondylosyndesis** spon'di-lo-<u>sin</u>-de-sis Musculoskeletal System

between two contiguous joints and phalanges, e.g., between the fingers and toes	a flattened tendon, connecting a muscle with the parts it moves
holes in a bone through which large vessels and nerves pass	the cup-shaped cavity (socket) receiving the head of the femur
palm or face upward	a rounded process, such as the protuberance on either side of the ankle joint, at the lower end of the fibula or the tibia
a chronic inflammatory disease affecting many systems of the body	forward displacement of a vertebra over a lower segment; a type of dislocation
surgical creation of ankylosis between contiguous vertebrae; spinal fusion	puncture of a joint cavity to remove fluid

blepharoptosis blef′ar-op-<u>to</u>-sis Eyes and Ears	**keratoconus** ker′ah-to-<u>ko</u>-nus Eyes and Ears
retinoblastoma ret′i-no-blas-<u>to</u>-mah Eyes and Ears	**enucleation** e-nu′kle-<u>a</u>-shun Eyes and Ears
trabeculectomy trah-bek′u-<u>lec</u>-to-me Eyes and Ears	**emmetropia** em′e-<u>tro</u>-pe-ah Eyes and Ears
ophthalmoscope of′<u>thal</u>-mo-skop Eyes and Ears	**cerumen** se-<u>roo</u>-men Eyes and Ears
furunculosis fu-rung′ku-<u>lo</u>-sis Eyes and Ears	**enucleation** en-<u>nu</u>-cle′a-shun Eyes and Ears

conical protrusion of the central part of the cornea	drooping of upper eyelid
surgical removal of the eye	a tumor arising from the retinal cells
normal vision	excision of fibrous bands or connective tissue
earwax	instrument containing a perforated mirror and lenses used to examine the interior of the eye; also called funduscope
removal of the eye	a skin infection affecting the ear canal

pituitary (hypophysis) pi-<u>tu</u>-i-tar′e (hi-<u>pof</u>-i-sis) Endocrine System	**acromegaly** ak′ro-<u>meg</u>-ah-le Endocrine System
exophthalmic goiter ek′sof-<u>thal</u>-mic <u>goi</u>-ter Endocrine System	**myxedema** mik′se-<u>de</u>-mah Endocrine System
pheochromocytoma fe′o-kro′mo-si-<u>to</u>-mah Endocrine System	**anorexia** an′o-<u>rek</u>-se-ah Endocrine System
diaphoresis di′ah-fo-<u>re</u>-sis Endocrine System	**emaciation** e-ma′se-<u>a</u>-shun Endocrine System
hypoglycemia hi′po-gli-<u>se</u>-me-ah Endocrine System	**hypophysectomy** hi-pof′i-<u>sek</u>-to-me Endocrine System

abnormal enlargement of the extremities of the skeleton, nose, jaws, fingers, and toes; caused by hypersecretion of the pituitary growth hormone after maturity	an endocrine gland at the base of the brain attached by a stalk to the hypothalamus; secretes several important hormones to regulate the function of the thyroids, gonads, adrenal cortex, and other endocrine organs
a dry, waxy type of swelling with deposits of mucin in the skin, swollen lips, and thickened nose	toxic goiter; Graves' disease; protrusion of the eyeballs, swollen neck, weight loss, shaking, and mental deterioration are symptoms
lack or loss of appetite for food	"pheochromo" means dusky color; tumor of the medulla characterized by hypertension, weight loss, and personality changes
excessive leanness; a wasted condition	profuse perspiration
excision of the pituitary gland (hypophysis)	blood sugar (glucose) level is below normal

INDEX